VITAMINS AND HORMONES

VOLUME 37

VITAMINS AND HORMONES

ADVANCES IN RESEARCH AND APPLICATIONS

Edited by

PAUL L. MUNSON
University of North Carolina
Chapel Hill, North Carolina

EGON DICZFALUSY
Karolinska Sjukhuset
Stockholm, Sweden

JOHN GLOVER
University of Liverpool
Liverpool, England

ROBERT E. OLSON
St. Louis University
St. Louis, Missouri

Consulting Editors

ROBERT S. HARRIS
32 Dwhinda Road
Newton, Massachusetts

KENNETH V. THIMANN
University of California, Santa Cruz
Santa Cruz, California

JOHN A. LORAINE
University of Edinburgh
Edinburgh, Scotland

IRA G. WOOL
University of Chicago
Chicago, Illinois

Volume 37

1979

ACADEMIC PRESS   A Subsidiary of Harcourt Brace Jovanovich, Publishers

New York   London   Toronto   Sydney   San Francisco

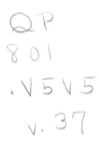

ACADEMIC PRESS, INC.
111 Fifth Avenue, New York, New York 10003

United Kingdom Edition published by
ACADEMIC PRESS, INC. (LONDON) LTD.
24/28 Oval Road, London NW1 7DX

LIBRARY OF CONGRESS CATALOG CARD NUMBER: 43–10535

ISBN 0–12–709837–2

PRINTED IN THE UNITED STATES OF AMERICA

79 80 81 82   9 8 7 6 5 4 3 2 1

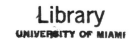

Contents

CONTRIBUTORS TO VOLUME 37 ix
PREFACE xi
ERRATUM xiii

Aspects of the Metabolism and Function of Vitamin D

D. E. M. LAWSON AND M. DAVIE

I.	Introduction	2
II.	7-Dehydrocholesterol in Skin	4
III.	Synthesis of Vitamin D by Irradiation	6
IV.	Vitamin D in Skin	11
V.	Factors Affecting the Cutaneous Synthesis of Vitamin D by Ultraviolet Light	14
VI.	Cutaneous Absorption of Vitamin D	19
VII.	Storage of Vitamin D	21
VIII.	Ultraviolet Light in the Management of Vitamin D Deficiency	26
IX.	Binding Proteins for Vitamin D Metabolites	28
X.	Physiological Mechanisms of the Intestinal Absorption of Calcium	43
XI.	Biochemical Responses in the Intestine to Vitamin D	46
XII.	Effect of Vitamin D on Bone Formation	59
	References	61

Epidermal Growth Factor–Urogastrone, a Polypeptide Acquiring Hormonal Status

MORLEY D. HOLLENBERG

I.	Introduction	69
II.	Isolation and Properties of Mouse and Human Epidermal Growth Factor–Urogastrone (EGF-URO)	72
III.	Biosynthesis, Storage, and Secretion of EGF-URO	75
IV.	Biological Actions of EGF-URO	78
V.	The Membrane Receptor for EGF-URO	83
VI.	Structure–Activity Relationships for Receptor Binding and Biological Activity	97
VII.	The EGF-URO Receptor, Cell Transformation, and Tumorigenesis	100
VIII.	Is EGF-URO a Hormone?	103
	References	106

Control of ACTH Secretion by Corticotropin-Releasing Factor(s)

ALVIN BRODISH

I.	Introduction	111
II.	Central Nervous System Activation of Corticotropin-Releasing Factor (CRF)	112
III.	Nature of Hypothalamic CRF	113
IV.	Dynamic Changes in ACTH Secretion	115
V.	CRF in Peripheral Blood	123
VI.	Hypothalamic Control Center for ACTH Release	125
VII.	Nature of the Functional Deficit in Rats with Hypothalamic Lesions	128
VIII.	Assays for CRF	132
IX.	Hypothalamic and Extrahypothalamic CRF in Peripheral Blood	138
X.	Tissue CRF	143
	References	150

Modulation of Memory by Pituitary Hormones and Related Peptides

HENK RIGTER AND JOHN C. CRABBE

I.	General Introduction	154
II.	Memory Processes	154
III.	Effects of Peptides on Memory—Introduction	162
IV.	Amelioration of Behavioral Deficits	165
V.	Effects in Normal Animals	182
VI.	Effects of Experimental Amnesia	196
VII.	The Endorphins: A New Field of Research	202
VIII.	Peptides and Memory Processes: Human Data	210
IX.	Possible Sites and Mechanisms of Actions	219
X.	Concluding Comments	231
	References	233

Inhibin: From Concept to Reality

P. FRANCHIMONT, J. VERSTRAELEN-PROYARD, M. T. HAZEE-HAGELSTEIN, CH. RENARD, A. DEMOULIN, J. P. BOURGUIGNON, AND J. HUSTIN

I.	Relationship between Gametogenesis and FSH Secretion: Definition of Inhibin	244
II.	Sources of Inhibin and Techniques for Purification	246
III.	Detection and Measurement of Inhibin	249
IV.	Physicochemical and Immunological Characteristics of Inhibin	260
V.	Biological Properties of Inhibin	267
VI.	Origin and Transport of Inhibin	287
VII.	Possible Roles of Inhibin	293
VIII.	Summary and Conclusions	298
	References	299

Hormonal Control of Calcium Metabolism in Lactation

Svein U. Toverud and Agna Boass

I.	Introduction	303
II.	Regulation of the Serum Calcium Concentration in Lactation	305
III.	Intestinal Calcium Absorption	321
IV.	Urinary Calcium Excretion in Lactation	331
V.	Calcium and Vitamin D in Milk	335
VI.	Skeletal Calcium Content	338
VII.	Conclusions and Hypotheses	341
	References	343

Subject Index 349

Contributors to Volume 37

Numbers in parentheses indicate the pages on which the authors' contributions begin.

AGNA BOASS, *Dental Research Center, University of North Carolina, Chapel Hill, North Carolina 27514* (303)

J. P. BOURGUIGNON, *Radioimmunoassay Laboratory, Institute of Medicine, University of Liège, Liège, Belgium* (243)

ALVIN BRODISH, *Department of Physiology and Pharmacology, Bowman Gray School of Medicine of Wake Forest University, Winston-Salem, North Carolina 27103* (111)

JOHN C. CRABBE,* *CNS Pharmacology Department, Scientific Development Group, Organon, Oss, The Netherlands* (153)

M. DAVIE, *Dunn Nutritional Laboratory, University of Cambridge and Medical Research Council, Cambridge, England* (1)

A. DEMOULIN, *Radioimmunoassay Laboratory, Institute of Medicine, University of Liège, Liège, Belgium* (243)

P. FRANCHIMONT, *Radioimmunoassay Laboratory, Institute of Medicine, University of Liège, Liège, Belgium* (243)

M. T. HAZEE-HAGELSTEIN, *Radioimmunoassay Laboratory, Institute of Medicine, University of Liège, Liège, Belgium* (243)

MORLEY D. HOLLENBERG, *Division of Pharmacology and Therapeutics, University of Calgary Faculty of Medicine, Calgary, Alberta, Canada T2N 1N4* (69)

J. HUSTIN, *Radioimmunoassay Laboratory, Institute of Medicine, University of Liège, Liège, Belgium* (243)

D. E. M. LAWSON, *Dunn Nutritional Laboratory, University of Cambridge and Medical Research Council, Cambridge, England* (1)

* Present address: Medical Research Service, Veterans Administration Medical Center, Portland, Oregon 97201.

CH. RENARD, *Radioimmunoassay Laboratory, Institute of Medicine, University of Liège, Liège, Belgium* (243)

HENK RIGTER, *CNS Pharmacology Department, Scientific Development Group, Organon, Oss, The Netherlands* (153)

SVEIN U. TOVERUD, *Department of Pharmacology, School of Medicine, University of North Carolina, Chapel Hill, North Carolina 27514* (303)

J. VERSTRAELEN-PROYARD, *Radioimmunoassay Laboratory, Institute of Medicine, University of Liège, Liège, Belgium* (243)

Preface

This year's "Vitamins and Hormones," Volume 37, presents six reviews. The first is about a vitamin, vitamin D, which is now regarded by many as a hormone precursor rather than as a dietary vitamin in the classic sense. The chapter by D. E. M. Lawson and M. Davie focuses on newer knowledge (since 1974) about vitamin D, with emphasis on biosynthesis in the skin, binding proteins in plasma and tissues, and mechanisms of calcium absorption by the intestine.

The article by Morley D. Hollenberg is on the chemistry, biochemistry, biological actions, and membrane receptor interactions of two chemically similar polypeptides, epidermal growth factor and urogastrone. Both are potent stimulants of cellular proliferation and inhibitors of gastric acid secretion. The author suggests that epidermal growth factor and urogastrone represent an emerging class of polypeptide modulating factors that may eventually achieve hormonal status.

The biologically well-established but chemically elusive hypothalamic corticotropin releasing factor (CRF) is reviewed by Alvin Brodish in relation to the evidence, for which he is mainly responsible, for a similar but more long-acting extrahypothalamic "tissue CRF." Brodish suggests that hypothalamic CRF provides a transient response to acute stress but that during continued stress of high intensity the needs of the organism may be met by tissue CRF.

Henk Rigter and John C. Crabbe address the intriguing question of the possible significance of pituitary hormones and related peptides, especially ACTH, vasopressin, and their analogs, in the modulation of memory, thereby providing an interdisciplinary chapter that relates psychology and endocrinology.

P. Franchimont and colleagues bring the tenuous 50-year-old "concept of a gonadal hormone regulating FSH secretion and related directly or indirectly to gametogenesis" up-to-date. The evidence they present and evaluate goes a long way toward convincing us that inhibin has indeed progressed "from concept to reality."

The final chapter in the volume, by Svein U. Toverud and Agna Boass, on hormonal control of calcium metabolism in lactation brings us again to vitamin D and its hormonal metabolite, 1,25-dihydroxycholecalciferol. This review is concerned with the integration of the effects of three hormones, parathyroid hormone, calcitonin, and 1,25-dihydroxycholecalciferol. They are all secreted in increased amounts during lactation, a physiological condition in which calcium homeostasis is subjected to intense stress.

The Editors join in thanking the authors of the reviews in this volume for their outstanding contributions.

It is with sadness that we record the death, on July 28, 1978, of Dwight J. Ingle, eminent endocrine physiologist, who was Coeditor of "Vitamins and Hormones" in 1960 and 1961.

PAUL L. MUNSON
EGON DICZFALUSY
JOHN GLOVER
ROBERT E. OLSON

Erratum

"Biological Effects of Antibodies to Gonadal Steroids" by Eberhard Nieschlag and E. Jean Wickings (Volume 36). The halftone on page 180 should appear with the legend for Fig. 10 (p. 181); the halftone on page 181 should appear with the legend for Fig. 9 (p. 180).

Aspects of the Metabolism and Function of Vitamin D

D. E. M. LAWSON AND M. DAVIE

Dunn Nutritional Laboratory,
University of Cambridge and Medical Research Council,
Cambridge, England

I. Introduction 2
II. 7-Dehydrocholesterol in Skin 4
    A. Distribution and Concentration 4
    B. Distribution according to Site, Age, Sex, Race, and Disease 5
    C. Effect of Ultraviolet Irradiation on Skin Lipids 6
III. Synthesis of Vitamin D by Irradiation 6
    A. Formation of Pre-vitamin D 6
    B. Conversion of Pre-vitamin D to Vitamin D 7
    C. Vitamin D Formation in Skin *in Vivo* 9
    D. Biological Activity of Pre-vitamin D 10
IV. Vitamin D in Skin 11
    A. Production of Vitamin D in Irradiated Skin 11
    B. Pattern of Vitamin D Response by Irradiated Skin 13
V. Factors Affecting the Cutaneous Synthesis of Vitamin D by Ultraviolet
    Light 14
    A. Physical and Environmental Factors 14
    B. Penetration of Ultraviolet Light into Skin 17
VI. Cutaneous Absorption of Vitamin D 19
    A. Absorption of Sterols 19
    B. Absorption of Vitamin D 20
VII. Storage of Vitamin D 21
    A. Sites of Vitamin D Storage 21
    B. Ultraviolet Light and Vitamin D Status 23
VIII. Ultraviolet Light in the Management of Vitamin D Deficiency 26
IX. Binding Proteins for Vitamin D Metabolites 28
    A. Binding Proteins in Plasma 28
    B. Tissue 25-Hydroxyvitamin D-Binding Proteins 39
    C. 1,25-Dihydroxyvitamin D-Binding Proteins in Tissues 40
X. Physiological Mechanisms of the Intestinal Absorption of
    Calcium 43
XI. Biochemical Responses in the Intestine to Vitamin D 46
    A. Introduction 46
    B. Response of Protein Synthesis 47
    C. Response of RNA Synthesis 52
    D. Response of Enzymes 54
    E. Cytological and Other Responses 56
    F. Summary 58
XII. Effect of Vitamin D on Bone Formation 59
    References 61

1

I. Introduction

In the 5 years since the last review of vitamin D appeared in "Vitamins and Hormones," progress in our understanding of vitamin D physiology and biochemistry has continued at a rapid rate, with indications that the study of these topics will be as rewarding in the future. Significant advances in the use of this knowledge for the successful treatment of metabolic bone disease may be forthcoming also. The position in 1974 may be briefly summarized as follows. The active form of vitamin D had been shown to be a metabolite 1,25-dihydroxyvitamin D [1, 25-$(OH)_2D_3$*] formed according to the scheme:

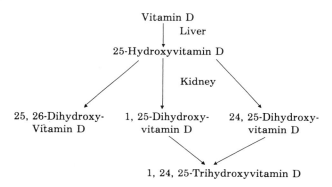

Although other metabolites were identified as 24,25-dihydroxyvitamin D, 25,26-dihydroxyvitamin D, and 1,24,25-trihydroxyvitamin D, the evidence available in 1974 pointed to 1,25-$(OH)_2D$ being the active form of vitamin D in the target tissues.

It was furthermore known that liver is the primary, and possibly sole, site of synthesis of 25-hydroxyvitamin D [25-$(OH)D$], but by a process that is not finely controlled. Also it had been shown that 1,25-$(OH)_2D$ synthesis occurs only at a single site, kidney, in a wide range of species by a process apparently carefully regulated by a number of factors. The plasma level of 1,25-$(OH)_2D$ is very low (< 50 pg per milliliter of plasma), and, as the substance acts on tissues

*The subscript 3 or 2 after D indicates the type of vitamin D or metabolite; it is inserted only if it is necessary to differentiate between the respective forms present.

remote from its site of synthesis, it was classified as a steroid hormone. In normal animals the main factor regulating the secretion of 1,25-(OH)$_2$D is parathyroid hormone, which is therefore the tropic hormone for this steroid. However, the control of 1,25-(OH)$_2$D synthesis is a very complex biochemical process with a range of factors involved in different physiological states. Naturally this aspect of vitamin D metabolism has been the subject of numerous papers, but it will not be covered further here since an extensive review of it is to appear elsewhere (Fraser, 1980).

With regard to the function of vitamin D, it has been known for some time that it has three main effects in animals: (a) to control calcium homeostasis; (b) to regulate the growth and development of bone; (c) to regulate phosphorus metabolism. The regulation of calcium homeostasis is achieved through the action of 1,25-(OH)$_2$D, parathyroid hormone, and calcitonin acting in conjunction. The 1,25-(OH)$_2$D acts on intestine, bone, and kidney so as to raise plasma calcium levels, and most investigations into the biochemical mechanisms by which this is achieved have involved the events in the intestine. In this chapter we review some of the recent studies on this aspect and of the related problem of the plasma and tissue binding proteins for the vitamin D metabolites.

Very little information was available in 1974 on the other two effects of vitamin D. Investigations of the growth and development of bone are technically difficult, and regulation of phosphorus metabolism had been relatively neglected up to 1974, but this latter situation may now be changing. Garabedian et al. (1976) have shown the important part played by 1,25-(OH)$_2$D in serum phosphorus homeostasis. We include also in this chapter a short account of the finding from a number of laboratories showing that the growth of bone requires metabolites of vitamin D other than 1,25-(OH)$_2$D. This promises to be one of the more exciting areas of vitamin D research in the future. However, we begin the chapter with an account of biochemistry of some skin lipids and of the events following exposure of skin to ultraviolet (UV) light. These topics have not been reviewed recently, but their importance becomes apparent with the finding that UV light, not diet, is the source of vitamin D in man. Consequently, the understanding of the etiology of rickets requires a more detailed knowledge than is currently available of the events occurring in skin in response to UV light and of the metabolism of the vitamin D so formed.

II. 7-Dehydrocholesterol in Skin

A. Distribution and Concentration

7-Dehydrocholesterol has been identified in the skin of many species including the rat (Gaylor and Sault, 1964), pig (Festenstein and Morton, 1955), mouse, guinea pig (Kandutsch et al., 1956), and man (Reinertson and Wheatly, 1959). 7-Dehydrocholesterol can be synthesized by skin (Gaylor and Sault, 1964; Semenov and Datsenko, 1976) from [^{14}C]acetate. Rat skin prepared by shaving skin and removing subcutaneous tissue had 103.8 μg of 7-dehydrocholesterol per gram of prepared skin (Yasumura et al., 1977), and in a study of 7-dehydrocholesterol in different layers of skin, the total in keratin, epidermal mucosa, and dermis plus sebaceous glands was 4.77 μg/cm^2 (Gaylor and Sault, 1964). Extraction of sterols from human skin taken at postmortem from abdomen, back, or thighs showed that total sterols were 1.33% and 1.44% of epidermal weight in males and females, respectively, and that 7-dehydrocholesterol was 3.8% and 2.7% of total sterols (Reinertson and Wheatley, 1959). The 7-dehydrocholesterol content of dorsal skin of normal male volunteers was 4.0% of total sterols (Reinertson and Wheatley, 1959). The 7-dehydrocholesterol level was 4.8 μg/gm (0.42 μg/cm^2) in the skin taken at postmortem of a female aged 70. Skin taken from a male aged 65 at postmortem had 9.6 μg/gm (1.4 μg/cm^2). Both specimens were taken in January in England, the skin examined being from the abdomen (D. R. Fraser, and M. Davie, unpublished observations).

Apart from the concentration, there are important differences in distribution of 7-dehydrocholesterol in the skin of rat and man. In the rat 45% exists in epidermal mucosa, sebaceous glands, and dermis whereas 55% occurs in dead keratin (see Section V,B). Moreover 65% of the 7-dehydrocholesterol in the live tissues is found in sebaceous glands (Gaylor and Sault, 1964). These also appear to be active sites of 7-dehydrocholesterol synthesis. In human skin a maximum of 0.0008% 7-dehydrocholesterol has been found in human skin surface lipids (Boughton and Wheatley, quoted in Wheatley and Reinertson, 1958). The epidermis contains the highest proportion of 7-dehydrocholesterol of total lipids, the dermal lipids containing about 10% of the epidermal content. 7-Dehydrocholesterol content in subcutaneous tissues is minimal (Wheatley and Reinertson, 1958). More detailed analysis of the various layers of skin shows that only 0.06% of total lipids is 7-dehydrocholesterol in stratum corneum and 0.35% in the Malpighian layer. The figure for the total epidermis is 0.27% (Reinertson and Wheatley, 1959). Most of the sterol in skin exists as cholesterol (Reinertson and Wheatley, 1959).

In man, therefore, most of the cutaneous 7-dehydrocholesterol resides in the Malpighian layer. Although surface 7-dehydrocholesterol may not be stable in the presence of oxygen (DeLuca *et al.*, 1971), it would be of more value in the rat, since absorption of cutaneous sterols occurs more readily in rats than in man (see Section VI). It is likely that there is adequate penetration of ultraviolet light to the Malpighian layer, and it has been shown that washing of human skin does not affect the response to UV light (Stamp, 1975).

B. Distribution according to Site, Age, Sex, Race, and Disease

Epidermis taken from abdomen, back, and thigh all show similar proportions of 7-dehydrocholesterol in the lipids extracted (1.6–4.9% of total sterols in adults). However, in epidermis from the sole of the foot, 7-dehydrocholesterol comprised only 0.7% of total sterols (Reinertson and Wheatley, 1959). With such uniform proportions of 7-dehydrocholesterol in skin, apart from the sole, there is no reason to suspect low levels in the skin of the face and hands. The proportion of 7-dehydrocholesterol in skin is relatively stable from late childhood to old age. In an infant of 2 weeks, however, 7-dehydrocholesterol constituted 8.8% of total sterols (Reinertson and Wheatley, 1959). There do not appear to be significant differences between males and females or Whites and Negroes (Reinertson and Wheatley, 1959).

Probably because of the considerable amount of 7-dehydrocholesterol in the skin, little attention has been paid to the level in disease. Patients with psoriasis, in which skin turnover time is increased, have been investigated, but estimation proved to be difficult because of an interfering sterol (Reinertson and Wheatley, 1959). One condition in which low levels of 7-dehydrocholesterol are found is rickets. Rats fed a rachitogenic diet for 14 weeks had levels of 7-dehydrocholesterol about 50% lower than levels of control animals (Yasumura *et al.*, 1977), and rachitogenic diets inhibit incorporation of [^{14}C]acetate into cholesterol precursors, including 7-dehydrocholesterol, and reduce cholesterol synthesis (Semenov and Datsenko, 1976). This reduction in cholesterol is not necessarily found in other tissues (Cruess and Clark, 1971).

C. Effect of Ultraviolet Irradiation on Skin Lipids

Ultraviolet irradiation of human skin leads to a reduction in skin cholesterol (Rauschkolb *et al.,* 1967), both Negro and Caucasian skin showing the same response. Incubation of human skin slices which had been exposed to UV light demonstrated a reduced incorporation of [^{14}C]acetate into total lipid, phospholipid, free sterol, and neutral fat fractions. If, however, [^{14}C]mevalonate was substituted for [^{14}C]acetate no inhibition was seen (Black and Rauschkolb, 1971). In contrast to these studies, UV light has been found to increase skin surface lipids and the cholesterol content therein in man (Bloor and Karenfield, 1977).

In the rat UV irradiation leads to an increase in skin sterols (Wells and Baumann, 1954; Simko *et al.,* 1969). Irradiation of rat skin *in vivo* does not lead to a change in 7-dehydrocholesterol levels in either normal or vitamin D-deficient rats (Yasumura *et al.,* 1977) although an increase in cholesterol and 7-dehydrocholesterol synthesis has been reported (Semenov and Datsenko, 1976). Irradiation does not appear to influence 7-dehydrocholesterol levels in human skin obtained at postmortem during the winter months (D. R. Fraser and M. Davie, unpublished observations). These results are not unexpected, since the amount of vitamin D produced in skin by UV light is little compared with the available 7-dehydrocholesterol, and the change may well be within the experimental error of the method (see Section IV).

III. Synthesis of Vitamin D by Irradiation

A. Formation of Pre-vitamin D

Figure 1 demonstrates that a large number of products may be formed by the action of UV light on 7-dehydrocholesterol or ergosterol (referred to collectively as provitamin D). Several of these compounds, however, are of no importance in animals owing to the high temperature required for their formation. Moreover, much of the chemistry of vitamin D production from provitamin D has been performed in organic solvents, and it is only in recent years that attempts have been made to study the process in skin.

The first important step involves the cleavage of the 9-C–10-C bond of provitamin D. The role of UV light in promoting this reaction was appreciated 40 years ago (Windaus *et al.,* 1938, 1939), but the pathway to vitamin D was not fully understood for a further 20 years. The important compound pre-vitamin D, the essential precursor for all other products (Fig. 1) (Sanders *et al.*, 1969), was isolated by Velluz and Amiard (1949). The products of irradiation of provitamin D vary according to temperature and wavelength. The pyrocalciferol and isopyrocalciferol series are produced at temperatures in excess of 100°C. The wavelength used to irradiate provitamin D has important consequences on the photostationary state. To minimize vitamin D formation from pre-vitamin D, the irradiation must be performed below 20°C (Rappoldt and Havinga, 1960). The optimum wavelength for formation of pre-vitamin D is 296.5 nm (Havinga *et al.*, 1960; Abillon and Mermet–Bouvier, 1973), and a substantial decline in pre-vitamin D production occurs on either side of this wavelength. Irradiation of ergosterol in organic solutions results in a maximum pre-vitamin D_2 concentration after 1–2 hours (Rappoldt and Havinga, 1960). The time for maximum pre-vitamin D_2 production is less than 1 second using light up to 300 nm with 10^{18} photons per square centimeter per second (Abillon and Mermet–Bouvier, 1973). The quantity of UV energy delivered to ergosterol in organic solvents is also important in determining pre-vitamin D production. Kobayashi, having established that irradiation with UV light of 295 nm wavelength gave an optimal recovery, further showed that the maximal yield of potential vitamin D_2 occurred with an energy of 2.1–6.4 × 18^8 ergs/cm^2. Further energy led to a decline in potential vitamin D_2 recovery (Kobayashi and Yasumura, 1973). This observation may explain the decline in rachitic healing potency of rat skin when irradiated for long periods (Knudson and Benford, 1938), though whether this represents conversion of pre-vitamin D to toxisterols and of vitamin D to suprasterols (Fig. 1) remains to be established. In a normal animal, the ambient temperature of skin is likely to be such that any pre-vitamin D formed will be converted to vitamin D (see later). Furthermore, many of the substances that are derived from pre-vitamin D *in vitro* are unstable or formed only in certain solvents. Tachysterol undergoes rapid oxidation to a compound of molecular weight 800, and the photochemical formation of toxisterols A and B from pre-vitamin D depends upon the solvent used (Sanders *et al.*, 1969).

B. CONVERSION OF PRE-VITAMIN D TO VITAMIN D

The formation of pre-vitamin D is a photochemical reaction, whereas the formation of vitamin D from pre-vitamin D is heat dependent (Hanewald *et al.*, 1961). Table I (adapted from Hanewald *et al.*,

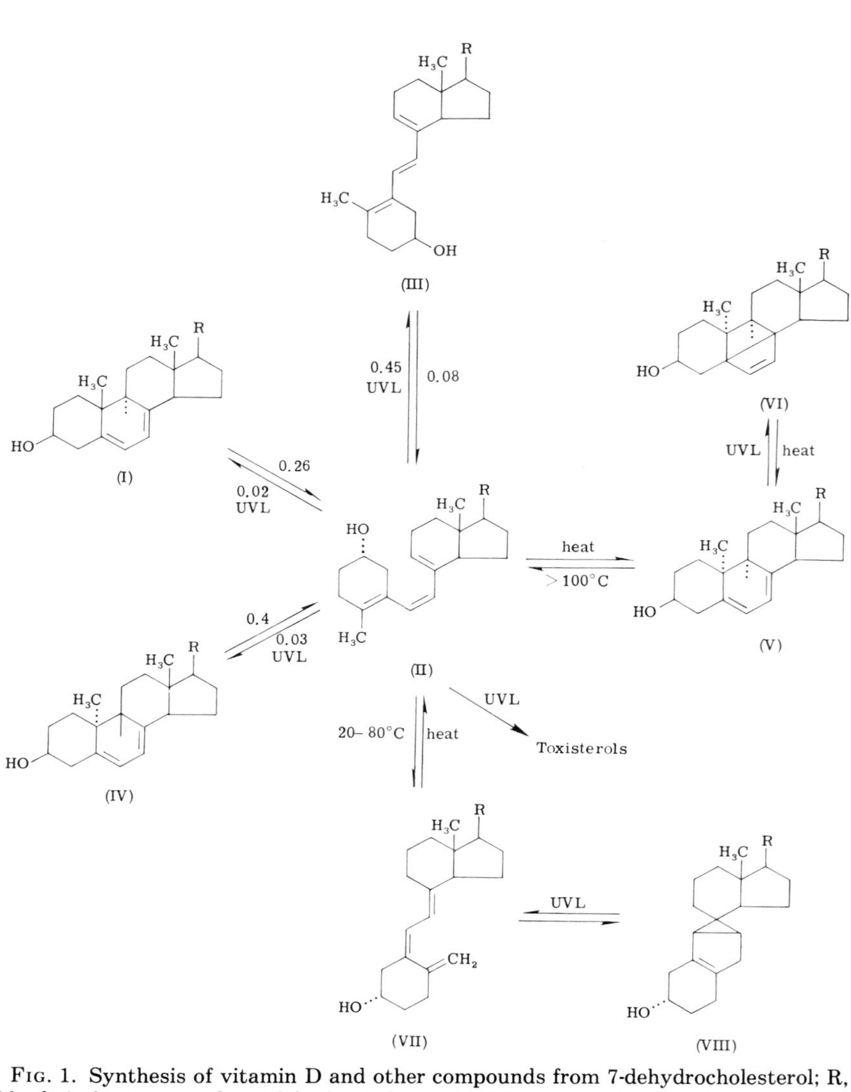

FIG. 1. Synthesis of vitamin D and other compounds from 7-dehydrocholesterol; R, side chain for ergosterol or 7-dehydrocholesterol; UVL, Ultraviolet light. Figures alongside photoreaction arrows indicate quantum yields. Structures: (I) 7-dehydrocholesterol, (II) pre-vitamin D, (III) tachysterol (*trans, cis*), (IV) lumisterol, (V) pyrocalciferol or isopyrocalciferol, (VI) photopyrocalciferol or isophotopyrocalciferol, (VII) calciferol, (VIII) suprasterol. Structural formulas were taken from Sanders *et al.* (1969).

TABLE I

TIME FOR CONVERSION OF VITAMIN D_3 FROM PRE-VITAMIN D_3[a]

| Percentage of D_3 formed | Temperature[b] | | |
	$-20°C$	$20°C$	$40°C$
5	68	0.4	0.05
20	269	1.6	0.1
40	681	3.8	0.5

[a] Adapted from Hanewald et al. (1961).
[b] Data given in days.

1961) shows the time required to form various amounts of vitamin D_3 from pre-vitamin D_3. The reaction is relatively rapid at 40°C. Conversely, as temperature increases, the proportion of pre-vitamin D_3 in the equilibrium mixture rises from 4% at 0°C to 11% at 40°C (Hanewald et al., 1961). Havinga has pointed out that the finding of vitamin D existing as the predominant form in the equilibrium mixture was initially unexpected in chemical terms. Further work on this point emphasized the importance of the trans-attached 5-membered D ring in moving the equilibrium away from pre-vitamin D (Havinga, 1973).

C. VITAMIN D FORMATION IN SKIN *in Vivo*

Much of the work leading to the elucidation of the chemistry of vitamin D has been performed in organic solvents. Recently there has been renewed interest in the reaction occurring *in vivo*. The reaction in skin requires about 1000 times as much energy to form vitamin D than is required in organic solvents (Bekemeier, 1966). The response of skin to ultraviolet light depends upon the species investigated (Section IV, A) and suggests caution in applying results from the widely used laboratory rat to other species. Unirradiated skin does not contain pre-vitamin D (Holick et al., 1977). If all extractions are performed at low temperature to prevent conversion of pre-vitamin D to vitamin D, pre-vitamin D can be identified in skin after UV irradiation (Petrova et al., 1976; Holick et al., 1977). On warming, the characteristics of this metabolite change to those of vitamin D (Holick et al., 1977). Pre-vitamin D_4 has also been identified in the skin of rats given [³H]22,23-dihydroergosterol intravenously and subsequently irradiated (Petrova *et al.*, 1976), raising the possibility that 7-dehy-drocholesterol synthesized in sites other than skin may be available for conversion to vitamin D. Although vitamin D has been identified in skin (Okano *et al.*, 1977; Esvelt *et al.*, 1978), the extraction procedure used may have promoted the reaction pre-vitamin D → vitamin D *in vitro*. It still therefore remains to be established that this conversion occurs primarily in skin and that the kinetics established *in vitro* are applicable *in vivo*. Recent work suggests that pre-vitamin D may have less affinity than vitamin D for the plasma vitamin D-binding protein, and it has been proposed that vitamin D accumulates in skin and is released only slowly (Holick and Clark, 1978). However, the increase in plasma 25-(OH)D concentration per minute of exposure is maximal after the initial exposures and gradually declines (Davie and Lawson, 1980). This, together with the finding that plasma 25-(OH)D levels reach a plateau during irradiation of a limited area (see Section IV,B), suggests that release is most rapid after the initial exposures.

D. BIOLOGICAL ACTIVITY OF PRE-VITAMIN D

Assessment of the biological activity of pre-vitamin D is complicated by the necessity for pre-vitamin D to enter a warm environment prior to reaching any theoretical sites of action. Thus the heat-dependent conversion of pre-vitamin D to vitamin D will start immediately. The antirachitogenic properties of pre-vitamin D administered orally have been compared with those of vitamin D (Hanewald *et al.*, 1961). Pre-vitamin D was considerably less active than vitamin D assessed radiologically in 9-day-old rachitic chicks, the activity ratio of provitamin D: vitamin D being 0.35. This activity ratio could, as Hanewald *et al.* (1961) stated, be due to the conversion of pre-vitamin D to vitamin D, but at body temperature this percentage conversion should be achieved after about 9 hours (Table I). If all the pre-vitamin D remained in the body until it was converted to vitamin D, an activity ratio closer to the equilibrium ratio (11:89, pre-vitamin D:vitamin D) would be expected. It is not yet clear why the observed activity is different from that expected. It is possible that pre-vitamin D administered orally is not metabolized in the same way as that originating in skin or that the lack of affinity for the plasma vitamin D binding protein (see above) affects its biological activity.

The properties of irradiated rat skin in healing rickets are well established (Knudson and Benford, 1938). Extracts of sterols of irradiated rat skin have been partially purified, and two substances were found to have antirachitic activity (Datsenko, 1969). It is possible that these correspond to pre-vitamin D and vitamin D, but the nature of the substances was not determined.

IV. Vitamin D in Skin

A. Production of Vitamin D in Irradiated Skin

1. *In Vitro Studies*

This was first studied comprehensively using a biological assay in rats (Bekemeier, 1966) and more recently by high-pressure liquid chromatography (Okano *et al.*, 1977; Esvelt *et al.*, 1978). In addition, indirect assessments have been made (Stamp *et al.*, 1977; Davie and Lawson, 1980). The amount of vitamin D formed in isolated skin exposed to ultraviolet light is shown in Table II (Bekemeier, 1966). There are considerable differences among species, some, such as the dog, apparently forming very little vitamin D. In man 3.2 μg per gram of abdominal skin has been found (Rauschkolb *et al.*, 1969), but this seems rather high either for unirradiated skin or for irradiated skin, as it is difficult to detect any change in skin 7-dehydrocholesterol levels when isolated skin is irradiated (Section II). The differences may, however, indicate that the importance of vitamin D from cutaneous or dietary sources varies among different species.

The level of vitamin D achieved in irradiated isolated skin may not, however, be a physiological response. Using small amounts of UV

TABLE II

Vitamin D Produced in Isolated Skin
of Various Species in Response
to Ultraviolet Light[a]

Species	Vitamin D (ng/cm^2)
Pig	1525 ± 483
Man	385 ± 230
Rat	193 ± 75
Rabbit	90 ± 50
Guinea pig	90 ± 50
Dog	< 25
Poultry	Very low

[a]From Bekemeier (1966).

energy (1.42 μW/cm^2 per second for 120 minutes, total 10^{-2} J) similar quantities of vitamin D (12.5–14.7 ng per gram of skin) were found in isolated skin or skin *in vivo* (Okano *et al.*, 1977). A larger quantity of UV energy (630 J to dorsal and lateral skin of 120 gm rats) yielded 325 ng of vitamin D per gram of isolated rat skin (Esvelt *et al.*, 1978), but such a yield is seen only in isolated skin exposed to considerable energy. The irradiation of human skin *in vivo* yielded about 25 ng of vitamin D per square centimeter, considerably less than the value seen in isolated skin (Table II).

2. *In Vivo Studies*

The estimation of vitamin D produced in skin has yielded useful information about its potential capacity for vitamin D synthesis. The possible difference of response of skin *in vivo* and after isolation has caused investigators to use other indices to compare with direct cutaneous measurements. These assessments of vitamin D action or metabolites of vitamin D introduce a number of other variables, such as cutaneous absorption, but may be of value in following the amount of vitamin D formed that is of physiological value. A comparison of the effects of whole-body UV irradiation of human subjects and of oral vitamin D administration on plasma 25-(OH)D response showed that daily whole-body irradiation was equivalent to 250 μg of vitamin D daily by mouth (Stamp *et al.*, 1977), although if observations on the UV-irradiated group had been prolonged the daily oral equivalent might have been higher. The rise in serum calcium seen in epileptic children observed during 3 months of oral vitamin D therapy or 3 months of UV light 3 times per week over 600 cm^2 of dorsal skin in the winter months showed that under these conditions UV irradiation was equivalent to about 75 μg of vitamin D orally per day (M. Davie, unpublished observations). In addition to comparing the effects of UV light and oral vitamin D upon plasma 25-(OH)D and serum calcium, it is also possible to estimate directly the vitamin D produced in skin from the product of plasma volume times increase in plasma 25-(OH)D concentration. [At the levels of plasma 25-(OH)D normally achieved during these experiements, there is virtually no cholecalciferol in plasma (M. Davie and D. E. M. Lawson, unpublished observations).] This product gives the total increase in plasma 25-(OH)D and, if divided by the area irradiated, yields a figure of 9.3 ng/cm^2 (Davie and Lawson, 1980), a value close to that found in skin under similar conditions by Bekemeier (1966). Such data as are available indicate that cutaneous vitamin D synthesis is equivalent to quite high oral intakes, but whether this reflects differences in availability or metabolism is uncertain.

B. Pattern of Vitamin D Response by Irradiated Skin

The appearance of vitamin D after UV irradiation of skin is rapid (Bekemeier, 1966; Stamp, 1975; Davie and Lawson, 1980). However, using isolated skin Bekemeier (1966) found that, after the peak vitamin D concentration was reached (under conditions employed, 1.5 μg/cm^2 after 60 minutes of irradiation) the level began to fall during further irradiation, declining to less than 50% of maximum value after 24 hours. *In vivo,* however, the level reaches a plateau (Bekemeier, 1966). In other studies the vitamin D response of skin *in vivo* has been followed by measuring plasma 25-(OH)D. This reaches a plateau after 5–12 exposures (9–27 minutes over 10–22 days; total power at λ265, λ297, λ303 nm = 220 μW/cm^2) of 600 cm^2 dorsal skin; continued irradiation three times weekly (3 minutes per exposure) for 2 more months was not accompanied by a further increase in plasma 25-(OH)D levels (M. Davie, D. E. M. Lawson, and J. O. Barnes, unpublished observations). The rise in plasma 25-(OH)D level shows an inverse correlation with plasma volume. In contrast to irradiating a limited body area, plasma 25-(OH)D shows a continued rise during whole-body irradiation, although a plateau eventually occurs. The initial rapid rise of plasma 25-(OH)D suggests that there is a pool of 7-dehydrocholesterol that can easily be converted to pre-vitamin D, but that thereafter much less is made. The continued rise during the whole-body irradiation demonstrated that higher levels of plasma 25-(OH)D can be achieved if sufficient substrate is made available. Thus it is lack of substrate rather than inhibition of 25-(OH)D formation that prevents a further rise in plasma 25-(OH)D during limited exposure to UV light (Davie and Lawson, 1980). By implication it also indicates that most of the vitamin D is formed in the initial exposures and can be stored—either as vitamin D or pre-vitamin D—before conversion to 25-(OH)D. Knowledge about storage is limited and is discussed later. Whether the vitamin remains in the skin and is slowly, or immediately, transferred elsewhere requires investigation. During the plateau period of vitamin D in skin or 25-(OH)D in plasma, it is probable that sufficient vitamin D is continuously formed in skin to sustain the vitamin level, since plasma 25-(OH)D levels have been observed to fall rapidly after cessation of artificial UV light (Davie,

1980). Further studies are required on the ability of various sites to form pre-vitamin D and on the biological availability of formed vitamin. Data at present available suggest that dorsal skin responds better than abdominal skin (Bekemeier, 1966).

V. Factors Affecting the Cutaneous Synthesis of Vitamin D by Ultraviolet Light

A. Physical and Environmental Factors

In normal circumstances UV light is derived from the solar spectrum. Fluorescent bulbs emit ultraviolet irradiation, but this is usually absorbed by the glass and other fittings (Neer et al., 1971). On reaching the earth's atmosphere, UV light is affected by several factors. Attenuation due to gaseous molecules in the atmosphere (Rayleigh scattering) is inversely proportional to the fourth power of the wavelength. In the UV spectrum it achieves some importance and would be the most important attenuating factor were it not for the existence of the ozone layer. This layer exists between 10,000 and 40,000 ft and is maximal at 20,000 ft, but it is usually expressed as a layer of 3 mm at normal temperature and pressure. The most concentrated region of ozone contains about 6×10^{12} molecules/cm^3 (Koller, 1969; London, 1969). In common with other sources of light, UV power is reduced if the incident light from the illuminating source reaches a surface at an angle other than 90°, the power being spread over a greater area. Power declines proportionally to the curve of the angle from normal (θ) (illumination of angled surface = illumination of perpendicular surface times $\cos \theta$). Thus power is halved when $\cos \theta = 0.5$ (60°), and further deviation from normal has a proportionally greater effect. The power reaching the earth's surface when the above factors are considered has been computed (Schulze and Gräfe, 1969). Table III (taken from their work) shows the marked reduction due to ozone at the wavelengths optimal for vitamin D synthesis. Atmospheric ozone has been monitored at Oxford (UK) over the last 25 years, and the ozone layer has been found to increase by about 10% per annum. The possible effects on vitamin D production calculated by these authors merit further investigation (Leach et al., 1976). Other factors of importance include aerosol scattering and cloud.

Aerosols, with particles 10^2 to 10^{-3} μm in size, exist in the atmosphere when conditions are below saturation. This quantity is of

TABLE III

ATTENUATION OF ULTRAVIOLET POWER BY OZONE[a]

Wavelength (nm)	Extraterrestrial radiation[b] (W/m²)	UV global radiation[c] (W/m²)		Percent UV global radiation after ozone absorption	
		90°	37°	90°	37°
290	5.2	3.1	1.5	10^{-8}	10^{-15}
300	6.1	3.8	1.8	6	0.96
310	7.6	5.5	2.7	43	24

[a] UV global solar radiation (watts per square meter) was measured at wavelengths 290, 300, and 310 nm for sun altitudes 90° and 37° (after Schulze and Gräfe, 1969).

[b] Extraterrestrial irradiation refers to the power that would reach the earth's surface in the absence of the atmosphere.

[c] UV global radiation is the sum of direct solar and sky radiation (after Rayleigh scattering).

course variable, but in the "clear standard atmosphere" at sea level the attenuation coefficient due to aerosol at 300 nm is about 0.3/km compared to 0.15/km due to Rayleigh scattering (Koller, 1969). The effect of cloud density is seen in Fig. 2 (Schulze and Gräfe, 1969). Even on a cloudy day, attenuation reaches only 50%.

One important consequence of the scattering of UV radiation is that shade does not diminish UV power as much as might be expected (Amelung and Kuhnke, 1939). Quantitative estimations of UV power reaching a woman placed on an unshaded lawn support this contention, since the power reaching the side that received no direct sunlight was over 60% of that reaching the side facing the sun (Challoner et al., 1976).

Since little UV light reaches the earth's surface, it is obviously of importance for the body to be exposed if benefit is to accrue. It is important to go outside, but also of great importance to be outside at the critical time of day and at the right time of the year. The opportunity to go outside may be limited because of work, gardeners receiving about six times as much power as laboratory workers (Challoner et al., 1976). Old people may be unable to go outside owing to illness (Pittet et al., 1979). Laboratory workers receive about 16 times more energy than patients in a hospital ward (Challoner et al., 1976). The lack of exposure may account for the reduced variation of plasma 25-(OH)D seen in the elderly (Lester et al., 1977), since the elderly appear to respond as well as younger persons (Davie and Lawson, 1980).

Ultraviolet light power varies considerably with latitude, time of

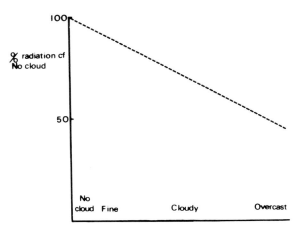

FIG. 2. Effect of cloud cover on the intensity of radiation (280–315 nm) reaching the earth's surface. After Schulze and Gräfe (1969).

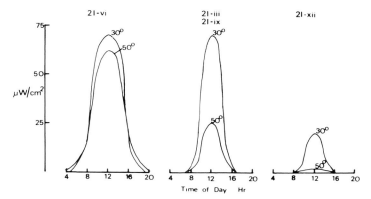

FIG. 3. Ultraviolet global solar radiation at wavelength 307.5 nm (Northern hemisphere) showing the power according to time of day and time of year at latitudes 30° and 50° (21-vi=June 21; 21-iii=March 21; 21-ix=September 21; 21-xii=December 21). After Schulze and Gräfe (1969).

year, and time of day. Figure 3 (adapted from Shulze and Gräfe, 1969) shows these variations. The rapid decline of power at latitude 50° after midsummer compared to the power at 30° is notable. Furthermore, most of this UV power is available between the hours of 8 AM and 4 PM (different times may apply locally when energy saving times are in force). Third, it is seen that the power at latitude 50° is negligible in winter. Data on daily UV energy and yearly energy at various latitudes for different wavelengths of light have been published (Johnson et al., 1976). At latitude 50° the months June through August contain most of the energy (Fig. 4).

B. PENETRATION OF ULTRAVIOLET LIGHT INTO SKIN

Studies on the optics of skin in relation to UV light and vitamin D were begun soon after the discovery of the healing power of UV light in rickets (Bachem and Reed, 1929; Lucas, 1933). The structure of a typical area of skin from the human back is shown in Fig. 5 (Bloom and Fawcett, 1975; Johnson et al., 1968). The stratum corneum varies in thickness according to the site from which it is taken. The stratum lucidum is a thin layer from which all cell nuclei have disappeared. The stratum granulosum is only 3–5 cells thick and lies superficial to the stratum spinosum which is composed of cuboidal cells. The stratum germanitivum is a single layer just above the dermis. The latter two layers are known as the Malpighian layer. The thickness of this layer

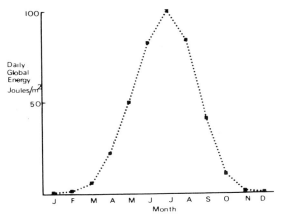

Fɪɢ. 4. Calculated integrated daily global ultraviolet irradiation at sea level (direct solar energy and scattered energy) for 300 nm at latitude of 50°. The values for the middle of each month are shown from January to December. The total annual radiation at this wavelength and latitude is 1.2×10^4 J/m^2.

varies, since the dermal–epidermal junction is undulating. It is not yet certain how far UV light has to penetrate to synthesize vitamin D that is biologically available. Although some vitamin D would be made in the stratum corneum, it seems unlikely that enough is made here or that it is available (see Sections II and VII), leaving the Malpighian layer as the most important site of synthesis. The ability of the stratum corneum to impede the transmission of UV light therefore assumes considerable interest. Various techniques of separating the layers, such as cantharidin, heat, and vacuum, have been used. Using the cantharidin method, White human skin (stratum corneum) was found to be 9.5 μm thick compared to 11.1 μm for African skin (from hip). Transmission of erythemal rays (290–340 nm) was about 50% in White skin, but only 21% in African skin. Pigmentation contributed substantially to this, but the thickness of the horny

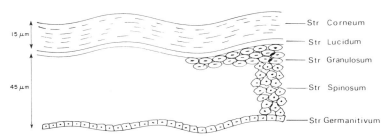

Fɪɢ. 5. Diagram of skin from human back.

layer was also important in the African (Thomson, 1955). The light passing through skin is not all directly transmitted. Light may be scattered or absorbed as well as transmitted, and investigations of these factors have been undertaken. It seems probable, however, that total transmission is the important quantity to measure, and there may be a substantial difference between direct and total transmission (Everett *et al.*, 1966). Studies with monochromatic light source indicate that, at 300 nm, total transmission through stratum corneum is between 25 and 50%, if areas with a notably thick stratum corneum are excluded (Everett *et al.*, 1966). About 10–25% reaches the dermis, nearly all of this light being scattered radiation (Everett *et al.*, 1966). Erythema, induced by UV light could reduce transmission, but it remains to be established that repeated suberythemal doses of UV light affect transmission.

Although pigmentation leads to reduced transmission of UV light, it does not appear to reduce plasma 25-(OH)D response in whole-body irradiation (Stamp, 1975) or controlled irradiation to a known area (Davie and Lawson, 1980). Most artificial UV light work has been undertaken with relatively powerful lights in comparison to sunlight and further studies are required to investigate the possibility of dark-skinned persons exhibiting a higher response threshold.

It has been claimed that male sex hormones promote the production of 25-(OH)D after UV light in rats (Ohata *et al.*, 1977), but it is not clear at what stage testosterone was working. No evidence for a difference according to sex was found in man (Davie and Lawson, 1980).

VI. CUTANEOUS ABSORPTION OF VITAMIN D

A. ABSORPTION OF STEROLS

A wide variation in skin penetration by various sterols has been described (Feldmann and Maibach, 1969). A simple technique using urinary excretion of [^{14}C]cortisol as an indication of total absorption was used to determine the absorption from various skin sites (Feldmann and Maibach, 1967). The least absorption occurred from the plantar aspect of the foot, and the greatest from the scrotum (Table IV) (Feldmann and Maibach, 1967). Areas with a considerable thickness of stratum corneum showed a diminished absorptive capacity, but areas with substantial amounts of hair showed increased

TABLE IV

Skin Absorption of [¹⁴C]Cortisol in Man:
Total Urinary Excretion of ¹⁴C over 5 Days as a Ratio
of Ventral Forearm[a]

Site	Urinary excretion ¹⁴C
Ventral forearm	1.0
Plantar foot	0.14
Palm	0.83
Back	1.7
Scalp	3.5
Forehead	6.0
Scrotum	42.0

[a]Adapted from Feldmann and Maibach (1967).

penetration. Thus a thick stratum corneum is an effective absorptive barrier, but the presence of hair follicles enhances absorption.

In comparative work the differences in absorption in various species of animal are important. In general man appears to absorb steroids to a lesser extent than any other animal (Bartek et al., 1972). Table V, adapted from Bartek et al. (1972), demonstrates this for testosterone in man, rat, rabbit, and pig. Low skin penetration has also been found for steroids other than testosterone. Of 16 steroid preparations tested, absorption varied from 0.4% (dexamethasone) to 18.5% (dehydroepiandrosterone). The mean absorption over 5 days was 8% (Feldmann and Maibach, 1969).

B. Absorption of Vitamin D

The application of irradiated 7-dehydrocholesterol (Hume et al., 1927) or vitamin D (Shaeffer et al., 1956) to rachitic rats is known to induce healing. Indeed topical application of an alcoholic solution of

TABLE V

Percutaneous Absorption of Testosterone 5 Days
after Application[a]

Species	Percent absorbed
Man	10
Pig	25
Rat	45
Rabbit	70

[a]Adapted from Bartek et al. (1972).

TABLE VI

COMPARISON OF RADIOACTIVITY APPEARING IN HUMAN PLASMA AFTER
ADMINISTRATION OF [³H]CHOLECALCIFEROL BY EITHER
ORAL, INTRAVENOUS OR CUTANEOUS ROUTE

	Route				
	Oral	Intravenous (iv)	Cutaneous		
No. of subjects	12	13	3		
Radioactivity in plasma	dpm/ml/μCi	dpm/ml/μCi	dpm/ml/μg	% Oral	% iv
8 Hours after dosing	165	277	5.2	3.2	1.9
24 Hours after dosing	—	—	5.7	3.5	2.1

vitamin D appeared to be as effective as the same dose administered orally (Shaeffer et al., 1956). With a high concentration of 7-dehydrocholesterol in the upper epidermal layers and a high degree of cutaneous absorption, the rat will benefit considerably from UV light reaching the skin surface. In man the lower concentration of 7-dehydrocholesterol in upper epidermal layers means that pre-vitamin D synthesis below the stratum corneum is more important. However, the small amount of 7-dehydrocholesterol in the stratum corneum still has a greater opportunity for conversion. Moreover material with vitamin D activity has been extracted from washings of unbroken skin, presumably from the stratum corneum (Stamp, 1975). The absorption of such material in man would be expected to be low. Table VI shows the ³H-labeled vitamin D₃ (dpm/ml per microcurie of administered dose) in plasma of adult subjects given the vitamin orally, intravenously or cutaneously (M. Davie, unpublished observations). The total radioactivity appearing in plasma after application to dorsal skin in either ethyl ether or wool fat was considerably less than the radioactivity in plasma after oral or intravenous D₃ administration.

VII. STORAGE OF VITAMIN D

A. SITES OF VITAMIN D STORAGE

The distribution of vitamin D in body tissues has been the subject of much investigation since its discovery. Early work was concerned with the administration of large amounts of vitamin D and the use of biological assays to quantify antirachitic potency in different tissues. A dose of 200,000 units of Viosterol by stomach tube to rabbits led to high concentrations in liver and blood, these being the tissues that retained vitamin D for the longest time (Heyman, 1937). Canine tissues examined 3 days after oral dosage with 200,000 units of vitamin D per kilogram showed the highest concentration of vitamin D in kidney. Heart, lung, brain, liver, and spleen all had similar low concentrations, and muscle and fat had least (Morgan and Shimotori, 1943). In the pig, vitamin D activity in blood was the same as or greater than that in liver after oral dosing and took longer to fall after cessation of the supplement (Quarterman *et al.*, 1964a).

The results from studies using bioassays after administration of large amounts of vitamin D do not indicate that any one site selectively concentrates vitamin D. Blood may constitute the largest pool, but other tissues are capable of holding vitamin D. The difference between vitamin D and vitamins A and E, which are concentrated in liver, is well recognized (Quarterman *et al.*, 1964a).

The availability of radioactive vitamin D has enabled studies to be done with more physiological doses. A dose of ^{14}C-labeled vitamin D_3 in corn oil equivalent to 4000–5000 IU/kg was fed to rats for 12 days, when they were killed. Of the vitamin D_3 administered, only 22.2% could be accounted for in the tissues and only 46–75% in tissues and excreta. The highest concentration was found in kidney, but the largest pool was in fat by virtue of its weight. Blood and liver contained less vitamin D, and low concentrations were found in muscle. Of the radioactivity found in fat 60% was vitamin D_3, but much less of the radioactivity in muscle, kidney, and blood was vitamin D. Some animals were observed after cessation of vitamin D_3 administration, and radioactivity fell at similar rates in all tissues except fat, where the decline was slower (Rosenstreich *et al.*, 1971). When radioactive vitamin D suspended in Intralipid is administered intravenously to man, fat and skeletal muscle are the main sites of uptake (Mawer *et al.*, 1972). In fat, cholecalciferol was the principal form present, but in other tissues the proportion of 25-(OH)D_3 was higher. In a patient supplemented with vitamin D, all tissues examined for vitamin D activity had a higher vitamin D_3 activity than blood.

The existing data on the fate of exogenously administered vitamin D do not allow a definite statement to be made about storage. It may be inferred, however, that all tissues may take up vitamin D. In contrast to the many studies of exogenously administered vitamin D or orally administered radioactive vitamin D, there are no direct data concerning the fate of vitamin D synthesized in the skin. Some information may be obtained indirectly by analysis of tissues from farm animals. These investigations suggest that higher concentrations of vitamin D activity are found in blood than in any other tissue. In sheep the highest concentration of vitamin D activity occurred in blood (Quarterman *et al.*, 1964b, quoting New Zealand Department of Agriculture 1949–1950), and in sheep slaughtered in the autumn, vitamin D concentration in blood was twice that in the liver. Moreover, blood held 8–12 times the total quantity of vitamin D activity (Quarterman *et al.*, 1964b). Analysis of bovine tissues showed a level of 25-(OH)Dof 40–58 ng/gm in blood (Koshy and Vander Silk, 1976), whereas in muscle the level was 1.5–3.4 ng/gm in liver 2.7–5.3 ng/gm, and in kidney 5.1–9.8 ng/gm (Koshy and Van der Silk, 1977).

All tissues therefore appear to be able to take up vitamin D or 25-(OH)D and to release their vitamin D in times of need. Fat may differ from other tissues in releasing its vitamin D activity more slowly. The proportion of vitamin D and 25-(OH)D may depend on the state of vitamin D repletion, the method of administration of vitamin D, and the animal used.

B. ULTRAVIOLET LIGHT AND VITAMIN D STATUS

The effectiveness of UV light in the cure of rickets has been known since the work of Huldschinsky (1919) and Chick (1932). Despite these observations, clinical experience at the time made it clear that solar radiation at the appropriate wavelengths was inadequate in large areas of the world to prevent rickets, and consequently it was thought necessary to supplement the diet with vitamin D. Since 1945, however, it has been apparent that children over 2 years old, particularly European children, had very low dietary vitamin D intakes and yet rickets is nonexistent in this group in contrast to the early days of this century. Consequently, it appeared that solar UV light could make a significant contribution to maintenance of vitamin D status, although it has been difficult to measure this contribution. A seasonal variation in the incidence of rickets had been observed in the past, so that a rise in plasma vitamin D levels in animals (Quarterman *et al.*, 1964b) and in plasma 25-(OH)D levels in man (Stamp and Round, 1974) was not unexpected. During the summer, urinary calcium excretion increases (Morgan *et al.*, 1972) and sunlight exposure correlates with serum calcium and phosphate (Hodkinson *et al.*, 1973). However, a correlation between outdoor exposure and

plasma 25-(OH)D levels is less well established. Such a relationship
has been observed among Asian immigrants to Britain (Hunt *et al.*,
1976) but was not found among old people (Nayal *et al.*, 1976).
However, a correlation between dietary vitamin D and plasma
25-(OH)D, an indication of vitamin D status, has been reported (Hunt
et al., 1976, Nayal *et al.*, 1976). These correlations were observed in
subjects who had low levels of plasma 25-(OH)D, and thus significant
changes in plasma 25-(OH)D levels in response to the administration
of vitamin D would be more easily observed than if levels were high.
Under experimental conditions 5 μg or 12.5 μg of vitamin D daily by
mouth appear to make little impact on plasma 25-(OH)D levels
(Poskitt *et al.*, 1979; Somerville *et al.*, 1977). Since the intake of
vitamin D is about 2.5 μg/day in Britain, diet would not be expected to
contribute to vitamin D status in the United Kingdom.

There has not yet been any systematic prospective study investigating the role of summer ultraviolet light in maintaining
vitamin D status. The evidence at present available from epidemio-
logical (Poskitt *et al.*, 1979) or experimental observation (Davie, 1980)
indicates that cessation of ultraviolet power is accompanied by
a rapid decline of plasma 25-(OH)D levels. In keeping with these
observations, blood vitamin D activity in sheep fell rapidly after the
end of the summer (Quarterman *et al.*, 1964b). In the same study with
sheep, the peak summer level of 25-(OH)D achieved was highest in
those kept in southern England and lowest in the animals kept in
Scotland. However, by the following March all sheep had similar
plasma 25-(OH)D levels (Fig. 6). In contrast, elderly human subjects

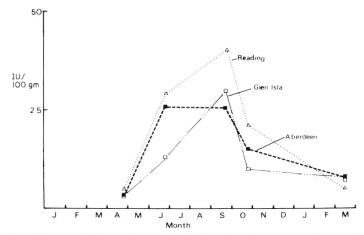

Fɪɢ. 6. Blood levels of vitamin D activity in sheep kept in southern England (Reading) or Scotland (Glen Isla and Aberdeen). Adapted from Quarterman *et al.* (1964b).

studied throughout a period of 12 months showed a positive, logarithmic correlation between plasma 25-(OH)D levels in late summer and late winter (Fig. 7) (Lawson et al., 1979).

The discrepancy between the observations in sheep and elderly human subjects is not easily explained, although the differences in vitamin D activity of sheep plasma in winter may not have been large enough to be detected on a biological assay. The data shown in Fig. 7 demonstrate two further points. First, the level of plasma 25-(OH)D in summer exceeds 10 ng/ml in less than 50% of this elderly population. Second, only about 25% have levels over 5 ng/ml at the end of winter, and if plasma 25-(OH)D levels are to reach 10 ng/ml at this time, then summer levels should exceed 15 ng/ml, a figure achieved by only 20% of this population. The ideal level of plasma 25-(OH)D, or a value below which calcium balance becomes negative, is not known, and there is not a good correlation between plasma 25-(OH)D levels and osteomalacia (Davie et al., 1978). The available data, however, do allow several conclusions to be reached. Plasma 25-(OH)D levels rise in summer, but fall rapidly when UV exposure ceases; the higher the level of plasma 25-(OH)D achieved in summer, the higher will be the late winter level. However, there is considerable fall between summer

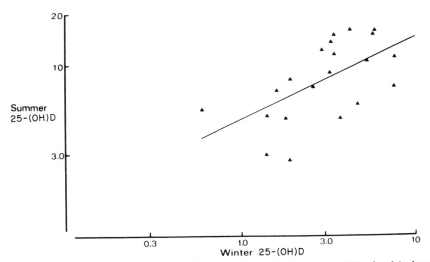

FIG. 7. Plasma 25-(OH)D levels in elderly subjects in the north of England in late summer plotted against the value (in the same individual) at the end of the following winter. The winter level of 25-(OH)D appears to be dependent upon the summer level, and the graph demonstrates that very few elderly subjects achieve summer levels of plasma 25-(OH)D adequate to maintain levels above 5 ng/ml in winter. The correlation coefficient (+0.58) is significant at the 1% level. Data from Lawson et al. (1979).

and winter, and higher summer 25-(OH)D levels than are usually found in the elderly are required to reflect winter levels that might be considered adequate.

Apart from rickets, low plasma 25-(OH)D levels and indeed osteomalacia may exist in a number of conditions associated with impaired intestinal fat absorption. Low plasma 25-(OH)D levels in such conditions as postgastrectomy osteomalacia, idiopathic steatorrhea, and primary biliary cirrhosis are generally ascribed to malabsorption of vitamin D. As discussed in Section VIII, all these conditions respond to UV light with a prompt rise of plasma 25-(OH)D levels. It would therefore be surprising to find low plasma 25-(OH)D levels in these conditions if UV exposure were adequate. This, however, may not be the case (Pittet *et al.*, 1979) and a number of other factors, such as skin threshold response to UV light in the presence of jaundice and the enterohepatic circulation (Arnaud *et al.*, 1975), may also have to be considered. The finding, therefore, that low plasma 25-(OH)D levels occur in the presence of fat malabsorption does not necessarily indicate that malabsorption of dietary vitamin D is directly responsible for the low 25-(OH)D levels observed.

In all these studies there is an assumption that 25-(OH)D levels in plasma reflect vitamin D status. This is consistent with the limited information currently available (Quarterman *et al.*, 1964b; Edelstein *et al.*, 1974), but only with full knowledge of the pattern of formation of vitamin D itself by UV light and of its metabolites and their distribution in the body can we confidently assess the contribution of solar UV light to vitamin D status.

VIII. Ultraviolet Light in the Management of Vitamin D Deficiency

Since the synthesis of vitamin D_2 is simple and the administration of oral vitamin D_2 convenient and cheap, most conditions associated with vitamin D deficiency, though not necessarily vitamin D resistance, have been treated with oral vitamin D_2. In cases where malabsorption of vitamin D occurs, intramuscular injection of vitamin D has been used although the release of vitamin D from the injection site is very slow.

Impaired vitamin D deficiency is frequently found in patients with poor ability to absorb nutrients, as occurs following a partial gastrectomy (Morgan *et al.*, 1965) and in idiopathic steatorrhea (Badenoch and Fourman, 1954) and chronic cholestasis (Atkinson *et al.*, 1956). Furthermore, resistance to the action of oral or intramuscular vitamin D may exist in gluten-sensitive enteropathy (Nassim *et al.*, 1959). Whole-body UV light has been used in the latter condition to effect a rapid improvement of symptoms of osteomalacia (Jung *et al.*, 1978). Similarly, a patient with postgastrectomy osteomalacia experienced a rapid improvement of serum calcium, phosphate, and alkaline phosphatase after only 50 J of UV light (Pittet *et al.*, 1979). In chronic cholestasis due to primary biliary cirrhosis, the rise of plasma 25-(OH)D was similar to that of normal persons in response to whole-body UV light (Jung *et al.*, 1979). These observations testify to the effectiveness of ultraviolet light in healing osteomalacia or raising plasma 25-(OH)D in conditions associated with malabsorption. There are few data, however, concerning the duration and frequency of therapy required to maintain a response. The data reviewed in Section IV suggest that short but fairly frequent courses are required.

Osteomalacia is also found among patients on anticonvulsant drugs (Kruse, 1968), but the appealing hypothesis of microsomal enzyme induction and increased destruction of vitamin D (Dent *et al.*, 1970) to explain this association has not been proved (Stanbury and Mawer, 1978). Ultraviolet light administered to the whole body or a small area of the back led to a rapid response of serum calcium, phosphate, alkaline phosphatase, and 25-(OH)D (Stamp, 1974; Davie, 1980). In both cases healing of osteomalacia occurred with UV light treatment.

Vitamin D deficiency is also a problem in the elderly population (Chalmers *et al.*, 1967). Ultraviolet light is as effective in raising plasma 25-(OH)D levels in elderly as it is in a younger population (Davie and Lawson, 1980). Irradiation from an artificial light source appears to be capable of inducing calcium absorption in the elderly (Neer *et al.*, 1971). These considerations have led to a suggestion that a natural sunlight source of low intensity might be of value in maintaining vitamin D status in the elderly (Corless *et al.*, 1978).

Although ultraviolet light is effective in raising plasma 25-(OH)D levels and initiating healing of osteomalacia in vitamin D deficiency, it appears that the plasma 25-(OH)D levels will start to fall if exposure is not continued. Such prolonged exposure to ultraviolet light may not be hazardous in the elderly when life expectation is limited. Ultraviolet light is, however, a skin carcinogen (*Lancet*, 1978), and were it not for the ozone layer considerable quantities of short wavelength irradiation would reach the earth's surface. Many available ultraviolet lamps emit light wavelengths of less than 290 nm. Ultraviolet light may be of value in healing osteomalacia and possibly is more effective than oral therapy. Its value in the long term in managing patients at risk of osteomalacia, when compared with oral or parenteral vitamin D supplements, is yet to be proved, and the risk of short wavelength irradiation must be taken into account.

IX. Binding Proteins for Vitamin D Metabolites

A. Binding Proteins in Plasma

1. *Introduction*

There is in plasma of all animals a protein of the α- or occasionally β-globulin family with a high affinity for the vitamin D metabolites (reviewed by Lawson, 1978). This protein has the highest affinity for 25-(OH)D, perhaps not unexpectedly in view of the concentration of this steroid in plasma. Several studies have shown that *in vivo* vitamin D and 25-(OH)D are bound to this specific binding protein but at short time intervals after intravenous dosing with vitamin D a portion of the steroid is transported in association with the plasma lipoproteins and occasionally albumin. The properties of the α-globulin are typical of this class of steroid-binding proteins. The presence of high-affinity sites is indicated by the high association constant ($> 10^9 \ M^{-1}$), and the low number of sites per protein molecule by the saturable nature of the binding activity. The features of the steroid molecule necessary for binding activity are the three conjugated double bonds, those at C-7–C-8 and C-10–C-19 being cis relative to the C-5–C-6 double bond (VII, Fig. 1). A hydroxyl group at C-25 is also required, but there is only a small reduction in binding if hydroxyl groups at adjacent carbons are introduced into the 25-(OH)D molecule. The importance of the hydroxyl group at C-3 for binding activity to the plasma binding protein has not yet been assessed.

While these studies of the vitamin D-binding protein were progressing, Daiger and his colleagues (1975), studying the genetic variation in the binding of radioactive ligands to plasma proteins, observed that vitamin D and 25-(OH)D were associated with G_c protein. It is now accepted that the vitamin D-binding protein is in fact the well known group-specific component (G_c) system. As a result there was an immediate and substantial increase in our knowledge of vitamin

D-binding protein resulting from the 16 years of studies on the G_c protein, particularly on its polymorphic electrophoretic variants found in all human populations. In this chapter reference will be made to the protein by both names, depending upon the investigator whose findings are being reviewed.

2. G_c Protein Phenotypes and Their Genetic Variation

There are three common G_c phenotypes detectable electrophoretically, either by immunoelectrophoresis or by electrophoresis on starch or acrylamide gels (Fig. 8) (Hirschfeld, 1959). Some plasma samples contain a fast migrating band denoting the G_c1-1 phenotype, whereas plasma samples of a second type contain a slower migrating band representing the G_c2-2 phenotype. The third type of plasma contains both components in approximately equal amounts and is known as G_c2-1 phenotype. In appropriate electrophoretic systems (e.g., starch gel), it is possible to separate both the G_c1-1 and the G_c2-2 types into two components, of which the slower moving band of G_c1-1 and the faster moving band of G_c2-2 have the same mobility (Reinskou, 1963; Ackfors and Beckman, 1963; Bearn et al., 1964). Thus three bands are present in the heterozygote pattern for G_c2-1. Inheritance characteristics of these proteins have shown that the three G_c types are determined by a pair of autosomal alleles, G_c^1 and G_c^2, neither of which is dominant (Cleve and Bearn, 1962; Reinskou, 1965). A number of rare G_c phenotypes differing from the usual patterns have been identified arising from mutations in the G_c^1 and G_c^2 alleles (for review, see Cleve, 1973). Some of these mutations are extremely rare; for example, G_c^2 allele has been found in only four families (Sorgo, 1975), and G_c Bangkok has been found in a Thai family (Rucknagel et al., 1968). Polymorphism arising from the involvement of a third G_c allele is found in Chippewa Indians in the United States and Australian and Papauan aborigines (G_c Chip and G_c^{Ab}, respectively). The G_c system has proved to be of value as a genetic marker useful in population genetics and in forensic medicine (Reinskou 1968; Giblett, 1969). Gene frequencies of G_c in Caucasians are on the average 0.75 for G_c^1 and 0.25 for G_c^2. Analysis of 80 plasma samples containing bound ^{14}C-labeled vitamin D_3 showed the radioactivity to be associated with proteins that gave an electrophoretic pattern identical with the G_c protein for that sample (Daiger et al., 1975). The gene frequencies for the vitamin D_3-binding genotype of these subjects was calculated to be 0.73 and 0.27, a finding that provided the first indication that the vitamin

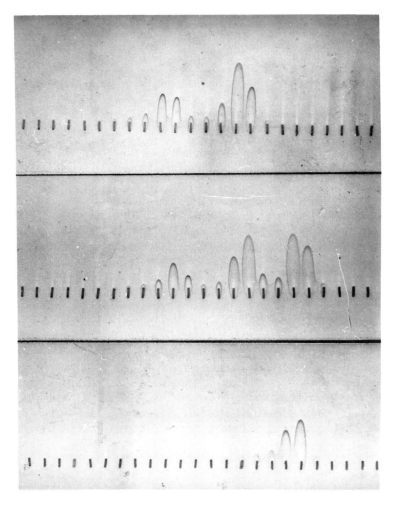

FIG. 8. Analysis of G_c protein phenotypes. The proteins in three different samples of plasma were separated by isoelectric focusing in agarose with Ampholines pH 4–7 at 4°C, current 400 V, and 15 A initially. After 2 hours the gel was sliced along its length in 1-mm sections, and the protein was transferred by electrophoresis into agarose containing antihuman G_c protein. The presence of G_c protein is indicated by rockets. Phenotypes: top, G_c1-1; middle, G_c2-1; bottom, G_c2-2. This system resolves two components in the G_c1-1 samples, but shows only one component in G_c2-2 samples. G_c2-1 contains a mixture of the others in approximately equal amounts. The focusing system was run from the right toward the positive pole. In the electrophoresis system the positive pole is at the top of the plate.

D_3-binding protein and the G_c proteins were identical. Further evidence to support this conclusion is reviewed in the next section, but it is perhaps worth noting that no individual has so far been discovered without G_c protein although over 75,000 individuals have been examined (Cleve, 1973). The vitamin D-binding properties of the rare G_c variants have also been studied, but no differences were found in the following: G_c Darmstadt, G_cY/AB, G_c Toulouse, G_c Norway, G_c Wien, C_c Chippewa, G_c Opava, G_cZ, G_c Pygmy, G_c Caucasian, G_cB1 (American Negro), G_cOr (Chinese and Japanese) and G_c Eskimo (Cleve and Patutschnick, 1977; Daiger and Cavalli-Sforza, 1977). These studies were made using mainly the labeled vitamin, and it was subsequently shown that the three forms $G_c1\text{-}1$, $G_c2\text{-}2$, $G_c2\text{-}1$ bind 25-(OH)D equally well and in this laboratory we have found that this applies also to the other metabolites $1,25\text{-}(OH)_2D_3$ and $24,25\text{-}(OH)_2D_3$.

3. G_c-Protein/Vitamin D-Binding Protein

  a. *Isolation.* Human G_c protein was isolated, and certain physical properties were recorded some time ago (for review, see Putnam, 1977). Perhaps with the successful isolation of human vitamin D-binding protein and the demonstration that these are the same protein (Bouillon *et al.*, 1976a; Haddad and Walgate, 1976a; Imawari *et al.*, 1976), the further analysis of this protein will be resumed with added impetus. The isolation of these proteins in a pure form has not posed any particular problems or involved the use of novel techniques. The procedures adopted have usually involved a precipitation step with, for example, $(NH_4)_2SO_4$ and the use of a number of ion exchange and gel filtration steps. Some investigators have found chromatography on hydroxyapatite columns to be a useful step, and several procedures have involved preparative electrophoresis to complete the purification.

  b. *Evidence for Coidentity of G_c Protein and Vitamin D-Binding Protein.* The first evidence that G_c protein and vitamin D-binding protein are identical came from genetic studies referred to above and from comparison of the immunological characteristics of these two proteins.

  Antibodies have been raised against the pure vitamin D-binding protein and used with antihuman G_c to show that the two antigens are immunologically identical (Haddad and Walgate, 1976a; Bouillon *et al.*, 1976a; Imawari and Goodman, 1977). The vitamin D-binding protein to which the ^{14}C-labeled vitamin has been attached either *in vivo* or *in vitro* is precipitated by anti-G_c protein; in addition, after immunoelectrophoresis of vitamin D-binding protein with ^{14}C-labeled vitamin D bound to it, the resulting precipitation line contained the radioactivity. Anti-G_c protein removes all vitamin D-binding activity from plasma, and anti-vitamin D binding protein depletes plasma of immunoreactivity against anti-G_c protein. Finally, the two precipitin lines formed with anti-vitamin D binding protein and anti-G_c protein of immunodiffusion against whole plasma show complete reaction of identity. Although these results are explicable on the basis that both G_c protein and vitamin D-binding protein as isolated could contain a quantity of the other protein as a contaminant, the results of Daiger *et al.* (1975) eliminate this possibility, as they found the genotypes of these two proteins to have identical gene frequencies.

   c. *Chemical and Physical Properties.* Comparison of the chemical and physical properties of the pure G_c protein and vitamin D-binding protein from human plasma have confirmed the view that the proteins are identical. Thus the amino acid composition of the two proteins is extremely close (Table VII), with about 20% of the amino acid residues as dicarboxylic acids. There are only 2 or 3 tryptophan residues in the molecule but there are relatively large amounts of histidine and cystine (7 and about 25 residues per mole, respectively). It is reported that the N-terminal amino acid is blocked. The question of the quantity and type of carbohydrates attached to the protein is uncertain. The preparations of those investigators regarding the protein as a vitamin D-binding protein appeared to contain about 1% carbohydrate, whereas as much as 4% carbohydrate was found in the earlier G_c preparations (Schultze *et al.*, 1962). Although originally sialic acid was not found in the carbohydrate moiety of the G_c protein, a recent report, utilizing more sensitive techniques, found about 1.2% of this molecule on G_c protein (Svasti and Bowman, 1978). Furthermore, evidence was provided that the different electrophoretic mobilities of the two G_c1-1 proteins result from a difference in their sialic acid content (Svasti and Bowman, 1978; Van Baelen *et al.*, 1978). The faster moving band contains 10-fold more sialic acid than the slower band. The molecular weight of the vitamin D-binding protein of human plasma was reported as 52,000, 56,000, and 59,000 for the three preparations so far obtained, whereas a value of 51,000 was obtained by two groups for G_c protein. Most investigators find the sedimentation coefficient to be 4.15 S and the isoelectric point to be 4.9. The association constant of the protein for the reaction with 25-(OH)D is 10^9 to 10^{10} M^{-1} with one binding site per mole.

TABLE VII
AMINO ACID COMPOSITION OF G_c AND VITAMIN D-BINDING PROTEINS[a]

Amino acid	Vitamin D-binding protein	G_c protein
Lysine	45	40
Histidine	7	8
Arginine	13	13
Aspartic acid	45	44
Threonine	30	28
Serine	40	38
Glutamic acid	65	55
Proline	35	27
Glycine	19	22
Alanine	33	34
Half-cystine	27	17
Valine	26	27
Methionine	9	5
Isoleucine	9	9
Leucine	55	50
Tyrosine	18	11
Phenylalanine	20	17
Tryptophan	2	—
	498	445

[a]Amino acid composition is given as moles per mole of protein and is taken from Bouillon et al. (1976a) for the vitamin D-binding protein and from Simons and Bearn (1967) for G_c protein.

4. Vitamin D-Binding Protein Concentration in Human Plasma

By immunological techniques the plasma concentrations of vitamin D-binding protein have been measured in a wide range of clinical conditions and also in normal men, women, and children (Table VIII). Not only is this protein present in all plasma samples so far analyzed but its concentration is remarkably constant (Haddad and Walgate, 1976b; Imawari and Goodman, 1977; Bouillon et al., 1977). The amount of protein present in plasma is unaffected by sex, age, or conditions of vitamin D sensitivity (sarcoidosis) or of resistance. The concentration of the protein is also unchanged in plasma of patients with Paget's disease, primary hyperparathyroidism, and hypoparathyroidism (Imawari and Goodman, 1977). However, the levels of the protein are lowered in patients with primary biliary cirrhosis

TABLE VIII

CONCENTRATION OF VITAMIN D-BINDING PROTEIN LEVELS IN NORMAL SUBJECTS
AND IN VARIOUS DISEASES[a]

	No. of subjects			Concentration (μg/ml)		
	A	B	C	A	B	C
Normals: Adults	40	35	181	525	421	340
Children	12	—	15	524	—	346
Vitamin D deficient	11	—	—	576	—	329
Vitamin D therapy	12	—	—	496	—	—
Cord, term	10	—	30	558	—	268
Cord, premature	9	—	—	359	—	—
Pregnant women	11	—	—	1524	—	574
Oral contraceptive therapy	10	—	—	824	—	396
Sarcoidosis	6	—	—	492	—	—
Hypoproteinema	10	—	—	234	—	—
Anticonvulsant therapy	5	—	—	485	—	—
Sex-linked hypophosphatemic rickets	14	—	—	551	—	—
Adrenocorticosteroid therapy	6	—	—	660	—	—
Paget's disease	—	6	—	—	432	—
Hyperlipidemic	—	66	—	—	446	—
Osteoporosis	—	—	16	—	—	351
Acromegaly	—	—	9	—	—	404
Growth hormone deficiency	—	—	22	—	—	348

[a] The values quoted are taken from Haddad and Walgate (1976b) for group A; Imawari and Goodman. (1977) for group B; Bouillon et al. for group C.

(223 ± 54 μg/ml in 8 patients) and in those with obstructive jaundice (235 ± 17μg/ml in 6 patients). In these assays the control range was 300–550 μg of vitamin D binding protein per milliliter of plasma Jung et al., 1978). This result is perhaps not expected, as parenchymal cells in culture are able to synthesize this protein (Prunier et al., 1964), and the effect is not specific to the vitamin D-binding protein as albumin concentrations are also reduced. A significant correlation was found between the concentration of the vitamin D-binding protein and of albumin in chronic liver disease ($r = 0.78$, $P < 0.001$).

Apparently the placenta is impermeable to the vitamin D-binding protein so that the fetus produces its own phenotypical protein. The levels of the protein in pregnant women are increased from week 10 of gestation presumably under the influence of estrogens as the levels in women receiving oral contraceptives are also raised. In contrast the levels in the fetus are somewhat below the level in adults (Reinskou, 1968).

No connection has been found between the plasma level of 25-(OH)D and the level of vitamin D-binding protein. Subjects studied have ranged from those with vitamin D deficiency to those with intoxication symptoms and consequently very high plasma levels of 25-(OH)D, but no cases were found in which the concentration of the binding protein varied with changes occurring in the plasma 25-(OH)D levels. Furthermore the plasma levels of the protein are unaffected by changes in plasma Ca concentrations. In molar terms the mean vitamin D-binding protein concentration ranges from 7 to 9 μM (depending upon which of the published data are accepted) compared to normal plasma 25-(OH)D levels of about 50 nM. Even at the highest 25-(OH)D concentrations observed in normal individuals not receiving vitamin D treatment (about 100 ng/ml) about 90% of the plasma vitamin-binding protein is circulating primarily without any steroid bound to it.

The reason for the large excess of this protein is unclear but the view that it is required to protect the animal from overproduction of 25-(OH)D following over-exposure to sunshine seems unlikely since at the highest natural concentration of this steroid over 90% of the binding sites are still empty. The presence in plasma of a high concentration of a protein with a high affinity for 25-(OH)D will result in the accumulation of this steroid in plasma rather than in the tissues when vitamin D status is low. This will ensure the most economic use of the vitamin D available. Many investigators feel that the plasma transporting proteins for steroids have no function being required only to maintain a low plasma concentration of the unbound form of the steroid. The concentration of the free form of the vitamin D metabolites would presumably increase under certain conditions without a large reserve of the protein readily available. If this protein has a function perhaps additional to those considered above it must be concerned with its presence in tissues. Investigations of the vitamin D-binding proteins in tissues have been made through a study in rabbits of the form in plasma (Haddad *et al.*, 1980). Plasma vitamin D-binding protein is metabolized faster than albumin and is rapidly taken up by the tissues including kidney, liver, skeletal muscle, heart, lung, intestine, testis, and bone. There is about twice the amount of vitamin D-binding protein in the extravascular pool as in the intravascular pool—25-(OH)D is cleared much more slowly than vitamin D-binding protein so that significant recirculation occurs. The molar excess of this protein relative to 25-(OH)D in plasma, and the relatively rapid turnover of vitamin D-binding protein suggests its function is to deliver 25-(OH)D to a wide range of cell types.

5. *Species Distribution of Vitamin D-Binding Proteins*

Vitamin D-binding activity has been found in the plasma of every class of vertebrate so far examined, the most extensive survey being conducted by Hay and Watson (1976a,b). In cartilagenous fish and amphibia binding activity is associated with a protein having the electrophoretic mobility of a lipoprotein possibly an α-lipoprotein as the binding activity is not precipitated by heparin and $MnCl_2$.

The plasma of bony fish, reptiles, birds, and mammals contains a protein with binding activity for vitamin D and metabolites having electrophoretic mobilities that range from albumin to α- and β-globulins (Table IX). Although the vitamin D-binding protein in seven species of mammals including elephant, dolphin, whale and some New World monkeys comigrates with albumin on gel electrophoresis, it can be distinguished from albumin by its different sedimentation coefficient (Bouillon *et al.*, 1976b).

Consequently the majority of vertebrates use a specific binding protein to transport vitamin D and metabolites rather than more general carriers such as albumin and lipoproteins.

Birds show the largest variation in the type of protein used as carrier for 25-(OH)D since proteins with the electrophoretic mobility of α- and β-globulins and of albumin are used. Some species of birds, including the domestic chicken, have in their plasma, as carriers of vitamin D and metabolites, two proteins that possess β-globulin mobility on gel electrophoresis. These two proteins should not be confused with the polymorphism shown by the human vitamin D-binding protein discussed previously, since the analytical systems used have insufficient resolving power to separate the polymorphic forms of

TABLE IX

CLASSES OF VERTEBRATE 25-HYDROXYCHOLECALCIFEROL-BINDING PROTEINS

Class	Electrophoretic mobility zone[a]
Fish	
Cartilaginous	Lipoproteins-(4)
Bony	α-Globulin (18)
Amphibians	Lipoproteins (12)
Reptiles	α-Globulin (5)
Birds	α-(3) and β-Globulins (12)
Mammals	α-Globulin (65)
	Albumin (7)

[a]Figures in parentheses indicate the number of species in each class. Data taken from Hay and Watson (1976a,b).

these proteins. Evidence has been presented showing that one of the two chick plasma proteins is a cholecalciferol-binding protein, although with a high affinity *in vitro* for 25-(OH)D also, whereas the second protein is the 25-(OH)D-binding protein similar to that found in other animals (Edelstein *et al.*, 1973). The former protein has a molecular weight of about 60,000, a sedimentation constant of 3.5–4.0 S, and an association constant of $3 \times 10^8 M^{-1}$. Other studies have led to proposals of a specific function for the cholecalciferol-binding protein in relation to vitamin D metabolism and egg yolk formation (Fraser and Emtage, 1976). Since only cholecalciferol, but not 25-(OH)D, readily enters the egg yolk *in vivo*, and as an association of the cholecalciferol-binding protein and phosvitin can readily be demonstrated, it has been proposed that the role of this protein is concerned with ensuring the specific uptake by the egg of cholecalciferol, but not of 25-(OH)D.

The 25-(OH)D-binding protein in chick plasma has a molecular weight of about 54,000; otherwise its physical properties are very similar to those of the cholecalciferol-binding protein (Edelstein *et al.*, 1973). The vitamin D-binding protein from rat plasma has also been isolated in pure form (Bouillon *et al.*, 1978).

6. *Metabolite Specificity of the Vitamin D-Binding Protein*

The specificity of the vitamin D-binding protein from some species for the vitamin D metabolites has been the subject of several studies. The relative insolubility of vitamin D in aqueous solution and its tendency to form micelles or adhere to the surface of the apparatus has hindered the study of the interaction between vitamin D and any possible binding protein. Thus displacement curves for the vitamin with potential binding proteins cannot be readily constructed to reveal proteins able to bind vitamin D specifically, using this technique. As mentioned previously only a few species of birds have a plasma protein for which there is some evidence that the protein can bind vitamin D specifically (Edelstein *et al.*, 1973). This was demonstrated by *in vivo* studies using radioactive vitamin D and metabolites.

The plasma of most species contains only a single protein able to bind vitamin D metabolites, and of these the protein has the highest affinity for 25-(OH)D; reference has already been made to the features of this latter molecule necessary for binding to the protein. The high affinity of the protein for 25-(OH)D has allowed the development of a competitive protein binding assay for this steroid (for review see Lawson, 1980), which has proved of great value in a number of clinical studies of vitamin D metabolism because the major form of the vitamin D activity in plasma is 25-(OH)D. Other metabolites of vitamin D with a C-25 hydroxyl group also have a high affinity for this protein, so that a competitive protein binding assay for 24,24-(OH)D has also been developed (Taylor *et al.*, 1976; Haddad *et al.*, 1977; Kremer and Guillemant, 1978).

The association constant for the binding of 1,25-(OH)$_2$D$_3$ to the plasma protein is relatively low (about $5 \times 10^7 M^{-1}$), and this binding activity is apparently not saturable by this steroid, implying perhaps that the binding is nonspecific. Yet 1,25-(OH)$_2$D is associated with plasma vitamin D-binding protein when plasma proteins are fractionated and the distribution of the hormone on the proteins is recorded. Attempts in this laboratory to show by the equilibrium dialysis technique that 1,25(0H)$_2$D in plasma is protein bound have been unsuccessful, however, since at the end of the dialysis procedure the hormone is always found attached to the dialysis bag or membrane.

7. Relationship to Inhibitor of 25-(OH)D- 1-hydroxylase

The hydroxylation at C-1 of 25-(OH)D to produce 1,25-(OH)$_2$D occurs only in kidney mitochondria by a mixed-function oxidase. The characteristics of the reaction and cofactors necessary for activity have been established for the enzyme from chick kidney mitochondria (for review, see Fraser, 1980). Although the enzyme activity can be readily detected in the kidneys of chicks and quails (Montecuccoli *et al.*, 1977), in general very little activity is detectable in mammalian kidneys (Henry and Norman, 1975). Thus in rat kidneys the enzyme is undectectable and in adult pig kidneys a very low level of activity was found, but in contrast 3-month-old pigs have a level of this enzyme similar to that in chick kidneys (Sommerville *et al.*, 1978).

The ineffectiveness of rat kidney preparations in forming 1,25-(OH)$_2$D *in vitro* has been the subject of a number of investigations, from which it has emerged that rat kidney contains a relatively high concentration of an inhibitor of the 1-hydroxylase enzyme. This inhibitory factor is present in a number of tissues including intestine, liver, and to some extent muscle, and it has been isolated from rat serum (Botham *et al.*, 1974). The factor from rat serum inhibits the 25-(OH)D-1-hydroxylase activity when added to chick kidney preparations *in vitro*. The serum factor was shown to be a protein with physical characteristics indistinguishable from the rat plasma vitamin D-binding protein (Botham *et al.*, 1976). An antibody was raised in rabbits against the rat serum inhibitor and separated from the endogenous inhibitor present in rabbit plasma. The addition of antibody to the rat serum inhibitor of 25-(OH)D-1-hydroxylase confirmed that the inhibition was due to plasma vitamin D-binding protein. Again, antibody added to rat kidney mitochondrial preparations increased their 1-hydroxylase activity (Ghazarian *et al.*, 1978). The inhibitory effect of the plasma protein on the 1-hydroxylase enzyme in chick kidney mitochondria could be partially reversed by addition of the antibody. Although this reversal was minimal, their results are useful in reaching a fuller understanding of the nature of the inhibitory agent(s) of the 1-hydroxylase in rat kidney.

B. TISSUE 25-HYDROXYVITAMIN D-BINDING PROTEINS

One of the curious features of the binding proteins for 25-(OH)D is their apparent presence in tissues despite the lack of evidence that this steroid has a function at any site that would necessitate the presence of such a protein. Binding activity for 25-(OH)D has been found in all nucleated cells in tissues of rats and chicks (Haddad and Birge, 1975; Lawson and Emtage, 1974a; Ulmann *et al.*, 1977; Oku *et al.*, 1974). This activity is due to a protein with a high affinity ($K_a >$ $10^9 \ M^{-1}$) and high specificity for 25-(OH)D. At first it was thought to be a binding protein different from that in plasma since it was significantly larger (sedimentation constant of 5–6 S) and the two proteins could be separated by ion-exchange and gel-filtration chromatography and by polyacrylamide gel electrophoresis (Lawson *et al.*, 1976). However, it subsequently emerged that the binding activity for 25-(OH)D in tissues was due to a complex formed between the plasma vitamin D-binding protein and a protein present in the cytoplasm of all nucleated cells. Thus tissue 25-(OH)D-binding proteins react with anti-plasma vitamin D-binding protein, and after incubation of tissue cytosols with plasma containing [26-^{3}H]25-(OH)D$_3$, the radioactivity is associated with a fraction having a sedimentation constant of 5–6 S (Van Baelan *et al.*, 1977). This fraction is not formed if the cytosol is first heated to 60°C for 60 minutes. The cytosolic component involved in the formation of this complex is heat sensitive and has a sedimentation constant about 4 S. The 5–6 S binding protein is reported not to be present in human and rat kidney cells and human fibroblasts cultured in the presence of serum. These cells, however, contained the 4 S cytosolic protein, since the cytosol fraction formed a complex with added plasma 25-(OH)D-binding protein. The suggestion has been made (Van Baelen *et al.*, 1977) that the 5–6 S tissue 25-(OH)D-binding protein is an artifact formed on homogenization of the tissue when the plasma and cytosolic proteins come into contact but other interpretations of all of the available data are possible (Cooke *et al.*, 1979a). The question of the function of the 4 S cytosol protein still remains. A fortuitous association without a biological function between the latter protein and the plasma protein seems unlikely and further investigation of this tissue protein with a high specificity and affinity for the 25-(OH)D-binding protein (Cooke *et al.*, 1979b) seems desirable.

C. 1,25-DIHYDROXYVITAMIN D-BINDING PROTEIN IN TISSUES

1. *Intestine*

In common with the other steroid hormones 1,25-$(OH)_2$D is found at only two sites, nuclei and cytoplasm, in the cells of its target tissues, and in the intestine at least it is transferred by a temperature-dependent process from the cytoplasm into the nucleus (Brumbaugh and Haussler, 1974). 1,25-$(OH)_2$D is associated with a protein at both sites and the characteristics of these proteins have been the subject of a number of studies. Although attempts have been made to purify these proteins by the use of a variety of chromatographic techniques (Lawson and Emtage, 1974b; Frolick and DeLuca, 1976; McCain *et al.*, 1978; Wecksler and Norman, 1979) this aim will not readily be accomplished owing to the low levels at which the proteins are present in the intestine and the current inability to prevent their structural decomposition. The stability of the proteins is improved if they are kept at as low a temperature as possible and by the inclusion in the solution of extraneous sulfydryl groups and saturating levels of the hormone.

Storage of the nuclear protein at 4°C results in complete loss of binding activity for the hormone over 3–4 days, but at −20°C some activity is still present after 7 days. The addition of 20% (w/v) glycerol to the storage solution decreases the rate of decline in this binding activity (Lawson and Wilson, 1974; McCain *et al.*, 1978). Because of the instability of the intestinal 1,25-$(OH)_2$D-binding proteins all studies of their characteristics have so far used whole intestinal cytosol or crude extracts of the nuclei. A word of caution is perhaps appropriate at this point. The cytosols of the target tissues of 1,25-(OH)$_2$D including intestine contain a number of proteins able to bind to varying extents the hydroxylated metabolites of cholecalciferol. These proteins include the 25-(OH)D-binding proteins from plasma and from tissues, and in addition 1,25-(OH)$_2$D will bind to other components of the cytosol unless care is taken to wash the intestinal mucosal cells thoroughly before homogenization (Kream *et al.*, 1976, 1977a). These proteins can be distinguished by their sedimentation constants in a sucrose gradient. The cytosols of chick intestinal mucosal cells bind 1,25-(OH)$_2$D to a 3.0 S macromolecule having a high affinity and low capacity for the hormone. However, if the tissues are washed before homogenization, the cytosol binds the hormone to a 3.7 S protein having a high affinity (K_a 10^9 M^{-1}) and low capacity for the hormone.

Consideration has been given to the effect of replacing one of the three hydroxyl groups of 1,25-(OH)$_2$D on the affinity of the protein for the steroid. The hydroxyl group at C-1 is the most important feature of the 1,25-(OH)$_2$D molecule influencing binding to the cytosolic protein, but all three hydroxyl groups are involved in the binding to the active site on the protein (Kream *et al.*, 1977b; Eisman and DeLuca, 1977). The hydroxyl at C-3 makes the least contribution toward maintenance of this binding activity. The importance of the contribution of the three conjugated double bonds of 1,25-(OH)$_2$D has not yet been fully assessed. Rotation of the A ring of the molecule to place the C-19 methylene group on the opposite side of the molecule to its usual position (i.e., trans series of vitamin D isomers) reduces binding activity considerably. Interestingly, 1,25-(OH)$_2$D$_2$ and 1,25-(OH)$_2$D$_3$ bind to the chick intestinal cytosol protein with equal affinity (Hughes *et al.*, 1976; Kream *et al.*, 1977b), although the former steroid has 10–20% of the biological activity of 1,25-(OH)$_2$D$_3$ *in vivo* in the chicken (Chen and Bosmann, 1964). In a series of studies into the cause of the relative ineffectiveness of vitamin D$_2$ and its metabolites compared to the vitamin D$_3$ compounds, DeLuca and colleagues have found that the only difference lies in the low binding activity between the binding protein in plasma and 25-(OH)D$_2$ compared to 25-(OH)D$_3$ (Belsey *et al.*, 1974) and is presumably the cause of the more rapid metabolism of vitamin D$_2$ observed in chicks compared to rats.

An alternative approach to the study of the intestinal receptor proteins has involved a system by which the transfer of steroid from cytosolic protein to a nuclear extract (called chromatin by the investigators) could be studied *in vitro* (Procsal *et al.*, 1975). The findings on the structural requirements of the steroid for its interaction with chick intestinal receptor proteins in this system were in essential agreement with those observed for the binding to the cytosolic protein alone.

1,25-$(OH)_2$D is found in intestinal nuclei in association with an acidic protein that can be solubilized from the nuclei by extraction with buffers at pH 9 or solutions containing up to 0.6 M KC1. Analysis of such extracts prepared from nuclei preloaded with radioactive 1,25-$(OH)_2$D showed the hormone to be bound to a protein with a sedimentation constant of about 3.5 S. KC1 extracts of intestinal nuclei from untreated vitamin D-deficient chicks showed saturable binding activity for 1,25-$(OH)_2$D when incubated with the hormone *in vitro* (Lawson and Wilson, 1974). This finding was unexpected, as most steroid hormones are bound by nuclear components only when the nuclei are incubated with the hormone in the presence of the cytosolic receptor protein. Nevertheless this particular nuclear component showing binding activity for 1,25-$(OH)_2$D seems to have the characteristics expected of one involved in the physiological response of the intestine to the hormone. The protein nature of this nuclear component was indicated by a number of properties including loss of binding activity following treatment with proteolytic enzymes whereas RNase and DNase had no effect on binding activity. The sedimentation constant of this protein was about 3.5 S, and the protein has a high affinity for 1,25-$(OH)_2$D (K_a 1.5 × 10^9 M^{-1}). Analysis of the high-affinity binding activity for the 1,25-$(OH)_2$D showed that the number of sites in the intestinal nuclei due to this high-affinity receptor was sufficient to bind the hormone up to a concentration of 2.4 pmol per gram of tissue. This is the amount of the hormone bound to the receptor when saturated and is close to the maximum amount of 1,25-$(OH)_2$D that intestinal nuclei can accumulate *in vivo*.

2. *1,25-Dihydroxyvitamin D Receptors in Tissues Other Than Intestine*

In addition to the intestine other tissues also have receptors for 1,25-$(OH)_2$D. These tissues are known to accumulate the hormone and transfer it to their nuclei; they include bone, parathyroid glands, and kidney. Although vitamin D is thought to have an action in muscle, no receptor for 1,25$(OH)_2$D has yet been described for this tissue. Other tissues, such as liver, testes, adrenal glands, and spleen, which are not traditionally regarded as target tissues for vitamin D, do not contain 1,25-$(OH)_2$D receptor proteins (Tsai and Norman, 1973; Brumbaugh *et al.*, 1975). The cytosols of fetal rat or embyronic chick calvaria contain a 3.5 S protein able to bind 1,25-(OH)$_2$D specifically (Kream *et al.*, 1977c). Chick parathyroid glands have been shown to accumulate 1,25-(OH)$_2$D and to localize the hormone between the cytosol fraction and the nucleus (Henry and Norman, 1976). Perhaps not unexpectedly, therefore, 1,25-(OH)$_2$D receptor proteins have been found at both these sites in the parathyroid glands (Brumbaugh *et al.*, 1975; Cloix *et al.*, 1976). Chick kidney nuclei also contain a protein extractable by dilute salt solutions, which binds 1,25-(OH)$_2$D. The receptors from all these tissues have very similar physical characteristics to the intestinal receptors.

3. *Conclusion*

1,25-(OH)$_2$D receptors exist in tissues known to respond to the hormone, i.e., intestine, kidney, bone, and parathyroid gland. The proteins are present in both the nuclei and cytoplasm of these tissues. Although they have some properties similar to those shown by the other steroid hormone receptors, for example, $K_a > 10^9 \ M^{-1}$ and a temperature-dependent transfer from cytoplasm to nucleus, they differ from the other receptors in that the protein from both cell sites has the same sedimentation constant (3.5–3.7 S). It is on the basis of this latter characteristic that this receptor can be distinguished from the 25-(OH)D-receptors in tissues and plasma. Further progress in defining the action of 1,25-(OH)$_2$D in the intestinal nuclei would be aided by the availability of pure receptor, but its instability creates severe problems. The similarity in physical characteristics between the receptors from the various tissues suggests that the proteins will be found to be very similar, if not identical, to each other.

X. PHYSIOLOGICAL MECHANISMS OF THE INTESTINAL ABSORPTION OF CALCIUM

The physiological processes involved in the absorption of calcium across intestinal mucosal cells involve complex mechanisms that have been surprisingly little studied compared to the mechanisms involved in the absorption of other nutrients. The movement of calcium across membranes occurs presumably by similar processes in all cells including mucosal cells, but only in recent years has it been appreciated that such movements are of importance in controlling a number of vital membrane-bound physiological processes, and consequently the interest in this subject should now increase. In general terms, calcium may be absorbed by an active transport process and/or by passive diffusion. The complexity of the calcium-absorbing system arises because the level of dietary calcium, and consequently of luminal calcium, can vary over very wide limits and also the level of activity of the different mechanisms for calcium absorption varies on passing from duodenum to jejunum and ileum. In addition the mechanism in the intestine for calcium absorption adapts to the level of dietary calcium. In adults about 30% of dietary calcium is absorbed, but this increases to about 60% if the level of dietary calcium falls or there is a physiological need to increase calcium uptake as occurs in growth, pregnancy, and lactation. Active transport occurs when the solute is absorbed against a chemical and electropotential gradient and involves the expenditure of metabolic energy. Diffusion may be of two types: one is called simple diffusion, in which the solute travels down a concentration gradient; the second type is known as facilitated or carrier-mediated diffusion, in which case the system shows saturation kinetics. In this latter case, the solute movement occurs without expenditure of energy.

Irrespective of the method used, all measurements of calcium absorption in rats and chicks show a net transfer of calcium from lumen to plasma. This transfer occurs against a positive potential difference on the serosal side (1–4 mV) and is blocked by metabolic inhibitors, so that the process occurring at low luminal calcium concentrations satisfies the criteria for classification as active transport. The mechanism is saturable and specific for calcium. At higher calcium concentrations (above 2–5 mM), calcium movement occurs by a diffusion process. It is not yet possible to assess the relative contribution of the two systems to the net calcium transport, but in general the active transport process declines in activity on passing from duodenum to ileum whereas diffusional calcium absorption is more detectable in the ileum. Active transport also occurs in the dog, sheep, and pigs (Cramer, 1968; Fox et al., 1978). Problems became apparent with this view of calcium transfer when attempts were made to show whether vitamin D acted at the mucosal or serosal surfaces (or both) of intestinal cells. Furthermore, Harrison and Harrison (1965) observed that in their everted intestinal sac system calcium was absorbed by a diffusional process, and they proposed that vitamin D altered the permeability of the intestinal mucosa to calcium. In a series of studies Wasserman and his colleagues have greatly extended our knowledge of the processes involved in calcium absorption (for reviews, see Wasserman, 1968; Wasserman and Taylor, 1969). An essential observation was that vitamin D increases the calcium flux from plasma to lumen in addition to the flux from lumen to plasma, a result confirmed subsequently by others (Holdsworth *et al.*, 1975). Movement in the direction plasma to lumen may result from stimulation by vitamin D of diffusional leaks or by an effect on pump P (Fig. 9). Net transfer of calcium could occur if both P_2 and P_1 are stimulated, but with a greater increase in P_2 and P_1. These alternatives were resolved by distinguishing between the two parts of calcium absorption, namely, uptake (movement across mucosal membrane) and calcium release from the cell (movement across serosal membrane). Calcium uptake by mucosal cells stimulated by vitamin D is not prevented by metabolic inhibitors such as N_2, cyanide, and low temperature. Consequently, the effect of vitamin D is not on the pumps, but rather it acts to increase the diffusional permeability of the intestine to calcium. The stimulation of the intestinal calcium pump in the direction of the plasma by vitamin D results in this view indirectly by raising cellular calcium concentration and exposing the pump to increased level of calcium ions. Further analysis of the calcium uptake and release processes by mucosal cells of rachitic chicks with time after a dose of vitamin D showed that the vitamin has three effects on the calcium absorption mechanism. It increases (*a*) the rate of uptake by mucosal tissue; (*b*) the mucosal calcium pool size; (*c*) the rate of release of calcium across the serosal surface of intestinal cells. Preparations of intestinal tissue have been developed that seem to allow calcium transport to proceed by similar physiological processes as occur in the whole animal (Adams and Norman, 1970).

The entry of calcium by facilitated diffusion into the mucosal cell can be stimulated by vitamin D and by calcium ionophores such as filipin (Adams *et al.*, 1970) and A23187 (S. M. Lane and D. E. M. Lawson, unpublished observations), providing that the ionophores are

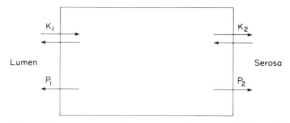

FIG. 9. Possible calcium movements across membranes of intestinal mucosal cells. P_1 and P_2 are pumps that must operate if intracellular calcium is to remain low. Transfer of calcium by diffusional processes K_1 and K_2 also occurs. From Wasserman and Taylor (1969).

placed in contact with the mucosal border of the cells, not the serosal border. Concomitant with an increased transport of calcium by the ionophores, there is an increase in Ca-stimulated ATPase activity. Inhibitors of the Ca-ATPase activity, such as quercetin, also prevent calcium from being transported, but only if added to the medium on the serosal side of the intestinal preparation. This suggests that the Ca-ATPase affected by vitamin D is on the serosal membrane—a view, however, that has not been rigorously established. It is still uncertain therefore whether vitamin D affects the serosal membrane directly or whether the calcium pump, possibly the ATPase, is stimulated indirectly. In addition to the ionophores one other substance, N,N-dicyclohexylcarbodiimide, is known to stimulate calcium transport (Holdsworth *et al.*, 1975). An effect is observed with this substance whether it is added to the serosal or to the mucosal medium bathing the intestinal preparation. It also differs from the ionophores in stimulating calcium transport only in intestines from vitamin D-treated birds, not from rachitic birds. N,N-Dicyclohexylcarbodiimide will be a most interesting substance for further study because it appears to act by supplementing, directly or indirectly, the rate-limiting step in calcium transport, i.e., passage across the serosal membrane (Wong and Norman, 1975). Whether this action is on the serosal membrane or on the mechanism for presenting the calcium to the serosal membrane pump awaits future information. The presence of phosphate is not essential for intestinal calcium transport although it may aid this process. However, most recent investigators seem to have found that the presence of Na^+ on the serosal membrane fluids in *in vitro* preparations is essential (Harrison and Harrison, 1969; Martin and DeLuca, 1969).

XI. BIOCHEMICAL RESPONSES IN THE INTESTINE TO VITAMIN D

A. INTRODUCTION

All the available evidence suggests that $1,25\text{-}(OH)_2D_3$ is the active form of vitamin D in the stimulation of intestinal calcium and phosphorus absorption. Thus it is the most potent form of the vitamin known to stimulate these processes, and the intestine can accumulate the hormone from plasma. After dosing of rachitic animals with vitamin D, the intestinal concentration of this steroid is higher than that of any other metabolite. Furthermore, changes in the calcium absorption activity in the intestine of rachitic chicks dosed with 1,25-(OH)$_2$D follow very closely the changes in the level of this substance in the intestine. Although 24,25-(OH)$_2$D stimulates calcium absorption in experimental animals *in vivo* the effect results from its conversion to 1,24,25-(OH)$_3$D since 24,25-(OH)$_2$D is inactive in anephric animals (Tanaka *et al.*, 1975). Not unexpectedly if 1,25-(OH)$_2$D is a steroid hormone, this metabolite is found at only two sites in the intestine, nucleus and cytoplasm, and specific binding proteins are present at both sites with the probable role of transporting 1,25-(OH)$_2$D into the nucleus (Lawson, 1978). Stimulation of calcium absorption by 1,25-(OH)$_2$D or vitamin D can be prevented by inhibitors of protein synthesis, such as actinomycin D, puromycin, and α-amanitin, suggesting that either the hormone acts to control protein synthesis or protein synthesis must continue for calcium to be absorbed.

B. Response of Protein Synthesis

1. *Calcium-Binding Protein*

One of the major responses of intestinal cells to vitamin D or 1,25-(OH)$_2$D is the synthesis of a protein known as calcium-binding protein (CaBP). In some species, such as chicks and calves, the protein is not present in vitamin D-deficient animals, but this vitamin D dependency cannot be so readily demonstrated in other species, such as pig (Harrison *et al.*, 1975) and guinea pig (Wasserman *et al.*, 1978). The vitamin D dependence of the protein, the increase in intestinal CaBP concentration in animals adapted to a low calcium intake, and the specificity of the protein for calcium are all indicative of a role for it in calcium absorption. Other tissues, such as kidney and uterus, in which extensive vitamin D-stimulated calcium movements occur also contain this protein

The CaBP is found in several tissues in addition to intestine and kidney, including thyroid, liver, pancreas, brain, parotid gland, and plasma (Arnold *et al.*, 1975; Taylor, 1974; Goodwin *et al.*, 1978). The concentrations of CaBP in these tissues is less than 1% of that in intestine. In addition, the antisera of the intestinal CaBP cross-reacts with the protein in the other tissues. Parathyroid glands of the pig contain a calcium-binding protein larger than that in the intestine and not reactive against anti-intestinal CaBP (Murray *et al.*, 1975).

Chick tissues and some mammalian kidneys contain a CaBP with a molecular weight of 27,000, but the protein in other mammalian tissues has a molecular weight of about 9000. Antisera raised against the larger 27,000 MW protein cross-reacts with the proteins of similar size from other tissues, suggesting that even if all the larger proteins are not identical they have antigenic determinants in common. In contrast, there is no cross-reaction between antisera to the 9000 MW protein in guinea pig intestine and bovine intestine with proteins of similar size from other sources (Wasserman *et al.*, 1978). Rat intestine appears to contain two calcium-binding proteins (MW 12,500 and 27,000), the smaller of which is more dependent on vitamin D (Moriuchi *et al.*, 1975). The larger protein was detected in rat intestine with a more sensitive assay for these proteins than is normally used, and it may well be that other tissues also contain it. It is of interest that the small protein is present primarily in the duodenum, and the larger protein in the ileum, of the rat.

The amino acid sequence of porcine intestinal calcium-binding protein is now known (Hofmann *et al.*, 1977) as well as the partial sequence of the bovine intestinal protein (Fullmer and Wasserman, 1977). The amino-terminal groups of these proteins are blocked with an acetyl group causing technical difficulties with sequence analysis, but it is apparent from Table X that of the first 50 residues of the two proteins only 6–8 differ from each other and each of these differences can be accounted for by a single base change within each codon. Proteins with such a degree of invariance in their amino acid sequence could be expected to have a critical physiological role. The mammalian

TABLE X

AMINO ACID SEQUENCE OF PORCINE CALCIUM-BINDING PROTEIN (CaBP) AND PARTIAL
SEQUENCE OF BOVINE CaBP[a]

```
        1                                      10
Ac- Ser-Ala-Glu-Lys-Ser-Pro-Ala-Glu-Leu-Lys-Ser-Ile-Phe-Glu-Lys-Tyr-
    (Ac-Ala-Lys)              (Glu)            (Gly)
            20                                          30
Ala-Ala-Lys-Glu-Gly-Asp-Pro-Asn-Glu-Leu-Ser-Lys-Glu-Glu-Leu-Lys-Gln-
                        40                              (Leu)
Leu-Ile-Gln-Ala-Glu-Phe-Pro-Ser-Leu-Leu-Lys-Gly-Pro-Arg-Thr-Leu-
    (Leu)    (Thr)
    50                                  60
Asp-Asp-Leu-Phe-Gln-Glu-Leu-Asp-Lys-Asn-Gly-Asp-Gly-Glu-Val-Ser-
    (Glx)
              70                              80
Phe-Glu-Glu-Phe-Gln-Val-Leu-Val-Lys-Lys-Ile-Ser-Glu-Lys-Gln-OH
```

[a]The amino acid sequence given is that found for pig CaBP, and the amino acids in parentheses are those present in that position in bovine CaBP.

intestinal CaBP of 9000 MW has only a single tyrosine residue and, at least for the protein in pig intestine, this amino acid is located at the calcium-binding site, as shown by circular dichroism and ultraviolet light studies (Dorrington et al., 1974).

It is of interest that pig intestinal CaBP contains a sequence of residues (57–68) very similar to the sequence in a number of other proteins, including parvalbumin, the light chain of myosin, and troponin C, which are known to bind calcium strongly. The confirmation of this sequence in parvalbumin consists of a helix, a loop in which the calcium is bound, and another helical region. Whether the sequence of amino acids from 57 to 68 of intestinal CaBP contains this conformation remains to be shown, but the views of Kretsinger (1976) on the similarity of structure and basic function of these proteins may suggest a new hypothesis for the mechanism of action of CaBP.

Obviously a complete understanding of the function of CaBP requires a knowledge of its intracellular location. Immunofluorescent localization procedures used by Wasserman and colleagues have shown that CaBP is present in goblet cells of chick intestine and is associated with the absorptive surface of intestinal epithelial cells (Taylor and Wasserman, 1970). Such a distribution has not been found in other studies. In two cases the protein has been reported as present in the cytoplasm of the intestinal mucosal cells of the chick and pig (Morrissey et al., 1976, 1978a; Arnold et al., 1976). Some CaBP also seemed to be associated with intestinal nuclei, but in neither case was the protein found in goblet cells. Support for a plasma-membrane localization has come recently from the use of scanning microscopy of intestinal cells labeled with a fluorescent CaBP antibody (Noda et al., 1978). However, after homogenization of the intestine from any animal and fractionation by the usual techniques to yield the various cell organelles, the CaBP is always found in the cytoplasmic fraction. Recently Feher and Wasserman (1978) have reported that 10% of the CaBP is associated with a membrane fraction, but one that is not derived from the plasma membrane.

Inhibitors of protein synthesis either in vivo or in vitro prevent vitamin D from stimulating not only calcium absorption but also CaBP formation (Lawson and Emtage, 1974c). CaBP synthesis results from the translation of a new mRNA for this protein and does not involve its formation from a precursor (Emtage et al., 1973). The protein is synthesized on free rather than membrane-bound polyribosomes, suggesting that it is an intracellular protein. Consistent with this view is the finding that the size of the protein synthesized on the polyribosomes is the same as that found in the cell, whereas membrane and extracellular proteins are synthesized as larger forms (Spencer *et al.,* 1978a,b).

The relationship with time between the increase in the synthesis of CaBP and in calcium transport in response to vitamin D and 1,25-(OH)₂D has emphasized the importance of the other intestinal responses to 1,25-(OH)₂D in the process of calcium absorption. After a dose of vitamin D, the changes in calcium absorption and in the synthesis and tissue concentration of CaBP occur coincidently about 8 hours after dosing. In response to 1,25-(OH)₂D, however, increased calcium transport can be detected 1 hour after dosing, but the difference from the untreated controls becomes significant only after 2 hours (Fig. 10). Immunologically detectable CaBP is found in the intestine only 5–7 hours after 1,25-(OH)₂D dosing, although synthesis on polysomes or mRNA activity for CaBP can be seen after about 3.5 hours. Thus unless CaBP is active in chick intestine in concentrations about 0.1% of that normally present, these results show that this protein is not essential for calcium transport at least in the early stages after 1,25-(OH)₂D dosing (Spencer *et al.,* 1976a, 1978a; Morrissey *et al.,* 1978b). The maximum increase in calcium transport observed after 125 ng of 1,25-(OH)₂D is attained by 8 hours and is similar in extent to that observed after 1.25 μg of vitamin D, but the stimulation in the former case is short-lived. At later times after administering the hormone, however, when calcium transport has declined to its basal rate, the cellular content of CaBP remains raised. Presumably, therefore,

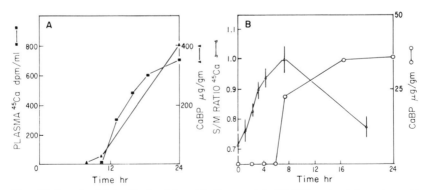

FIG. 10. Levels of intestinal calcium-binding protein (CaBP) and calcium absorption in rachitic chicks after dosing with either vitamin D (panel A) or 1,25-(OH)D (panel B). Groups of chicks were dosed intracardially with vitamin D (5 μg), and calcium absorption was measured *in vivo* from the amount of ⁴⁵Ca from test dose appearing in plasma after 1 hour. Other chicks received 1,25-(OH)₂D (125 μg), and calcium absorption was measured with everted intestinal sacs. CaBP was measured by immunoelectrophoresis.

other factors essential for calcium transport are affected by the hormone besides CaBP, and these factors have a high turnover.

2. *Brush-Border Membrane Proteins*

With the exception of CaBP, it has not been possible to demonstrate an increased synthesis of any other chick intestinal cytoplasmic protein at any time interval after a dose of either viamin D or 1,25-(OH)$_2$D to rachitic chicks (Lawson, 1978). The synthesis of up to three proteins in the brush border of the chick intestine may be increased at various times after 1,25-(OH)$_2$D administration (Wilson and Lawson, 1977). The molecular weights of two of these proteins have been estimated by sodium dodecyl sulfate (SDS) gel electrophoresis to be about 45,000 and 84,000. The incorporation of [^{3}H]leucine into these two proteins occurs at a sufficiently rapid rate for them to be candidates for a role in calcium absorption (Fig. 11). The increase in the synthesis of the third protein occurs at a much slower rate than the other two and has not been studied further.

Brush borders can be readily divided into a membrane fraction and a core fraction. The 45,000 MW protein is located in this latter fraction, whereas the 84,000 MW protein is primarily in the membrane fraction. The smaller protein is the major protein component of the core of the brush border and has been identified as actin (Tilney and Mooseker, 1971). The protein whose synthesis is stimulated by 1,25-(OH)$_2$D has all the properties of actin, including an identical mobility on SDS gel electrophoresis and on isoelectric focusing and

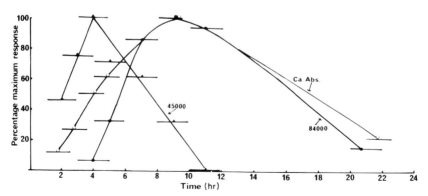

FIG. 11. Changes in the rate of synthesis of two brush border proteins and in calcium absorption in the intestine of rachitic chicks in response to 1,25-(OH)$_2$D (125 ng). ▲ Actin-like protein of 45,000 molecular weight; ●, 84,000 molecular weight protein; □, ^{45}Ca absorption (Ca Abs.) measured by *in vitro* everted intestinal sac method. For experimental details, see Wilson and Lawson (1977).

solubility in low-ionic strength solutions (Wilson and Lawson, 1978). Intestinal brush borders contain approximately equal amounts of β and γ forms of actin (α-actin is present exclusively in skeletal muscle).

C. RESPONSE OF RNA SYNTHESIS

After the rapid accumulation of 1,25-(OH)$_2$D in chick intestinal nuclei, the synthesis of nuclear RNA is stimulated, as is RNA polymerase activity and DNA template capacity, and the physiological response is inhibited *in vitro* by α-amanitin and actinomycin D, implicating RNA transcription and protein synthesis in the mechanism of action of the hormone (for review, see Lawson, 1978). The time sequence of changes in the activity of the mRNA coding for CaBP in chick intestinal polyribosomes has been followed in response to 1,25-(OH)$_2$D. About 2 hours after dosing with the hormone, chick intestinal polysomes contained a trace amount of CaBP as a nascent polypeptide chain (Spencer *et al.*, 1976b). The mRNA has been extracted from the intestinal polysomes of 1,25(OH)$_2$D-treated chicks and translated in a wheat germ extract system, and the CaBP synthesized was identified immunologically. At the same time that this mRNA was obtained from polysomes it was found in the intestinal cell nuclei also (Spencer *et al.*, 1978b). The mRNA was not detected in either the polysomes or nuclei of the vitamin D-deficient chick intestine. It is clear therefore that 1,25-(OH)$_2$D, either directly or indirectly, is involved in regulating transcriptional or maturational events in the intestinal nucleus required for the formation of CaBP mRNA. Spencer *et al.*, (1978b) found that during periods when CaBP synthesis on polysomes occurs at a significant rate, only about 5% of the total extranuclear mRNA was not being translated by the polysomes. The decrease in the mRNA coding for CaBP occurring after the maximum translation rate is reached (Fig. 12) suggests that both the synthesis and translation of this mRNA require the continued presence of the hormone in the intestine. The activity of the mRNA in the cytoplasm must be regulated either by a very short half-life of the RNA (3–4 hours) in the absence of hormone or by fine translational control of the RNA exerted by another 1,25-(OH)$_2$D-dependent factor. The same conclusion can be deduced from other observations. Thus nuclear mRNA activity in the intestine of birds dosed with vitamin D for 48–72 hours was the same as that observed after a pulse dose of the hormone. Hence the pool size of mature CaBP mRNA in the nucleus observed 10–12 hours after dosing with the hormone is the largest attainable and at this time gene

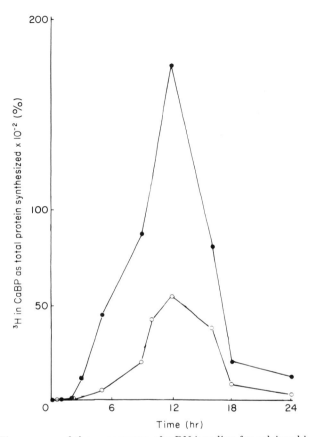

FIG. 12. Time course of the appearance of mRNA coding for calcium-binding protein (CaBP) in polyribosomes and nuclei from chicks dosed with 1,25-(OH)₂D (125 ng). Groups of four rachitic chicks were dosed intracardially with the hormone and killed at the indicated times. Polyribosomes prepared from pooled duodenal mucosas and RNA extracted from nuclei prepared from ileal mucosas of the same birds were translated *in vitro* and in the wheat germ system, respectively. ³H radioactivity in immuno-precipitable CaBP at each time interval is expressed as percentage of total acid-precipitable radioactivity. CaBP mRNA activity: ●, polyribosomal; ○, nuclear.

transcription is occurring at its maximum rate. Despite this, after doses of vitamin D polysomal synthesis of CaBP increases up to 72 hours, showing that vitamin D-dependent factors are present in the intestine which influence the turnover of this RNA. Finally, these studies of the sequence of events in chick intestinal nuclei in response to 1,25-(OH)₂D showed that reactions must be occurring that are additional to those directly affecting formation of nuclear mRNA coding for CaBP, since there is a delay of 6–8 hours between maximal accumulation of the hormone and maximal translation of the cytoplasmic mRNA. In other systems the newly transcribed mRNA is processed very rapidly, with a half-life of minutes, into mature mRNA (Curtis and Weissmann, 1976; Bastos and Aviv, 1977). The explanation of this delay and the identification of the factors regulating the formation and translation of mRNA coding for CaBP are currently under investigation.

D. RESPONSE OF ENZYMES

1. *Adenylcyclase*

Some years ago now it was shown that the activity of this enzyme in the intestinal brush borders of vitamin D-treated rats was higher than that of untreated vitamin D-deficient rats. In addition, cAMP stimulated the absorption of calcium measured *in vivo* or *in vitro*. In the latter case dibutyryl cAMP was added to the medium in which the intestinal loop was incubated (Neville and Holdsworth, 1969). These observations were extended by Corradino (1974), using his organ culture system of embryonic chick duodenum. With this technique an increase in calcium transport across the cultured intestine can be shown in response to the presence of 1,25-$(OH)_2$D in the culture medium. In this system vitamin D_3 increases the intestinal cAMP level after 3 hours, but the concentration declines to control levels at 6 hours. Thereafter there is a continued rise in cAMP levels. Dibutyryl cAMP when added to the culture medium raises calcium transport but does not induce CaBP synthesis. In addition, the effect of 1,25-$(OH)_2$D and dibutyryl cAMP on calcium transport is additive (Corradino, 1974, 1977). In contrast to these findings Walling *et al.*, (1976) observed that 1,25-$(OH)_2$D administered to vitamin D-deficient rats raised cAMP levels only in the duodenum but not in jejunum or ileum, although calcium transport was increased in all three sections. Furthermore, the increase in calcium transport was observed 3 hours before an increase in cAMP levels was found. It is apparent, therefore, that further information is required before the role of adenylcyclase, if any, in vitamin D action in the intestine is understood.

2. *Alkaline Phosphatase/Ca-ATPase*

Since the report by Pileggi *et al.* (1955) that alkaline phosphatase is related to vitamin D status, there have been numerous attempts to involve this enzyme in the vitamin D-sensitive portion of calcium absorption. The activity of the related enzyme Ca-ATPase is also increased by vitamin D, and there have been suggestions that the two activities are simply different manifestations of the same enzyme (Russel et al., 1972; Haussler et al., 1970). But on the basis of the detailed enzymtic characteristics of alkaline phosphatase and Ca-ATPase, other investigators have drawn the opposite conclusion (Felix and Fleisch, 1974; Wass and Butterworth, 1972). In recent years, however, increasing evidence has accumulated that intestinal alkaline phosphatase is not involved in the vitamin D-stimulated calcium transport process. Although calcium is absorbed in the duodenal, jejunal, and ileal regions of the intestine there is only a trace of alkaline phosphatase activity in the ileum. The adaptive response of the intestine to calcium deprivation is seen throughout the whole of the small intestine, but alkaline phosphatase is increased in the duodenum only (Krawitt et al., 1973). Histochemically demonstrable alkaline phosphatase activity has been found in the microvillar and basolateral regions of the duodenum and in the microvillar region of the jejunum, but not at all in the ileum (Ono, 1974). Finally the increase in alkaline phosphatase activity in the intestine of rachitic chicks in response to $1,25\text{-}(OH)_2D$ is slower than the increase in calcium absorption (Norman et al., 1970).

Recently attention has been drawn to the close correlation that exists between the changes in alkaline phosphatase activity and in phosphate absorption in response to $1,25\text{-}(OH)_2D$ (Morrissey et al., 1978b). That this enzyme may be involved in phosphate absorption is an intriguing possibility. Other investigators have shown that the electrophoretic mobility of alkaline phosphatase for vitamin D-deficient birds differs from that of normal birds owing to the absence of sialic acid (Moriuchi et al., 1977). Dosing the animals with vitamin D or metabolites increases the activity of the microsomal enzyme sialyltransferase, which adds sialic acid to the alkaline phosphatase. The calcium content of the microsomes also increased at the same time so that the changes in sialyltransferase activity may not be directly attributable to an effect of $1,25\text{-}(OH)_2D$ on microsomes.

The correlation that exists between the changes in calcium absorption and in Ca/Mg-ATPase in response to vitamin D (Melancon and DeLuca, 1970) has not received the attention it deserves. Results obtained in this laboratory seem to show that there are two ATPase enzymes stimulated by vitamin D, only one of which is magnesium dependent. The Ca/Mg-ATPase responds to $1,25\text{-}(OH)_2D$ in a similar manner as alkaline phosphatase which seems to rule out this enzyme for an important role in calcium transport. In contrast the response of the other Ca-ATPase to 1,25-(OH)$_2$D very closely follows that of calcium absorption (S. Lane and D. E. M. Lawson, unpublished observations) (Fig. 13). Further investigation of the relationship between this latter enzyme and calcium absorption are in progress.

Reference has already been made to the effect of ATPase inhibitors, such as quercetin, that confirm that Ca-ATPase is involved in calcium transport. As with the physiological studies (Section X), direct evidence is required that vitamin D stimulates this enzyme directly and that its activity is not increased after entry of calcium into the cell.

E. CYTOLOGICAL AND OTHER RESPONSES

The ultrastructure of the intestine of animals is altered in vitamin D deficiency; the microvilli are shorter, the Golgi complex is decreased in size, the amount of rough endoplasmic reticulum and the number of lysosomes are reduced. These changes are quite rapidly reversed in response to vitamin D (Jande and Brewer, 1974). An effect of vitamin D on the length of microvilli has been observed by others (Spielvogel *et al.*, 1972; Birge and Alpers, 1973; Bikle *et al.*, 1977), and the ultrastructural appearance of the zonula occludens emphasizes the importance of a normal vitamin D status for the integrity of the intestinal microvilli (Jande, 1978). Plasma membranes of mucosal absorptive cells of chick intestine contain structures that take up calcium. These structures are not present in embryonic intestine but are particularly common in normal birds treated with 1,25(OH)$_2$D (Jande, 1977). These structures are present in axons, and unconvincing claims have been made that they are sites of CaBP localization.

Attempts have been made to assess the distribution of calcium within the cells of the intestine and shell gland. The highest concentration of calcium is found in the mitochondria followed by the nuclear fraction (Sugisaki *et al.*, 1975; Hohman and Schraer, 1966). The high level found in the mitochondria of vitamin D-deficient rat intestine is lowered by treatment with vitamin D whereas the level in microsomes is raised. The nuclear and cytoplasmic calcium in both intestine and shell gland are not involved in the translocation of calcium across these tissues. Interesting comparisons have been made of the calcium content of the mitochondrial and microsomal fractions of the shell gland before and during egg shell formation. Comparison was also made of the calcium levels of the mitochondrial and micrososomal fractions of shell gland with those of liver. During eggshell formation

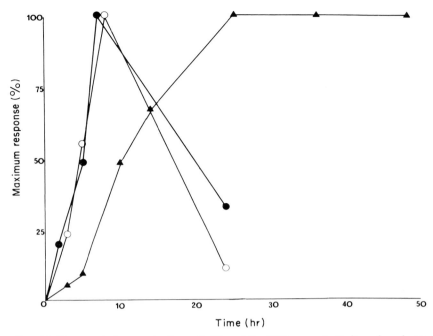

FIG. 13. Temporal changes in the activities of Ca-ATPase and alkaline phosphatase and in calcium absorption in the intestine of vitamin D-deficient chicks after a pulse dose of 1,25-(OH)$_2$D (125 ng). Results are expressed as percentage of the maximum value obtained for each of the three parameters irrespective of the time interval at which this was reached. For experimental details, see Lane and Lawson (1978). ▲, Alkaline phosphatase activity; ●, calcium-stimulated ATPase activity; ○, ^{45}Ca absorption.

there was a reduction specifically in shell gland mitochondrial calcium; this could imply that egg shell calcium has come via mitochondria. The increases in calcium levels of the shell gland microsomal fraction were such that they also could be involved in the formation of the shell.

Suggestions for a role for mitochondria in calcium absorption have been made before (Rasmussen and Bordier, 1974). Mitochondria take up and release large quantities of calcium very rapidly and vitamin D has been shown to stimulate the release of calcium from kidney mitochondria (Engstrom and DeLuca, 1964). However, the same effect can be observed with liver mitochondria. Recently, electron microscopic evidence has been provided showing that intestinal mitochondria in fasted animals are localized underneath the microvilli, but on exposing the intestine to calcium the mitochondria seem to move toward the basal surface of the cell. These mitochondria also appear to be loaded with calcium, whereas those in the intestine of fasted animals were not (Weringer *et al.,* 1978). Before these findings are incorporated into any proposals for a mechanism of calcium absorption, a number of control studies are necessary, such as studies on the effect of other nutrients and of vitamin D deficiency on mitochondrial distribution within intestinal cells.

In other electron micrographs, calcium deposits have been seen in intestinal microvilli from vitamin D-deficient rats; those microvilli decrease in number on treatment of the rats with vitamin D, the deposits subsequently being observed in the mitochondria (Sampson *et al.,* 1970). Intestinal mitochondria are also reported to release calcium more rapidly *in vitro* if suspended in a medium containing CaBP (Hamilton and Holdsworth, 1970, 1976). However, before mitochondria can seriously be considered to be involved in calcium absorption, there is a need for information on the specificity of the calcium movements *in vitro* in intestinal mitochondria under conditions in which pH and osmolarity are controlled.

F. SUMMARY

The conclusion from physiological studies of vitamin D-stimulated calcium absorption is that the understanding of this process in biochemical terms requires the identification of components of the system at two, or possibly three, sites in the mucosal cells. The localization of 1,25-(OH)$_2$D in intestinal nuclei and the effect of protein synthesis inhibitors imply that the hormone controls transcriptional steps in the synthesis of at least one protein—previously assumed to be CaBP. However, this effect is too slow to explain calcium absorption, and the pattern of formation of mRNA coding for CaBP is such that other vitamin D-deficient factors must regulate this process. Consequently, the basic action of 1,25-(OH)$_2$D is still unknown. Since nuclei and cytoplasm are the only fractions known to contain the hormone (despite several attempts in this laboratory, 1,25-(OH)$_2$D has never been detected in brush-border fractions), it is tempting to assume that 1,25-(OH)$_2$D must act on a transcriptional event in protein synthesis. The synthesis of two other proteins, located in the microvilli, one of which is most probably actin is also stimulated by 1,25-(OH)$_2$D, but whether the mechanism involves controlling their synthesis at the transcriptional stage is unknown. The effect of 1,25-(OH)$_2$D on these two proteins is additional to its regulation of CaBP formation mentioned above. The involvement of these two proteins in the facilitated diffusion of calcium across the microvillar membrane is a possibility, and they remain the only recognized vitamin D-sensitive components of this membrane. The reduction in the synthesis of these two proteins may account for the smaller size of the intestinal brush borders in vitamin D-deficient animals.

With regard to the components of the cytoplasmic compartment there are two contenders for the site of 1,25-(OH)$_2$D action, but no satisfactory conclusion can be reached until the location of CaBP in the intestine is settled. Support for a membrane location is as strong as for a cytoplasmic one. Finally, evidence is accumulating that calcium-stimulated ATPase is at least one of the components of the calcium pump mechanism in the basolateral membrane but whether directly affected by 1,25-(OH)$_2$D is unclear. It may also be possible for calcium to be transported across this membrane via a counterion transport mechanism involving Na$^+$ and the Na-ATPase. The findings reviewed here suggest that 1,25-(OH)$_2$D will be found to have more than one site of action in the intestine.

XII. Effect of Vitamin D on Bone Formation

Vitamin D has two actions in animals, one being the control of calcium homeostasis and the other regulation of bone growth. The homeostatic mechanism involves 1,25-(OH)$_2$D acting in intestine, kidney, and bone to increase serum calcium and phosphorus levels. This effect of 1,25-(OH)$_2$D in bone occurs through an increase in osteoclastic activity (Aaron, 1978). Originally bone mineralization was thought to follow the increase in calcium and phosphate levels, but this mineralization was shown not to involve true bone formation (Eastwood, et al., 1974; Rasmussen and Bordier, 1974). It is now almost certain that 1,25-(OH)$_2$D is not involved in the formation of bone but is responsible only for the calcium homeostatic action of vitamin D. In man, rats, and chicks with vitamin D deficiency, 1,25-(OH)$_2$D does not improve the degree of mineralization as assessed histologically (Bordier et al., 1978; Ornoy et al., 1978; Gallagher and Lawson, 1979). In contrast, the combined administration of 1,25-(OH)$_2$D and 24,25-(OH)$_2$D to rachitic chicks and vitamin D-deficient adults improves the degree of mineralization significantly. 24,25-(OH)$_2$D administered to rachitic animals alone has no effect on

serum calcium levels and only a small effect on mineralization. Consequently, the complete effect of vitamin D bone can be observed only
when the bone contains 24,25-(OH)$_2$D and 1,25-(OH)$_2$D is available to
maintain calcium and phosphorus levels in plasma and extracellular
fluids in general. In other studies, 1-hydroxyvitamin D [1-(OH)D], an
analog of 1,25-(OH)$_2$D, was not able to mineralize normally, relative to
vitamin D itself, the collar of cartilage formed around a fracture of the
tibia of a vitamin D-deficient chick (Dekel *et al.*, 1979). In the
1-(OH)D-treated birds the fracture callus was primarily cartilaginous
with very thin trabeculae. After a dose of radioactive cholecalciferol
there is a preferential accumulation of 25-(OH)D and 24,25-(OH)$_2$D in
the callus tissue with very little 1,25-(OH)$_2$D present. The possibility
that the ineffectiveness of 1,25-(OH)$_2$D is due to rapid metabolism, so
that the concentration in bone is not maintained at an adequate level,
has been eliminated (Gallagher and Lawson, 1979).

These findings have only now been obtained because in the past
estimates of potency of 1,25-(OH)$_2$D in bone were not made histologically, which is the only means of measuring true mineralization in
bone.

The metabolism in chicks of radioactive 24,25-(OH)$_2$D in the
presence of 1-(OH)D showed plasma to contain the highest level of
24,25(OH)D, followed by bone. The periosteal and metaphysial portions of bone contained the highest concentration of 24,25(OH)$_2$D, and
the activity of this metabolite was not due to 1,24,25-(OH)$_3$D (Noff *et
al.*, 1978). Support for an essential role of metabolites of vitamin D
other than 1,25-(OH)$_2$D comes from the finding that chick embryos
from hens maintained on 1,25-(OH)$_2$D are not viable compared to
those from hens maintained on 25-(OH)D or a combination of
1,25(OH)$_2$D and 24,25-(OH)$_2$D (Sunde *et al.*, 1978; Henry and Norman,
1978).

The findings reviewed in this last section show that all the actions
of vitamin D cannot be explained by 1,25-(OH)$_2$D, but which of the
other metabolites of vitamin D is active in bone formation awaits further information. The difficulty in ascribing the mineralizing activity
of vitamin D to 24,25-(OH)$_2$D is its very low concentration in bone
relative to 25-(OH)D. It should be appreciated that these findings do
not change previous observations that the Ca^{2+} mobilizing action of
vitamin D is affected by 1,25-(OH)$_2$D acting in conjunction with
parathyroid hormone. Bone formation requires not only the laying
down of new mineral and maintenance of osteoid material, but also the
removal (or mobilization) or existing bone salt, and an understanding
of the interrelationship of these two processes will be nearer with a
fuller appreciation of the nature of all the controlling substances.

REFERENCES

Aaron, J. E. (1978). *In* "Vitamin D" (D. E. M. Lawson, ed.), p. 201. Academic Press, New York.

Abillon, E., and Mermet-Bouvier, R. (1973). *J. Pharm. Sci.* **62**, 1688.

Ackfors, K. E., and Beckman, L. (1963). *Acta Genet. Statist. Med.* **13**, 231.

Adams, T. H., and Norman, A. W. (1970). *J. Biol. Chem.* **245**, 4421.

Adams, T. H., Wong, R. G., and Norman, A. W. (1970). *J. Biol. Chem.* **245**, 4432.

Amelung, W., and Kuhnke, W. (1939). *Dtsch. Med. Wochenschr.* **65**, 997.

Arnaud, S. B., Goldsmith, R. S., Lambert, P. W., and Go, V. L. W. (1975). *Proc. Soc. Exp. Biol. Med.* **149**, 570.

Arnold, B. M., Kovacs, K., and Murray, T. M., (1976). *Digestion* **14**, 77.

Arnold, B. M., Kuttner, M., Willis, D. M., Hitchman, A. J. W., Harrison, J. E., and Murray, T. M. (1975). *Can. J. Physiol. Pharmacol.* **53**, 1135.

Atkinson, M., Nordin, B. E. C., and Sherlock, S. (1956). *Quart. J. Med.* **25**, 229.

Bachem, A., and Reed, C. I. (1929). *Am. J. Physiol.* **90**, 600.

Badenoch, J., and Fourman, P. (1954). *Quart. J. Med.* **23**, 165.

Bartek, M. J., LaBudde, J. A., and Maibach, H. L. (1972). *J. Invest. Dermatol.* **58**, 114.

Bastos, R. N., and Aviv, H. (1977). *Cell* **11**, 641.

Bearn, A. G., Kitchin, F. D., and Bowman, B. H. (1964). *J. Exp. Med.* **120**, 83.

Bekemeier, H. (1966). *Int. Z. Vitaminforsch.* **10**.

Belsey, R. E., DeLuca, H. F., and Potts, J. T. (1974). *Nature (London)* **247**, 208.

Bikle, D. D., Empson, R. N., Herman, R. H., Morrissey, R. L., and Zolock, D. R. (1977). *Biochim. Biophys. Acta* **499**, 61.

Birge, S. J., and Alpers, D. H. (1973). *Gastroenterology* **64**, 977.

Black, H. S., and Rauschkolb, E. W. (1971). *J. Invest. Dermatol.* **56**, 387.

Bloom, W., and Fawcett, D. W. (1975). "A Textbook of Histology," 10th ed. Saunders, Philadelphia.

Bloor, M., and Karenfield, A. (1977). *Dermatologica* **154**, 5.

Bordier, P., Rasmussen, H., Marie, P., Miravet, L., Gueris, J., and Ryckwoert, A. (1978). *J. Clin. Endocrinol. Metab.* **46**, 284.

Botham, K. M., Tanaka, Y., and DeLuca, H. F. (1974). *Biochemistry.* **15**, 4961.

Botham, K. M., Ghazarian, J. G., Kream, B. E., and DeLuca, H. F. (1976). *Biochemistry* **15**, 2130.

Bouillon, R., Van Baelen, H., Rombauts, W., and de Moor, P. (1976a). *Eur. J. Biochem.* **66**, 285.

Bouillon, R., Van Baelen, H., and de Moor P. (1976b). *Biochem. J.* **159**, 463.

Bouillon, R., Van Baelen, H., and de Moor, P. (1977). *J. Clin. Endocrinol. Metab.* **45**, 225.

Bouillon, R., Van Baelen, H., Rombauts, W., and de Moor, P. (1978). *J. Biol. Chem.* **253**, 4426.

Brumbaugh, P. F., and Haussler, M. R. (1974). *J. Biol. Chem.* **249**, 1251.

Brumbaugh, P. F., Hughes, M. R., and Haussler, M. R. (1975). *Proc. Natl. Acad. Sci. U.S.A.* **72**, 4871.

Challoner, A. V. J., Corless, D., Davis, A., Deane, G. M. W., Diffey, B. L., Gupta, S. P., and Magnus, I. A. (1976). *Clin. Exp. Dermatol.* **1**, 175.

Chalmers, J., Conacher, W. D. H., Gardner, D. L., and Scott, P. J. (1967). *J. Bone Joint Surg. Br. Vol.* **49B**, 403.

Chick, H. (1932). *Lancet* **2**, 325, 377.

Chen, P. S., and Bosmann, H. B. (1964). *J. Nutr.* **83**, 133.

Cleve, H. (1973). *Isr. J. Med. Sci.* **9**, 1133.

Cleve, H., and Bearn, A. G. (1962). *Prog. Med. Genet.* **2**, 64.

Cleve, H., and Patutschnick, W. (1977). *Hum. Genet.* **38**, 289.

Cloix, J. F., Ulmann, A., Bachelet, M., and Funck-Brentano, J. L. (1976). *Steroids* **28**, 743.

Cooke, N. E., Walgate, J., and Haddad, J. G. (1979a) *J. Biol. Chem.* **254**, 5958.

Cooke, N. E., Walgate, J., and Haddad, J. G. (1979b). *J. Biol. Chem.* **254**, 5965.

Corless D., Gupta, S. P., Switala, S., Barragry, J. M., Boucher, B. J., Cohen, R. D., and Diffey, B. L. (1978). *Lancet*, **2**, 649.

Corradino, R. A. (1974). *Endocrinology* **94**, 1607.

Corradino, R. A. (1977). *In* "Vitamin D, Proceedings of 3rd Workshop" (A. W. Norman, ed.), p. 231. De Gruyter, Berlin.

Cramer, C. F. (1968). *Can. J. Physiol. Pharmacol.* **46**, 171.

Cruess, R. L., and Clark, G. (1971). *Proc. Soc. Exp. Biol. Med.* **136**, 415.

Curtis, P., and Weissmann, C. (1976). *J. Mol. Biol.* **106**, 1061.

Daiger, S. P., and Cavalli-Sforza, L. L. (1977). *Am. J. Hum. Genet.* **29**, 593.

Daiger, S. P., Schanfield, M. S., and Cavalli-Sforza, L. L. (1975). *Proc. Natl. Acad. Sci. U.S.A.* **72**, 2076.

Datsenko, Z. M. (1969). *Ukr. Biokhim. Zh.* **41**, 418.

Davie, M. (1980). M. D. Thesis, submitted, University of Cambridge.

Davie, M. and Lawson, D. E. M. (1980). *Clin. Sci.* In press.

Davie, M., Lawson, D. E. M., and Jung, R. T. (1978). *Lancet* **1**, 820.

Dekel, S., Ornoy, A., Sekeles, E., Noff, D., and Edelstein, S. (1979). *Calc. Tiss. Intl.* **28**, 245.

DeLuca, H. F., Blunt, J. W., and Rikkers, H. (1971). *In* "The Vitamins" (W. H. Sebrell and R. H. Harris, eds.), 2nd ed., Vol. 3 p. 225. Academic Press, New York.

Dent, C. E., Richens, A., Rowe, D. J. F., and Stamp, T. C. B. (1970). *Br. Med. J.* **4**, 69.

Dorrington, K. J., Hui, A., Hofmann, T., Hitchman, A. J. W., and Harrison, J. E. (1974) *J. Biol. Chem.* **249**, 199.

Eastwood, J. B., Bordier, P. S., Clarkson, E. M., Tun Chot, S., and De Wardener, H. E. (1974). *Clin. Sci. Mol. Med.* **47**, 23.

Edelstein, S., Lawson, D. E. M., and Kodicek, E. (1973). *Biochem. J.* **135**, 417.

Edelstein, S., Charman, M., Lawson, D. E. M., and Kodicek, E. (1974). *Clin. Sci. Mol. Med.* **46**, 231.

Eisman, J. A., and DeLuca, H. F. (1977). *Steroids.* **30**, 245.

Emtage, J. S., Lawson, D. E. M., and Kodicek, E. (1973). *Nature (London)* **246**, 100.

Engstrom, G. W., and DeLuca, H. F. (1964). *Biochemistry* **3**, 203.

Esvelt, R. P., Schnoes, H. K., and DeLuca, H. F. (1978). *Arch. Biochem. Biophys.* **188**, 282.

Everett, M. A., Yeargers, E., Sayre, R. M., and Olsen, R. L. (1966). *Photochem. Photobiol.* **5**, 533.

Feher, J. J., and Wasserman, R. H. (1978). *Biochim. Biophys. Acta* **540**, 134.

Feldmann, R. J., and Maibach, H. I. (1967). *J. Invest. Dermatol.* **48**, 181.

Feldmann, R. J., and Maibach, H. I. (1969). *J. Invest. Dermatol.* **52**, 89.

Felix, R., and Fleisch, H. (1974). *Biochim. Biophys. Acta* **350**, 84.

Festenstein, G. N., and Morton, R. A., (1955). *Biochem. J.* **60**, 22.

Fox, J., Care, A. D., and Swaminathan, R. (1978). *Br. J. Nutr.* **39**, 431.

Fraser, D. R. (1980). *Physiol. Rev.* In press.

Fraser, D. R., and Emtage, J. S. (1976). *Biochem. J.* **160**, 671.

Frolick, C. A., and DeLuca, H. F. (1976). *Steroids* **27**, 433.

Fullmer, C. S., and Wasserman, R. H. (1977). *In* "Calcium-binding Proteins and Calcium Function" (R. H. Wasserman, ed.), p. 303. Elsevier/North-Holland, Amsterdam

Gallagher, J., and Lawson, D. E. M. (1979). *In* "Proceedings of the 4th Workship on Vitamin D" (A. W. Norman, ed.), p. 399. de Gruyter, Berlin.

Garabedian, M., Pezant, E., Miravet, L., Fellot, C., and Balsan, S. (1976). *Endocrinology* **98**, 794.

Gaylor, J. L., and Sault, F. M. (1964), *J. Lipid Res.* **5**, 422.

Ghazarian, J. G., Kream, B., Botham, K. M., Nickells, M. W., and DeLuca, H. F. (1978). *Arch. Biochem. Biophys.* **189**, 212.

Giblett, E. R. (1969). "Genetic Markers in Human Blood." Blackwell, Oxford.

Goodwin, D., Noff, D., and Edelstein, S. (1978). *Biochim. Biophys. Acta* **539**, 249.

Haddad, J. G., and Birge, S. (1975). *J. Biol. Chem.* **250**, 299.

Haddad, J. G., and Walgate, J. (1976a). *J. Biol. Chem.* **251**, 4803.

Haddad, J. G., and Walgate, J. (1976b). *J. Clin. Invest.* **58**, 1217.

Haddad, J. G. Min, C., Mendelsohn, M., Slatopolsky, E., and Hahn, T. (1977). *Arch. Biochem. Biophys.* **182**, 390.

Haddad, J. G., Fraser, D. R., and Lawson, D. E. M. (1980). In preparation.

Hamilton, J. W., and Holdsworth, E. S. (1970). *Biochem. Biophys. Res. Commun.* **40**, 1325.

Hamilton, J. W., and Holdswoth, E. S. (1976). *Aust. J. Exp. Biol. Med. Sci.* **54**, 469.

Hanewald, K. H., Rappoldt, M. P., and Roborgh, J. R. (1961). *Recl. Trav. Chim. Pays-Bas* **80**, 1005.

Harrison, H. C., and Harrison, H. E. (1969). *Am. J. Physiol.* **217**, 121.

Harrison, H. E., and Harrison, H. C. (1965). *Am. J. Physiol.* **208**, 370.

Harrison, J. E., Hitchman, A. J. W., and Brown, R. G. (1975). *Can. J. Physiol. Pharm.* **53**, 144.

Haussler, M. R., Nagode, L. A., and Rasmussen, H. (1970). *Nature (London)* **228**, 1199.

Havinga, E. (1973). *Experientia*, **29**, 1181.

Havinga, E., deKock, R. J., and Rappoldt, M. P. (1960). *Tetrahedron* **11**, 276.

Hay, A. W. M., and Watson, G. (1976a). *Comp. Biochem. Physiol.* **53B**, 163.

Hay, A. W. M., and Watson, G. (1976b). *Comp. Biochem. Physiol.* **53B**, 167.

Henry, H. L., and Norman, A. W. (1975). *Comp. Biochem. Physiol.* **50B**, 431.

Henry, H. L., and Norman, A. W. (1976). *Biochem. Biophys. Res. Commun.* **62**, 781.

Henry, H. L., and Norman, A. W. (1978). *Science* **201**, 835.

Heyman, W. (1937). *J. Biol. Chem.* **118**, 371.

Hirschfeld, J. (1959). *Acta Pathol. Microbiol. Scand.* **47**, 160.

Hodkinson, H. M., Stanton, B. R., Round, P., and Morgan, C. (1973). *Lancet* **1** 910.

Hofmann, T., Kawakami, M., Morris, H., Hitchman, A. J. W., Harrison, J. E., and Dorrington, K. J. (1977). *In* "Calcium-Binding Proteins and Calcium Function" (R. H. Wasserman, ed.), p. 373. Elsevier/North-Holland, Amsterdam.

Hohman, W., and Schraer, H. (1966). *J. Cell Biol.* **30**, 317.

Holdsworth, E. S., Jordan, J. E., and Kaenan, E. (1975). *Biochem. J.* **152**, 181.

Holick, M. F., and Clark, M. B. (1978). *Fed. Proc., Fed. Am. Soc. Exp. Biol.* **37**, 2567.

Holick, M. F., Frommer, J. E., McNeil, S. C., Richtand, N. M., Henley, J. W., and Potts, J. T., Jr. (1977). *Biochem. Biophys. Res. Commun.* **76**, 107.

Hughes, M. R., Baylink, D. J., Jones, P. G., and Haussler, M. R. (1976). *J. Clin. Invest.* **58**, 61.

Huldschinsky, K. (1919). *Dtsch. Med. Wochenschr.* **45**, 712.

Hume, E. M., Lucas, N. S., and Smith, H. H. (1927). *Biochem. J.* **21**, 262.

Hunt, S. P., O'Riordan, J. L. H., Windo, J., and Truswell, A. S. (1976). *Br. Med. J.* **11**, 1351.

Imawari, M., and Goodman, D. S. (1977). *J. Clin. Invest.* **59**, 432

Imawari, M., Kida, K. S., and Goodman, D. S. (1976). *J. Clin. Invest.* **58**, 514.
Jande, S. S. (1977). *Anat. Embryol.* **150**, 155.
Jande, S. S. (1978). *Cytobios* **17**, 171.
Jande, S. S., and Brewer, L. M. (1974). *Z. Anat. Entwicklungsgesch.* **144**, 249.
Johnson, B. E., Daniels, F., and Magnus, I. A. (1968). "Photophysiology" (A. C. Geise, ed.), Vol. 4, p. 112. Academic Press, New York.
Johnson, F. S., Mo, T., and Green, A. E. S. (1976). *Photochem. Photobiol.* **23**, 179.
Jung, R. T., Davie, M., Hunter, J. O., and Chalmers, T. M. (1978). *Br. Med. J.* **1**, 1668.
Jung, R. T., Davie, M., Siklos, P., Chalmers, M., Hunter, J. O., and Lawson, D. E. M. (1979). *Gut* **20**, 840.
Kandutsch, A. A., Murphy, E. D., and Dreisbach, M. E. (1956). *Arch. Biochem. Biophys.* **61**, 450.
Knudson, A., and Benford, F. (1938). *J. Biol. Chem.* **124**, 287.
Kobayashi, T., and Yasumura, M. (1973). *J. Nutr. Sci. Vitaminol.* **19**, 123.
Koller, L. (1969). *In* "The Biological Effects of Ultraviolet Radiation" (F. Urbach, ed.), p. 329. Pergamon, Oxford.
Koshy, K. T., and Van der Silk, A. L. (1976). *Anal. Biochem.* **74**, 282.
Koshy, K. T., and Van der Silk, A. L. (1977). *Agric. Food Chem.* **25**, 3965.
Krawitt, E. L., Stubbert, P. A., and Ennis, P. H. (1973). *Am. J. Physiol.* **224**, 548.
Kream, B. E., Reynolds, R. D., Knutson, J. C., Eisman, J. A., and DeLuca, H. F. (1976). *Arch. Biochem. Biophys.* **176**, 779.
Kream, B. E., Yamada, S., Schnoes, H. K., and DeLuca, H. F. (1977a). *J. Biol. Chem.* **252**, 4501.
Kream, B. E., Jose, M. J. L., and DeLuca, H. F. (1977b). *Arch. Biochem. Biophys.* **179**, 462.
Kream, B. E., Jose, M. J. L., Yamada, S., and DeLuca, H. F. (1977c). *Science* **181**, 1086.
Kremer, R. and Guillemant, S. (1978). *Clin. Chim. Acta* **86**, 187.
Kretsinger, R. H. (1976). *Annu. Rev. Biochem.* **45**, 239.
Kruse, R. (1968). *Monatsschr. Kinderheilk.* **116**, 378.
Lancet (1978). **1**, 537.
Lane, S. M., and Lawson, D. E. M. (1978). *Biochem. J.* **174**, 1067.
Lawson, D. E. M. (1978). *In* "Vitamin D" (D. E. M. Lawson, ed.), p. 167. Academic Press, New York.
Lawson, D. E. M. (1980). *Methods Enzymol.* **67**, 459.
Lawson, D. E. M. and Emtage, J. S. (1974a). *In* "Calcium-Regulating Hormones" (R. V. Talmage, M. Owen, and J. A. Parsons, eds.), p. 330. *Excerpta Med. Found.*, Amsterdam.
Lawson, D. E. M., and Emtage, J. S. (1974b). *In* "The Metabolism and Function of Vitamin D" (D. R. Fraser, ed.), p. 75. Biochemical Society, London.
Lawson, D. E. M., and Emtage, J. S. (1974c). *Vitam. Horm. (New York)* **32**, 277.
Lawson, D. E. M., and Wilson, P. W. (1974). *Biochem. J.* **144**, 573.
Lawson, D. E. M., Charman, M., Wilson, P. W., and Edelstein, S. (1976). *Biochim. Biophys. Acta* **437**, 403.
Lawson, D. E. M., Paul, A. A., Black, A. E., Cole, T. J., Mandal, A. R., and Davie, M. (1979). *Br. Med. J.* **2**, 303.
Leach, J. F., Pingstone, A. R., Hall, K. A., Ensell, F. J., and Burton, J. L. (1976). *Aviat. Space Environ. Med.* **47**, 630.
Lester, E., Skinner, R. K., and Wills, M. R. (1977). *Lancet*, **1**, 979.
London, J. (1969). *In* "The Biological Effects of Ultraviolet Radiation" (F. Urbach, ed.), p. 335. Pergamon, Oxford.
Lucas, N. S. (1933). *Biochem. J.* **27**, 133.

McCain, T. A., Haussler, M. R., Okrent, D., and Hughes, M. R. (1978). *FEBS Lett.* **86**, 65.

Martin, D. L., and DeLuca, H. F. (1969). *Am. J. Physiol.* **217**, 1351.

Mawer, E. B., Backhouse, J., Holman, C. A., Lumb, G. A., and Stanbury, S. W. (1972). *Clin. Sci.* **43**, 413.

Melancon, M. J., and DeLuca, H. F. (1970). *Biochemistry* **9**, 1658.

Montecuccoli, G., Bar, A., Risenfeld, G., and Hurwitz, S. (1977). *Comp. Biochem. Physiol. A* **57**, 331.

Morgan, A. F., and Shimotori, N. (1943). *J. Biol. Chem.* **147**, 189.

Morgan, D. B., Paterson, C. R., Woods, C. G., Pulvertaft, C. N., and, Fourman, P. (1965). *Lancet* **2**, 1089.

Morgan, D. B., Rivlin, R. S., and Davis, R. H. (1972). *Am. J. Clin. Nutr.* **25**, 652.

Moriuchi, S.,Yamanouchi, T., and Hosoya, N. (1975). *J. Nutr. Sci. Vitaminol.* **21**, 251.

Moriuchi, S., Yoshizawa, S., and Hosoya, N. (1977). *J. Nutr. Sci. Vitaminol.* **23**, 497

Morrisey, R. L., Empson, R. N., Bucci, T. J., and Bickle, D. D. (1976). *Proc. Am. Soc. Exp. Biol.* **35**, 339.

Morrisey, R. L., Empson, R. N., Zolock, D. T., Bikle, D. D., and Bucci, T. J. (1978a). *Biochim. Biophys. Acta* **538**, 34.

Morrisey, R. L., Zolock, D. T., Bikle, D. D., Empson, R. N., and Bucci, T. J. (1978b). *Biochim. Biophys. Acta* **538**, 23.

Murray, T. M., Arnold, B. M., Kuttner, M., Kovcas, K., Hitchman, A. J. W., and Harrison, J. E. (1975). *In* "Calcium-Regulating Hormones" (R. V. Talmage, M. Owen, and J. A. Parsons, eds.), p. 371. *Excerpta Med. Found.* Amsterdam.

Nassim, J. R., Saville, P. D., Cook, P. B., and Mulligan, L. (1959). *Quart. J. Med.* **28**, 141.

Nayal, A. S., Maclennan, W. J., Hamilton, J. C., Rose, P., and Kong, M. (1976). *Gerontology* **24**, 117.

Neer, R. M., Davis, T. R. A., Walcott, A., Koski, S., Schepis, P., Taylor, I., Thorington, L., and Wurtman, R. J. (1971). *Nature (London)* **229**, 255.

Neville, E. S., and Holdsworth, E. S. (1969). *FEBS Lett.* **2**, 313.

Noda, S., Kubota, K., Yoshizawa, S., Moriuchi, S., and Hosoya, N. (1978). *J. Nutr. Sci. Vitaminol.* **24**, 331.

Noff, D., Goodwin, D., and Edelstein, S. (1979). *J. Mol. Med.* **3**, 147.

Norman, A. W., Mircheff, A. K., Adams, T. H., and Spielvogel, A. (1970). *Biochim. Biophys. Acta* **215**, 348.

Ohata, M., Sakagami, Y., and Fujita, T. (1977). *Endocrinol. Jpn.* **24**, 519.

Okano, T., Yasumura, M., Mizuno, K., and Kobayashi, T. (1977). *J. Nutr. Sci. Vitaminol.* **23**, 165.

Oku, T., Ooizumi, K., and Hosoya, N. (1974). *J. Nutr. Sci. Vitaminol.* **20**, 9.

Ono, K. (1974). *Acta Histochem.* **51**, 124.

Ornoy, A., Goodwin, D., Noff, D., and Edelstein, S. (1978). *Nature (London)* **276**, 517.

Petrova, E. A., Nikulicheva, S. I., and Khudadov, G. D. (1976). *Vopr. Pitan.* **12**, 8.

Pilleggi, V. J., DeLuca, H. F., and Steenbock, H. (1955). *Arch. Biochem. Biophys.* **58**, 194.

Pittet, P., Davie, M., and Lawson, D. E. M. (1979). *Nutr. Metab.* **23**, 109.

Poskitt, E. M. E., Cole, T. J., and Lawson, D. E. M. (1979;. *Br. Med. J.* **1**, 221.

Procsal, D. A., Okamura, W. H., and Norman, A. W. (1975). *J. Biol. Chem.* **250**, 8382.

Prunier, J. H., Bearn, A. G., and Cleve, H. (1964). *Proc. Soc. Exp. Biol. Med.* **115**, 1005.

Putnam, F. W. (1977). *In* "The Plasma Proteins" (F. W. Putnam, ed.), Vol. 3, p. 333. Academic Press, New York.

Quarterman, J., Dalgarno, A. C., Adam, A., Fell, B. F., and Boyne, R. (1964a). *Br. J. Nutr.* **18**, 65.

Quarterman, J., Dalgarno, A. C., and Adam, A. (1964b). *Br. J. Nutr.* **18**, 79.
Rappoldt, M. R., and Havinga, E. (1960). *Recl. Trav. Chim. Pays-Bas* **79**, 369.
Rasmussen, H., and Bordier, P. (1974). *In* "The Physiological and Cellular Basis of Metabolic Bone Disease," p. 243. Williams & Wilkins, Baltimore, Maryland.
Rauschkolb, E. W., Farrel, G., and Knox, J. M. (1967). *J. Invest. Dermatol.* **49**, 632.
Rauschkolb, E. W., Davis, H. W., Fenmore, D. C., Black, H. S., and Fabre, L. F. (1969). *J. Invest. Dermatol.* **53**, 289.
Reinertson, R. P., and Wheatley, V. R. (1959). *J. Invest. Dermatol.* **32**, 49.
Reinskou, T. (1963). *Acta Pathol. Microbiol. Scand. Sect. B* **59**, 526.
Reinskou, T. (1965). *Acta Genet. Statist. Med.* **15**, 234.
Reinskou, T. (1968). *Ser. Haematol.* **1**, 21.
Rosenstreich, S. J., Rich, C., and Volwiler, W. (1971). *J. Clin. Invest.* **50**, 679.
Rucknagel, D., Schreffler, D., and Halstead, S. (1968). *Am. J. Hum. Genet.* **20**, 418.
Russel, R. G. G., Monod, A., Bonjour, J. P., and Fleisch, H. (1972). *Nature (London)* **240**, 126.
Sampson, H. W., Mathews, J. L., Martin, J. H., and Kunin, A. S. (1970). *Calcif. Tissue Res.* **5**, 305.
Sanders, G. M., Pot, J., and Havinga, E. (1969). *Fortschr. Chem. Org. Naturst.* **27**, 131.
Schaeffer, A. E., Sassaman, H. L., Slocum, A., and Greene, R. D. (1956). *J. Nutr.* **59**, 171.
Schultze, H. E., Biel, H., Haupt, H., and Heide, K. (1962). *Naturwissenschaften* **49**, 108.
Schulze, R., and Gräfe, K. (1969). *In* "The Biological Effects of Ultra Violet Radiation" (F. Urbach, ed.), p. 359. Pergamon, Oxford.
Semenov, V. L., and Datsenko, Z. M. (1976). *Ukr. Biokhim. Zh.* **48**, 645.
Simko, V., Bovek, P., and Ginter, E. (1969). *Vintr. Lek.* **15**, 150.
Simons, K., and Bearn, A. G. (1967). *Biochim. Biophys. Acta* **133**, 499.
Somerville, P. J., Lien, J. W. K., and Kaye, M. (1977). *J. Gerontol.* **32**, 659.
Sommerville, B. A., Fox, J., Care, A. D., and Swaminathan, R. (1978). *Br. J. Nutr.* **40**, 159.
Sorgo, G. (1975). *Hum. Hered.* **25**, 305.
Spencer, R., Charman, M., Wilson, P. W., and Lawson, D. E. M. (1976a). *Nature (London)* **263**, 161.
Spencer, R., Charman, M., Emtage, J. S., and Lawson, D. E. M. (1976b). *Eur. J. Biochem.* **71**, 399.
Spencer, R., Charman, M., Wilson, P. W., and Lawson, D. E. M. (1978a). *Biochem. J.* **170**, 93.
Spencer, R., Charman, M., and Lawson, D. E. M. (1978b). *Biochem. J.* **175**, 1089.
Spielvogel, A. M., Farley, R. D., and Norman, A. W. (1972). *Exp. Cell. Res.* **74**, 359.
Stamp, T. C. B. (1974). *Proc. R. Soc. Med.* **67**, 2
Stamp, T. C. B. (1975). *Proc. Nutr. Soc.* **34**, 119.
Stamp, T. C. B., and Round, J. B. (1974). *Nature (London)* **247**, 563.
Stamp, T. C. B., Haddad, J. G., and Twigg, C. A. (1977). *Lancet* **1** 1341.
Stanbury, S. W., and Mawer, E. B. (1978). *In* "Vitamin D" (D. E. M. Lawson), p. 303. Academic Press, New York.
Sugisaki, N. I., Moriuchi, S., and Hosoya, N. (1975). *Science* **200**, 1067.
Sunde, M. L., Turk, C. M., and DeLuca, H. F. (1978). *Science* **200**, 1067.
Svasti, J., and Bowman, B. H.(1978). *J. Biol. Chem.* **253**, 4188.
Tanaka, Y., DeLuca, H. F., Ikekawa, N., Morisaki, M., and Koizumi, N. (1975). *Arch. Biochem. Biophys.* **170**, 620.
Taylor, A. N. (1974). *Arch. Biochem. Biophys.* **161**, 100.
Taylor, A. N., and Wasserman, R. H. (1970). *J. Histochem. Cytochem.* **18**, 107.

Taylor, C. M., Hughes, S. E., and de Silva, P. (1976). *Biochem, Biophys., Res. Commun.* **70**, 1243.

Thomson, M. L. (1955). *J. Physiol. (London).* **127**, 236.

Tilney, L. G., and Mooseker, M. (1971). *Proc. Natl. Acad. Sci. U.S.A.* **68**, 2611.

Tsai, H. C., and Norman, A. W. (1973). *J. Biol. Chem.* **248**, 5967.

Ulmann, A., Brami, M., Pezant, E., Garabedian, M., and Funck-Brentano, J. L. (1977). *Acta Endocrinol.* **84**, 439.

Van Baelen, H., Bouillon, R. and de Moor, P. (1977). *J. Biol. Chem.* **252**, 2515.

Van Baelen, H. Bouillon, R. and de Moor, P. (1978). *J. Biol. Chem.* **253**, 6344.

Velluz, L., and Amiard, G. (1949). *C. R. Acad. Sci.* **228**, 692.

Walling, M. W., Brastus, T. A., and Kimberg, D. V. (1976). *Endocrine Res. Commun.* **3**, 83.

Wass, M., and Butterworth, R. J. (1972). *Biochim. Biophys. Acta* **290**, 321.

Wasserman, R. H. (1968). *Calcif. Tissue Res.* **2**, 301.

Wasserman R. H., and Taylor, A. N. (1969). *In* "Mineral Metabolism" (C. Comar and F. Bronner, eds.), Vol. 3, p. 321. Academic Press, New York.

Wasserman, R. H., Fullmer, C. S., and Taylor, A. N. (1978). *In* "Vitamin D" (D. E. M. Lawson, ed.), p. 133. Academic Press, New York.

Wecksler, W. R., and Norman, A. W. (1979). *Anal. Biochem.* **92**, 314.

Wells, W. W., and Baumann, C. A. (1954). *Arch. Biochem. Biophys.* **53**, 471.

Weringer, E. J., Oldham, S. B., and Bethune, J. E. (1978). *Calcif. Tissue Res.* **26**, 71.

Wheatley, V. R., and Reinertson, R. P. (1958). *J. Invest. Dermatol.* **37**, 51.

Wilson, P. W., and Lawson, D. E. M. (1977). *Biochim. Biophys. Acta* **497**, 805.

Wilson, P. W., and Lawson, D. E. M. (1978). *Biochem. J.* **173**, 627.

Windaus, A., Deppe, M., and Wunderlich W. (1938). *Justus Liebigs Ann. Chem.* **533**, 118.

Windaus, A., Deppe, M., and Roosen-Punge, C. (1939). *Justus Liebigs Ann. Chem.* **537**,1.

Wong, R. G., and Norman, A. W. (1975). *J. Biol. Chem.* **250**, 2411.

Yasumura, M., Okano, T., Mizuno, K., and Kobayashi, T. (1977). *J. Nutr. Sci. Vitaminol.* **23**, 513.

VITAMINS AND HORMONES, VOL. 37

Epidermal Growth Factor–Urogastrone, a Polypeptide Acquiring Hormonal Status*

MORLEY D. HOLLENBERG†

Howard Hughes Medical Institute Laboratory, Division of Clinical Pharmacology, Departments of Medicine and of Pharmacology and Experimental Therapeutics, Johns Hopkins University School of Medicine, Baltimore, Maryland

I. Introduction 69
II. Isolation and Properties of Mouse and Human Epidermal Growth
    Factor–Urogastrone (EGF-URO)..................................... 72
    A. Mouse EGF-URO... 72
    B. Human EGF-URO.. 74
III. Biosynthesis, Storage, and Secretion of EGF-URO.................... 75
    A. Studies in the Mouse... 75
    B. Studies in Man.. 77
IV. Biological Actions of EGF-URO 78
    A. Actions *in Vivo*.. 78
    B. Effects *in Vitro*... 79
V. The Membrane Receptor for EGF-URO 83
    A. Characterization of the Receptor in Cultured Cells................ 83
    B. Receptor Mobility, Ligand Internalization, and the Mitogenic Action
       of EGF-URO 85
    C. Characterization of the Particulate and Soluble Receptor.......... 87
VI. Structure–Activity Relationships for Receptor Binding and Biological
    Activity.. 97
VII. The EGF-URO Receptor, Cell Transformation, and Tumorigenesis....... 100
VIII. Is EGF-URO a Hormone?... 103
    References 106

I. INTRODUCTION

Two remarkable, entirely independent stories document the discovery, isolation, and complete sequence determination of two related polypeptides, one from the mouse and the other from man, that are

*A portion of the work described in this review was supported by grants from the National Foundation March of Dimes and the National Institute of Arthritis, Metabolism, and Digestive Diseases (AM21921-01). Morley D. Hollenberg is an investigator of the Howard Hughes Medical Institute.

†Present address: Division of Pharmacology and Therapeutics, University of Calgary Faculty of Medicine, Calgary, Alberta, Canada.

both highly potent stimulators of cellular proliferation and inhibitors of gastric acid secretion. On the one hand, while work was in progress to purify nerve growth factor (NGF) from male mouse submaxillary glands (Cohen, 1960), it was observed that certain partially purified extracts of the glands produced biological effects distinct from those attributable to NGF. When injected daily into newborn mice, the fractions caused precocious opening of the eyelids (at 6–7 days instead of the normal 12–14 days) and premature eruption of the incisors (at 6–7 days instead of the normal 8–10 days). Using a bioassay based on the precocity of eyelid opening, Cohen (1962) was able to isolate a pure polypeptide, which, when administered to mice in microgram amounts, stimulates the proliferation and keratinization of epidermal tissue. Hence, the polypeptide was termed epidermal growth factor. In an elegant series of experiments, Cohen and co-workers established the complete amino acid sequence of this 53 amino acid single-chain polypeptide, including the location of the positions of the three disulfide bonds (Savage *et al.*, 1972, 1973).

Studies on the human polypeptide, on the other hand, date back to the late 1930s, when it was observed that human urine contains a potent inhibitor of gastric acid secretion (Gray *et al.*, 1939) and possibly other antiulcer factors (Sandweiss *et al.*, 1941). Using a bioassay that monitors the inhibition of acid secretion in either rats or dogs, Gregory and colleagues were able to isolate two closely related polypeptides (β- and γ-urogastrone) in amounts sufficient for structural studies (Gregory, 1975; Gregory and Willshire, 1975; Gregory and Preston, 1977). Once the sequence of the 53 amino acid single-chain β-urogastrone was determined, with assignment of the three disulfide bonds, the structural relationship to mouse epidermal growth factor was immediately apparent (Fig. 1); γ-urogastrone was found to be identical to β-urogastrone, except that it lacked the C-terminal arginine residue. Upon observing the structural similarity between the mouse and human polypeptides, Gregory and colleagues were quick to establish the gastric acid-inhibitory action of the mouse polypeptide and the proliferative action of the human polypeptide in the mouse bioassay (Gregory, 1975). Thus, both the human and mouse polypeptide possess the same intrinsic biological activities. Furthermore, it is evident that both polypeptides can share the same receptor sites with approximately equal affinities in human tissue (Hollenberg and Gregory, 1976).

At about the time that the structure of human urogastrone was determined, Cohen and colleagues were able to isolate two polypeptides from human urine concentrates, both of which were observed to

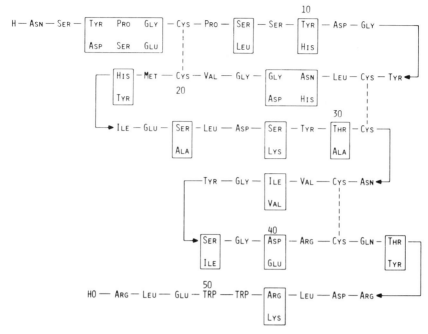

FIG. 1. The amino acid sequences of mouse (upper) and human (lower) epidermal growth factor–urogastrone. The sequence differences are indicated by the residues in boxes.

interact with the same membrane receptor and one of which was demonstrated to be an active mitogen both *in vivo* and *in vitro* (Starkey *et al.*, 1974; Cohen and Carpenter, 1975). The physicochemical data obtained by Cohen and colleagues suggest that the polypeptides isolated were the same as the urogastrones isolated by Gregory and co-workers.

Clearly the mouse and human polypeptides are chemically quite distinct, and it might be appropriate to retain the term urogastrone for the peptide(s) of human origin and the term epidermal growth factor to designate the polypeptide from the mouse. However, because the two polypeptides exhibit the same intrinsic biological activities and because they can share receptor sites with approximately equal affinities, it is likely that they are representative of a family of mitogenic acid-inhibitory polypeptides that, like insulin, may show appreciable interspecies structural variations. Therefore, for the purposes of this review, the combined term epidermal growth factor–

urogastrone (EGF-URO) will be used, thereby denoting the two apparently unrelated principal biological activities that the polypeptides exhibit. Although human EGF-URO (hEGF-URO) has not been compared with mouse EGF-URO (mEGF-URO) in all responsive systems, there is little reason to doubt that the polypeptide termed β-urogastrone is an epidermal growth factor of human origin.

Since the initial isolation in 1962, the actions of mEGF-URO have been extensively studied in a variety of responsive animals and cells both *in vivo* and *in vitro*. Much information concerning the isolation, structure, and action of mEGF-URO has already been comprehensively summarized in several relatively recent review articles (Carpenter, 1978; Carpenter and Cohen, 1978; Cohen, 1972; Cohen and Savage, 1974; Cohen and Taylor, 1974; Gregory *et al.*, 1978a; Hollenberg, 1976). Therefore, in this review, no attempt will be made to cover all aspects of the chemistry and physiology of EGF-URO. Rather, a summary of much of the previous work will be presented and more detailed attention will be given to some recent exciting developments in the studies of these very interesting polypeptides, with emphasis on the characterization of the membrane receptor. The reader is particularly encouraged to consult the reviews by Cohen and colleagues (see references cited above) and by Gregory *et al.* (1978a) for further detailed information.

II. Isolation and Properties of Mouse and Human Epidermal Growth Factor–Urogastrone (EGF-URO)

A. Mouse EGF-URO

The male mouse submaxillary gland is a remarkably rich source of mEGF-URO, which comprises approximately 0.5% (weight/dry weight) of the protein of the gland. In male mouse submaxillary gland homogenates, biological activity can be detected in both a high (MW approximately 74,000) and a low (MW approximately 6000) molecular weight fraction. By a variety of gentle procedures that do not lead to the hydrolysis of peptide bonds, the low molecular weight polypeptide responsible for the biological activity, mEGF-URO, can be dissociated from its binding protein. The high molecular weight complex comprises two molecules of mEGF-URO and two molecules of a binding protein (MW 29,300) that possesses arginine esterase activity (Taylor *et al.*, 1974). In many respects this property of EGF-URO is similar to the reversible association of the neurohypophysial polypeptides oxytocin and vasopressin to form "2 plus 2" complexes with the neurophysins (Acher *et al.*, 1955; Dean *et al.*, 1967; Hollenberg and Hope, 1968). There is also a striking parallel in the association of NGF with a protein complex of about 140,000 (Varon *et al.*, 1967). When separated from its binding protein, mEGF-URO is readily isolated by straightforward column chromatographic techniques (Cohen, 1962; Savage and Cohen, 1972). Advantage has been taken of the ability of mEGF-URO to adsorb to polyacrylamide (BioGel) at low pH, so as to permit a rapid and efficient isolation of the peptide from fresh-frozen submaxillary glands; on average, from an acid (pH 4.5) extract of submaxillary glands, about 0.6 mg of pure peptide can be recovered from each gram wet weight of tissue (Savage and Cohen, 1972). Using this efficient isolation procedure, Cohen and colleagues were able to obtain sufficient material for extensive physicochemical and structural studies (Holladay *et al.*, 1976; Savage *et al.*, 1972, 1973; Taylor *et al.*, 1972). The physicochemical properties of mEGF-URO are summarized in Table I; the amino acid sequence, with positioning of the disulfide bonds, is shown in Fig. 1. Topologically, the single-chain

TABLE I

PHYSICOCHEMICAL PROPERTIES OF MOUSE AND HUMAN EPIDERMAL
GROWTH FACTOR-UROGASTRONE (EGF-URO)[a]

Property	Mouse EGF	Human β-URO
Molecular weight (from amino acid sequence)	6041	6201
Sedimentation coefficient at pH 7.86, 4 mg/ml	1.25 S	NR[b]
Frictional ratio $(f+f_0)$	1.12[c]	NR
Partial specific volume (cm³/gm)	0.69	0.71[d]
Extinction coefficient $(E_{1\ cm}^{280\ nm})$	30.9	NR
Isoelectric point	pH 4.60	pH 4.5
Number of polypeptide chains	1	1
Amino terminus	Asparagine	Asparagine
Carboxy terminus	Arginine	Arginine
Disulfide bonds	3	3
Amino acids absent	Lys, Ala, Phe	Phe, Thr
Hexosamine	ND[b]	ND

[a]Adapted from Cohen and Taylor (1974) and from Gregory and co-workers (1978).
[b]NR, not reported; ND, not detected.
[c]Holladay, quoted by Carpenter and Cohen (1978).
[d]Calculated from amino acid composition.

structure comprises two interconnected loops (residues 1–31) joined
via an asparagine residue to a third loop formed by residues 33–42 of
the remaining 33–53 residue sequence. As will be discussed below, the
residues in the loop and "tail" portion of the sequence 33–53 probably play an important role in the interaction of EGF-URO with its
receptor.

B. Human EGF-URO

Human urine provides the richest convenient source of hEGF-URO.
By radioreceptor assay (Nexø *et al.*, 1977), it can be estimated that
random urine samples from male donors contain, on average, about
9.5 nmol/liter (about 60 μg/liter). By radioimmunoassay, it has been
determined that, on average, the 24-hour urinary output is from about
0.10 (males) to 0.13 (females) nmol/kg (600–800 ng/kg). Marked variation in individual urine samples is observed (Gregory *et al.*, 1977).
Compared to the isolation of mEGF-URO, the preparation of hEGF-
URO is relatively complex. The isolation requires the initial preparation from urine of either tannic acid–acetone (Gregory and Willshire,
1975) or benzoic acid–acetone powder of urinary proteins, followed
subsequently by multiple gel filtration and ion exchange steps. It is of
interest that both groups that isolated hEGF-URO obtained two active polypeptides by use of base ion-exchange resins; the polypeptide
lacking the terminal arginine residue (γ-urogastrone) is evidently
eluted last from the base ion exchange column (Gregory and Willshire,
1975). For an unknown reason, poor recoveries are encountered from
such base ion-exchange columns if the contact time between the sample and the column is long (H. Gregory, personal communication;
Gregory and Willshire, 1975). Affinity chromatography using anti-
EGF-URO antibody-agarose columns can also be used for the purification of hEGF-URO (Starkey *et al.*, 1974; H. Gregory, personal communication). There is sufficient cross-reactivity of anti-mEGF-URO
with hEGF-URO, such that affinity columns prepared with the antiserum to mEGF-URO can be used to isolate hEGF-URO. However,
such affinity columns are less efficient (about 10% yield) for the isolation of the human polypeptide from crude starting material (either
neutralized urine or tannic acid precipitate) than for the isolation of
the mouse polypeptide (approximately 80–100% yield) (E Nexø and
M. D. Hollenberg, unpublished observations). Furthermore, the problems of small column capacity and antibody leakage complicate the
use of affinity columns. Nevertheless, the antibody affinity columns

may prove to be extremely valuable for isolation by a rapid simple method of sufficient hEGF-URO for analytical purposes (e.g., for receptor studies or radioimmunoassay).

The physicochemical (Table I) and structural (Fig. 1) properties of hEGF-URO can be compared with those of mEGF-URO. Despite the over-all similarities, it is striking that the 16 differences in the amino acid sequence are distributed rather widely throughout the molecule; this is in contrast to the comparatively conservative species-to-species substitutions observed for insulin (Smith, 1966) wherein the mouse and human peptide differ at only nine positions. It may also be important that in the first two interconnected loops (residues 1–31), the amino acid substitutions (i.e., mouse human) comprise changes (e.g., neutral to acidic or basic residues) that would markedly alter the peptide microenvironment. In contrast, the differences between mouse and human EGF-URO in residues 33–53 (the "loop and tail" portion mentioned above) chemically represent conservative changes (e.g., $Ile_{35} \rightarrow Val_{35}$; $Asp_{40} \rightarrow Glu_{40}$; $Arg_{48} \rightarrow Lys_{48}$) in the molecule. This relative conservation in the sequence 33–53 may point to its importance in receptor–ligand interactions. It will be of considerable interest to determine whether this part of the molecule is also conserved in EGF-URO isolated from the rat (Moore,1978).

III. Biosynthesis, Storage, and Secretion of EGF-URO

A. Studies in the Mouse

In the mouse, the submaxillary gland represents a major site of synthesis, storage, and secretion of mEGF-URO. Both NGF and EGF-URO are present in the duct cells of the convoluted tubules of the gland, where mEGF-URO can be visualized by direct immunofluorescent methods (Turkington et al., 1971); in organ culture of submaxillary glands, it can be demonstrated that radioactive amino acid precursors are incorporated into mEGF-URO. As is the case for other polypeptides, mEGF-URO is stored in secretory granules (Pasquini et al., 1974) that can be visualized in the convoluted epithelial cells by refined electron microscopic techniques (Van Noorden et al., 1977).

Both the convoluted tubule architecture of the gland and the glandular content of mEGF-URO are androgen dependent (Bynny et al.,

1974). Thus, although mEGF-URO can be detected in the female submaxillary gland, both by immunoassay (approximately 70ng/mg wet
weight) (Bynny *et al.* 1972) and by immunofluorescence methods (Van
Noorden *et al.*, 1977), much more impressive amounts are stored in the
glands of male mice (approximately 1 μg/mg wet weight)(Bynny *et al.*,
1972). The amounts of mEGF-URO in the glands of female mice can
be elevated even above the male levels by administration of androgen
(Bynny *et al.*, 1972, 1974; Barthe *et al.*, 1974; Roberts, 1974); in castrated males, the gland levels fall to those of normal females (Bynny
et al., 1972, 1974). During development, the content of mEGF-URO is
very low in glands of immature animals (about 16 pg/mg wet weight in
15-day animals), reaches a half-maximal level (about 500 ng/mg) at approximately 35 days, and attains the adult level (1 μg/mg) at 50 days
or more (Bynny *et al.*, 1972). It is of interest that, despite the grossly
discrepant amounts of mEGF-URO found in the submaxillary glands
of the two sexes, little sex difference is detected in the serum (about 1
ng/ml) and urinary levels of immunoreactive mEGF-URO; the serum
levels also appear to be about 1 ng/ml in castrated males, androgen-
supplemented females, and immature (15–29 day) male mice (Bynny *et
al.*, 1974). Furthermore, in pregnant mice, the amount of mEGF-URO
detected in the submaxillary gland by immunofluorescence rises
markedly (Van Noorden *et al.*, 1977), and substantial amounts of
mEGF-URO can be detected in the milk (Bynny *et al.*, 1974). Surprisingly, no mEGF-URO could be detected by immunofluorescence in the
mammary glands at any stage of lactation (Van Noorden *et al.*, 1977).

Based on the above observations, it is likley that in the mouse there
is a source of mEGF-URO apart from the submaxillary gland. Organs
in which significant amounts of mEGF-URO have been detected
either by immunoassay (Bynny *et al.*, 1972) or by radioreceptor assay
(Frati *et al.*, 1976) include (in descending order of content) the kidney,
stomach, parotid, pancreas, small intestine, and liver. Additionally, it
appears that serum levels are under strict control, irrespective of the
hormonal (androgen) status of the animal.

Secretion of mEGF-URO from the mouse submaxillary gland is
under α-adrenergic control (Bynny *et al.*, 1974; Roberts, 1977). Both
the administration of α-adrenergic agonists and stimulation of the
superior cervical sympathetic ganglia lead to an elevation of serum
mEGF-URO levels (Bynny *et al.*, 1974). This response is blocked by
the α-adrenergic antagonist phenoxybenzamine. When mEGF-URO
enters the circulation, it is extremely rapidly cleared, appearing within
minutes in the stomach and urinary bladder, as estimated by whole-
body autoradiography of mice given ^{125}I-labeled hEGF-URO intravenously (H. Gregory, personal communication). Removal of the

superior cervical ganglia abolishes the circadian variation that can be observed in the levels of submaxillary gland mEGF-URO; in contrast, the plasma levels of mEGF-URO do not display a circadian variation (Krieger et al., 1976).

B. STUDIES IN MAN

Studies on the synthesis, storage, and secretion of hEGF-URO in man are as yet at a comparatively early stage. Using a fluorescence double-antibody technique, it has been possible to localize hEGF-URO in specialized cells of the human submandibular salivary gland and in cells of the glands of Brunner in the duodenum (Elder et al., 1978); tissues that did not yield fluorescence in that study include the parotid salivary glands, esophagus, antrum and fundus of the stomach, jejunum, colon, breast, pancreas, ovary, adrenal, thyroid, kidney, bladder, liver, prostate, smooth muscle, skeletal muscle, cardiac muscle, and thymus. It is not yet certain whether the duodenum and salivary glands are the sole sources of EGF-URO in man.

Remarkably large amounts of hEGF-URO are excreted daily in the urine (Gregory et al., 1977). The amounts recovered in the urine are even more impressive in view of the very short serum half-life of the polypeptide (about 1.5 minutes in test animals) (Gregory et al., 1978a); an extremely active process of biosynthesis and turnover is thereby implied. Immunoreactive hEGF-URO can also be detected in serum, saliva, and gastric juice (Gregory et al., 1978b), and appreciable amounts are thought to be present in amniotic fluid as early as 16–24 weeks of gestation (Barka et al., 1978). Most interestingly, in serum the major immunoreactive component is a comparatively large molecular weight species that gives rise to an hEGF-URO-like peptide upon trypsin treatment (Gregory et al., 1978b); Orth and co-workers have also obtained evidence that hEGF-URO exists in serum in a precursor form (Hirata and Orth, 1978). The occurrence in serum of the high molecular weight immunoreactive species that is apparently biologically inactive (as an inhibitor of acid secretion) (Gregory, et al., 1978a,b) complicates the interpretation of serum immunoassay data. It may thus be necessary to reevaluate the molecular form of the immunoreactive species previously detected in mouse serum (about 1 ng/ml mEGF-URO equivalent) (Bynny et al., 1974). It is indeed intriguing that hEGF-URO may circulate as a prohormone that can undergo proteolytic activation at a site of required action, e.g., in an area of tissue injury.

In man there does not appear to be a marked sex difference in the

urinary output of hEGF-URO; on average the amount excreted by
women is about 30% greater than that excreted by men (Gregory *et
al.*, 1977). As yet in humans it is not known whether the male submandibular gland content exceeds that of women or whether the gland
content of hEGF-URO can be altered either during pregnancy or
under the influence of α-adrenergic agents.

IV. BIOLOGICAL ACTIONS OF EGF-URO

A. ACTIONS *in Vivo*

As indicated in the Introduction, mEGF-URO was discovered
because of its ability to cause early incisor eruption and precocious
eye opening in newborn mice, as a consequence of increased epithelial
proliferation and keratinization (Cohen, 1962, 1965). These effects require the continued subcutaneous administration of comparatively
large amounts of peptide (0.5–6 μg/gm body weight), with a maximum
effect on the skin occurring at a dose of about 3 μg/gm per day (Mann
and Fenton, 1970). In skin, there is an increase in thickness of the
epidermis and a decrease in the thickness of the dermis accompanied
by a decrease in fat. These morphological effects can be correlated
with an early (4 hour) transient rise in the skin levels of both ornithine
and histidine decarboxylase upon administering mEGF-URO *in vivo*
(Stastny and Cohen, 1970; Blosse *et al.*, 1974). A number of other
tissues respond to mEGF-URO, including the kidney capsule, pericar-
dium, esophagus, tongue, and liver, which exhibits both bile duct proliferation (Farebrother and Mann, 1970) and an accumulation of fat
primarily as triglyceride (Heimberg *et al.*, 1965); the lung (Sundell *et
al.*, 1975) and testes (Carpenter and Cohen, 1978) are also targets for
mEGF-URO action. Presumably because of its proliferative action on
the skin, mEGF-URO enhances the topical carcinogenicity of
3-methylcholanthrene (Reynolds *et al.*, 1965; Rose *et al.*, 1976b); the
tumor-promoting activity of EGF-URO in other tissues has yet to be
studied. Upon topical administration, effects of mEGF-URO on the
proliferation of injured corneal epithelium can also be observed (Frati
et al., 1972; Savage and Cohen, 1973; Ho *et al.*, 1974).

The other principal action of EGF-URO, the inhibition of either
basal (Koffman *et al.*, 1977) or stimulated (Gregory *et al.*, 1978)
gastric acid secretion, can be observed in a variety of species (dog, cat,
rat, man, and rhesus monkey) in response to the intravenous ad-

ministration of doses (0.25 μg/kg) that are about 1/1000 of those required for causing eyelid opening (Gerring et al., 1974); the secretion of pepsin is also inhibited. As mentioned previously, both mouse and human EGF-URO produce an equivalent inhibitory action. The inhibitory effect upon acid secretion can be observed both in denervated Heidenhain pouch dogs as well as in innervated pouches and occurs to a similar extent whether the stimulus is histamine, pentagastrin, insulin, methacholine, or a test meal (Gerring et al., 1974). Whereas in normal subjects the secretion of intrinsic factor in response to histamine is also inhibited (Elder et al., 1975), in patients with Zollinger-Ellison syndrome, the secretion of intrinsic factor is augmented by hEGF-URO and acid secretion is inhibited (Elder et al., 1975). A differential effect of hEGF-URO on the parietal cell is thereby suggested. In contrast to the inhibition of acid and pepsin output, hEGF-URO at equivalent doses does not affect bile secretion, salivary secretion, gastric mucosal blood flow or the volume flow, bicarbonate output, and protein output of the pancreas (Gerring et al., 1974). It appears that EGF-URO exerts its inhibitory effect at the level of the gastric mucosa (Gregory et al., 1978a). In view of the effect of EGF-URO on the stomach, it is of interest that within 4 hours of the subcutaneous administration of mEGF-URO the levels of ornithine decarboxylase are elevated in the stomach and duodenum, but not in the midgut, colon, or heart, of neonatal mice (Feldman et al., 1978). In experimental animals (rats, guinea pigs), hEGF-URO prevents reserpine-induced gastric muscosal damage and promotes ulcer healing (Gregory et al., 1978a). The efficacy of EGF-URO as an antiulcer agent in man remains to be established.

B. Effects in Vitro

A large number of responses have been observed upon adding mEGF-URO to a variety of cell and organ culture systems derived from a number of different species. It is important that the proliferative action of EGF-URO can be observed both histologically and biochemically (accumulation of protein, RNA, and incorporation of [3H]thymidine into DNA) in organ cultures of chick embryo epidermis (Cohen, 1965; Hoober and Cohen, 1967a,b; Bertsch and Marks, 1974). Thus, the effects observed in vivo can be attributed to a direct effect of EGF-URO on the target tissues rather than to the effects of other hormones, possibly mobilized by the administration of EGF-URO. In concert with the changes in the synthesis of intracellular macro-

molecules, there is an early (1.5–4 hour) stimulation of polysome formation (Cohen and Stastny, 1968) and of ribosomal activity as
assayed in a cell-free protein synthesizing system (Hoober and Cohen,
1976b). Additionally, in cultured chick embryo epidermis, mEGF-
URO causes a rapid (within 15 minutes) increase in α-amino-
isobutyrate and uridine uptake, as well as a transient (maximum at 4
hours) but marked elevation of ornithine decarboxylase activity
(Stastny and Cohen, 1970). In cultured rabbit lens cells, it has also
been observed that mEFG-URO causes early (5 minute) transient
elevations of both cyclic AMP and cyclic GMP, long before the initiation of DNA synthesis (Hosam et al., 1976). mEGF-URO also causes
cellular proliferation in organ cultures of both chick and human cornea
(Savage and Cohen, 1973), mouse mammary glands (Turkington,
1969a), and mammary carcinomas (Turkington, 1969b) and in cultured
epithelial cells from benign mammary tumors (Stoker et al., 1976).
From the above discussion, it is evident that, like other mitogens,
EFG-URO in vitro causes a constellation of cellular effects associated
with the initiation of cell growth, a so-called "pleiotypic response"
(Hershko et al., 1971).

   Many types of cultured cells, derived from numerous species, can be
shown to respond to EGF-URO. In addition to the above-mentioned
studies, EGF-URO-mediated responses have been observed in cultures
of human fibroblasts [derived from skin, fetal lung (WI-38), and amniotic fluid] (Carpenter and Cohen, 1976b; Gospodarowicz et al.,
1977b; Hollenberg and Cuatrecasas, 1973, 1975; Hollenberg and Gregory, 1976), human tumor cells (HeLa and KB) (Covelli et al., 1972a),
human keratinocytes from skin, cornea, and conjunctive (Rheinwald
and Green, 1977; Sun and Green, 1976, 1977), human glial cells (Brunk
et al., 1976; Lindgren and Westermark, 1976; Westermark, 1976,
1977), human choriocarcinoma cells (Benveniste et al., 1978), both normal and SV 40-transformed mouse cells lines (3T3, 3T6, SV 40–3T3)
(Armelin, 1973; Carpenter and Cohen, 1978; Rose et al., 1976a), cells
from rabbit epidermis, kidney, cornea, and lens (Carpenter and Cohen,
1978; Hollenberg, 1975), Syrian hamster embryo fibroblasts
(Hollenberg et al., 1979), and cultures of bovine granulosa cells
(Gospodarowicz et al., 1977a). Studies of the binding of ^{125}I-labeled
EGF-URO provide evidence for the occurrence of receptors in cultured
fibroblasts for the cat and the mink as well (Todaro et al., 1976). The
studies in vitro on cultured cells testify to the remarkably widespread
tissue and species distribution of cell receptors for EGF-URO.

   It is important to note that the actions of EGF-URO in vitro may
also be observed in the absence of cell proliferation. For instance, as
already indicated, organ cultures of epidermal explants from 7–8-day

chick embryos proliferate in response to mEGF-URO (Cohen, 1965), whereas in explants from 8.5–9-day embryos no net accumulation of DNA can be demonstrated (Hoober and Cohen, 1967a). There appears to be a change in the proliferative response of the skin samples as the chick matures, although it can be shown that mEGF-URO does stimulate thymidine incorporation in explants from 9-day embryos (Bertsch and Marks, 1974). In analogous experiments using cultured rat hepatocytes, it has been shown that mEGF-URO markedly increases the cellular labeling index, [^{3}H]thymidine, but does not cause appreciable cell division (Richman et al., 1976). Thus, as indicated by a number of studies either with pure hormones (Baseman and Hayes, 1975) or with crude preparations of growth-promoting factors (Shodell, 1972; Leffert, 1974; Wolf et al., 1975) and as pointed out by Carpenter and Cohen (1978), the effects of EGF-URO in enhancing DNA synthesis and promoting cell division represent related but quite distinct actions of this polypeptide.

Effects of EGF-URO may also be observed *in vitro* in the absence of either enhanced DNA synthesis or cell division. A particularly striking effect of mEGF-URO in the absence of increased DNA synthesis in affected cells can be observed in the process of palate fusion, monitored in organ cultures of palatal shelves from 15-day-old rats (Hassell, 1975; Hassell and Pratt, 1977). In this preparation, mEGF-URO prevents the programmed death of the apposed medial-edge epithelium, a degenerative process necessary for the fusion of the two shelves. Labeling studies with [^{3}H]thymidine demonstrate that mEGF-URO, while maintaining the viability of the medial-edge epithelium, does not stimulate DNA synthesis (Hassell and Pratt, 1977). Other effects of EGF-URO that do not appear to require the enhancement of either DNA synthesis or proliferation per se include the stimulation of human chorionic gonadotropin secretion by cultured choriocarcinoma cells (Benveniste et al., 1978), the rapid inhibition of histamine-mediated acid secretion in short-term functional cultures of stomach mucosa (Gregory et al., 1978a), and the enhanced incorporation of ^{3}H-labeled glucosamine into both cellular and extracellular glycoproteins and glycosaminoglycans (Lembach, 1976). This effect on glycosylation may relate to the ability of EGF-URO to alter cellular viral infectivity (Knox et al., 1978), to stimulate the appearance of fibronectin (LETS protein) in mouse 3T3 cells (Chen et al., 1977), and to change the ability of 3T3 cells to interact with the mannoside-specific plant lectin concanavalin A (Con A) (Aharonov et al., 1978b). These latter effects presumably also represent events independent of DNA synthesis.

A most exciting recent observation concerns the ability of mEGF-

URO to stimulate the phosphorylation of membranes from mEGF-URO-responsive cells *in vitro* in the presence of [γ-^{32}P]ATP (Carpenter *et al.*, 1978). Within 10 minutes at $0°C$, EGF-URO causes the phosphorylation of a number of protein constituents having molecular weights 170,000, 150,000, 80,000, and 22,500. Although neither the identity nor the function of the phosphorylated proteins is known, the size of the largest constituent is very close to the molecular weights we (Sahyoun *et al.*, 1978; Hock et al., 1979) and others (Das *et al.*, 1977) have estimated for the EGF-URO receptor. One may thus posit that, like the nicotinic receptor for acetylcholine (Gordon *et al.*, 1977; Teichberg *et al.*, 1977), the EGF-URO receptor may be subject to phosphorylation-dephosphorylation reactions. The demonstration of an EGF-URO-modulated reaction in a membrane preparation adds a new dimension to the understanding of the mechanism whereby EGF-URO acts. The many actions of EGF-URO are summarized in Table II.

TABLE II

ACTIONS OF EPIDERMAL GROWTH FACTOR–UROGASTRONE (EGF-URO)[a]

In vivo	*In vitro*
Cell proliferation	Cell proliferation
Keratinization	Enhanced keratinocyte growth
Enhanced ornithine and histidine decarboxylase	Increased activity of ornithine decarboxylase
Incisor eruption	Enhanced metabolite transport (uridine, aminoisobutyrate glucose)
Inhibition of gastric acid secretion	Increased synthesis of DNA, RNA, and protein
Healing of ulcers	Increased membrane phosphorylation
Hepatic triglyceride accumulation	Increased cyclic nucleotide levels (both cAMP and cGMP)
	Enhanced hyaluronic acid synthesis
	Enhanced fibronectin synthesis
	Increased cell binding to insolubilized concanavalin A
	Altered viral growth (cytomegalovirus, reduced; herpes simplex type I increased)
	Inhibition of palate fusion
	Inhibition of acid secretion

[a]Data to substantiate the many actions of EGF-URO are found either in the specific text references or in references referred to in the reviews by Carpenter and Cohen (1978) and by Gregory *et al.* (1978a). For this table, it is assumed that mEGF-URO and hEGF-URO exhibit similar actions.

V. The Membrane Receptor for EGF-URO

A. Characterization of the Receptor in Cultured Cells

As with other polypeptides, the initial site of action of EGF-URO is a ligand-specific membrane-localized receptor. When administered *in vivo*, ^{131}I-labeled mEGF-URO is accumulated in target organs such as epidermis and cornea (Covelli *et al.*, 1972b), indicating the presence of specific binding sites in these tissues. In cultured fibroblast monolayers, the binding of ^{125}I-labeled EGF-URO can be characterized and correlated with the ability of EGF-URO to cause a biological response [e.g., stimulation of DNA synthesis or of α-aminoisobutyrate uptake (Fig. 2)]. As observed in several cultured cell systems (Aharonov *et al.*, 1978a; Carpenter *et al.*, 1975; Carpenter and Cohen, 1976a,b, 1978; Hollenberg, 1975; Hollenberg and Cuatrecasas, 1973, 1975; Holley *et al.*, 1977), the binding of ^{125}I-labeled EGF-URO is rapid, peptide-specific (in that other peptide hormones do not compete), saturable, and of high affinity (K_D about 5×10^{-10} M). In confluent human fibroblast monolayers, there are about 4 to 9×10^4 binding sites per cell (Hollenberg and Cuatrecasas, 1973, 1975; Carpenter *et al.*, 1975; Hollenberg and Schneider, 1979). In such fibroblasts, only a fraction of the available receptors need be occupied (about 20%) to elicit a maximum biological response. In other cells from about 1% (Vlodavsky *et al.*, 1978) to 75% (Hollenberg, 1975) of receptors must be occupied for a maximum response.

In many respects, the characteristics of EGF-URO binding in fibroblasts meet the criteria expected for a hormone–receptor interaction (Cuatrecasas and Hollenberg, 1976). However, the reversibility of binding exhibits important differences when the uptake of EGF-URO by intact cells is compared with the binding of EGF-URO by isolated membrane preparations (discussed later). Whereas in membranes the binding is readily reversible (half-life of dissociation, about 21 minutes at 24°C) (O'Keefe *et al.*, 1974), in intact cells binding is accompanied by a rapid (at 37°C) internalization of at least a portion of the receptor–peptide complexes, resulting in a degradation of EGF-URO by cells (Carpenter and Cohen, 1976a; Aharonov *et al.*, 1978a). At 37°C, bound ^{125}I-labeled EGF-URO is rapidly broken down into fragments of lower molecular weight (mainly iodotyrosine) (Carpenter and Cohen, 1978), which dissociate from the cell with an apparent half-life (about 20 minutes) close to that of the dissociation of intact EGF-URO from

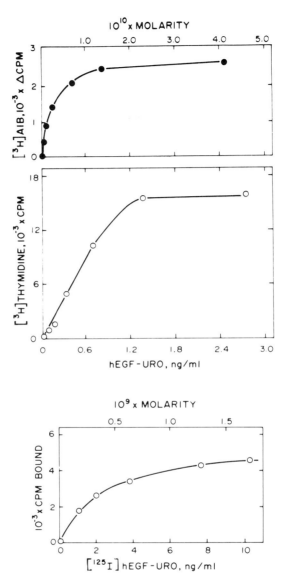

Fig. 2. Binding and action of human epidermal growth factor–urogastrone [hEGF-URO (β-urogastrone)] in human fibroblast monolayers. *Upper and middle:* The ability of hEGF-URO to stimulate either the uptake of ³H-labeled α-aminoisobutyric acid (³H-AIB) or the incorporation of ³H-labeled thymidine in contact-inhibited monolayers (1.5 cm in diameter) of human skin fibroblasts can be compared with (*lower*) the ability of replicate monolayers (36 μg of protein, approximately 120,000 cells) to bind ¹²⁵I-labeled hEGF-URO (124 cpm/pg). Data were adapted from Hollenberg and Gregory (1977).

isolated membranes. However, both at 24°C (M. D. Hollenberg and B. S. Beckman, unpublished) and at 0°C (Carpenter and Cohen, 1976a) the dissociation of labeled EGF-URO from intact cells is markedly prolonged; at room temperature and below, the cell-bound ligand remains intact and, upon extraction, can bind to receptors once again. It is not yet clear whether all the bound ligand becomes internalized, or whether a significant proportion of the bound ligand remains associated with the plasma membrane either in a cryptic form or in a high-affinity complex (Shechter *et al.*, 1978b). Interestingly, at 37°C a portion of the bound EGF-URO appears to become covalently attached to the receptor (Baker *et al.*, 1979; Linsley *et al.*, 1979).

The binding and (presumed) internalization of the receptor leads to a substantial reduction in the binding of EGF-URO by cells first preexposed to the native ligand and then subjected to binding studies with ^{125}I-labeled EGF-URO (so-called "down-regulation") (Carpenter and Cohen, 1976a; Aharonov *et al.*, 1978a). Other factors that affect the numbers of EGF-URO receptors in intact cultured cells include cell density (Pratt and Pastan, 1978; Holley *et al.*, 1977; Hollenberg *et al.*, 1979), the action of other hormones such as glucocorticoids (Baker *et al.*, 1978), and cell transformation by either viral (Todaro *et al.*, 1976) or chemical (Hollenberg *et al.*, 1979) carcinogens. Mutant cells that possess defects in glycosylation also exhibit reduced numbers of receptors for EGF-URO (Pratt and Pastan, 1978). Thus in cells, as opposed to isolated membrane preparations, the receptors for EGF-URO are in a dynamic state of regulation and turnover.

B. Receptor Mobility, Ligand Internalization, and the Mitogenic Action of EGF-URO

The apparent disappearance of EGF-URO binding sites from cells that have been previously exposed to the polypeptide is in keeping with early work on the shedding of antigen–antibody complexes from the cell surface (summarized briefly by Raff, 1976). The well recognized mobility of cell surface antigen–antibody complexes, measured by fluorescence techniques, has served as part of the stimulus for recent models of hormone action (see reviews by Cuatrecasas and Hollenberg, 1976; Hollenberg, 1978; Hollenberg and Cuatrecasas, 1978). The mobile receptor paradigm, developed independently in several laboratories (Cuatrecasas, 1974; Bennett *et al.*, 1975; Boeynaems and Dumont, 1977; DeHaen, 1976; Jacobs and Cuatrecasas, 1976), proposes that the ligand recognition molecule (receptor) is mobile and that once occupied it can associate with any of a number of membrane-localized substituents. Using highly fluorescent derivatives of mEGF-URO, it has been possible to monitor EGF-URO receptor mobility directly, both in mouse 3T3 cells (Shechter *et al.*, 1978a; Schlessinger *et al.*, 1978a,b; Maxfield *et al.*, 1978) and in cultured human carcinoma cells (A-431) (Haigler *et al.*, 1978). At room temperature, the receptor in 3T3 cells is mobile, with a diffusion coefficient of about 3 to 5 $\times$ 10^{-10} cm^2/per second, as determined by photobleaching–recovery measurements (Shechter *et al.*, 1978a; Schlessinger *et al.*, 1978a,b). Whereas the peptide binds in a diffuse pattern at 4°C, within 15 minutes of raising the temperature to 37°C the receptors aggregate into patches. At room temperature, the receptors can also be visualized in patches, even though the receptors are still clearly mobile. Surprisingly, within 20 minutes of raising the temperature from 23°C to 37°C there is a marked decrease in receptor mobility. This decrease of mobility is associated with an internalization of the fluorescent patches. In A-431 carcinoma cells, it was not possible to detect cell surface receptor patching by means of an indirect fluorescent antibody technique (Haigler *et al.*, 1978); the accumulation of fluorescent mEGF-URO in randomly distributed intracellular spheres could, however, be observed in these cells. The internalization of the EGF-URO receptor appears to occur at the same site(s) (the "coated pits") responsible for internalization of the low-density lipoprotein acceptor (Anderson *et al.*, 1977; Maxfield *et al.*, 1978).

The observations with fluorescent EGF-URO derivatives confirm by direct measurements some of the postulates of the mobile receptor paradigm, namely, that the receptors are mobile and that subsequent to ligand binding, the occupied receptor can form new complexes within the plane of the membrane. Further, the common site of internalization of several receptors suggests that there may be sequence homologies between receptors in those regions responsible for triggering internalization.

An important question to ask, however, is: How does the patching and internalization of the EGF-URO receptor relate to the mitogenic action of the peptide? In view of the delayed onset of DNA synthesis (maximum at 17–24 hours in human fibroblasts) compared with the rapid (within 1 hour at 37°C) binding and internalization and degradation of the EGF-URO receptor complex, it is not unreasonable to propose that a fragment of either EGF-URO or the receptor plays a role in the mitogenic process (Das and Fox, 1978; Hollenberg and Cuatrecasas, 1978). Indeed, experiments with insulin receptor antibodies (Jacobs and Cuatrecasas, 1978; Kahn *et al.*, 1978) suggest that the information for biological activity resides in the hormone receptor, not in the peptide per se. Das and Fox (1978), upon observing the rapid intracellular degradation of ^{125}I-labeled EGF-URO photoaffinity-labeled receptor, have underscored the possible importance of proteolytically cleaved receptor fragments in the mitogenic process.

Despite these reported observations, experiments from several laboratories indicate that the processes of receptor internalization and degradation, while potentially important, do not comprise a "trigger mechanism" for EGF-URO action. First, it can be shown that the addition of antibody to hEGF-URO-stimulated cells as long as 5 hours after the initial addition of peptide can substantially reverse DNA synthesis in human fibroblasts (Carpenter and Cohen, 1976b). This reversal occurs long after most cell-bound EGF-URO would have been internalized. Similarly, simply replacing the EGF-URO-containing medium with conditioned medium as long as 2–4 hours after the initial stimulus causes a marked diminution of response in cultured mouse 3T3 fibroblasts (Aharonov et al., 1978a). Likewise, in cultured human fibroblasts stimulated by mEGF-URO in a serum-free medium, the removal of mEGF-URO as long as 17 hours after the initial stimulus markedly diminishes the response that can be observed at 23 hours (Fig. 3). Finally, the cellular response (DNA synthesis) that can be detected even after removal of EGF-URO from the medium by washing can be reversed by the addition of EGF-URO antibody (Shechter et al., 1978b). It is thus evident that the mitogenic action of EGF-URO in fibroblasts requires that its presence in the incubation medium continue for prolonged periods of time and that the hormone–receptor complex responsible for this action be retained (possibly as a high-affinity or cryptic complex) at the cell surface so as to be accessible to antibody. It would appear that receptor internalization, degradation, and resynthesis are processes associated with, but separate from, the mitogenic action of EGF-URO. The relationship of receptor mobility and aggregation to the stimulation of cells remains to be determined.

C. CHARACTERIZATION OF THE PARTICULATE AND SOLUBLE RECEPTOR

1. The Receptor in Liver and Placental Membranes

Membranes from cultured fibroblasts bind EGF-URO with characteristics similar to those observed in the intact cell (Hollenberg and Cuatrecasas, 1973). However such membranes represent a rela-

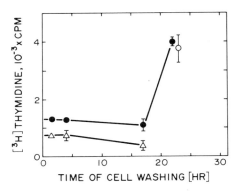

FIG. 3. Effect of removal of epidermal growth factor–urogastrone (EGF-URO) on the mitogenic response of fibroblasts. Human foreskin fibroblast monolayers were grown to confluency in multidish trays as described (Hollenberg and Cuatrecasas, 1975), and the growth medium was changed to serum-free Eagle's minimal essential medium containing 0.1% w/v bovine albumin (MEM/ALB). Cells were then incubated with (○, ●) or without (△) mEGF-URO (0.5 ng/ml); at the indicated times, the medium was replaced first with 2 ml (20 minutes, 37°C) and then with 1 ml of MEM/ALB. The culture of monolayers was then continued up to 23 hours after the initial addition of mEGF-URO, at which time the incorporation of [³H]thymidine during a 1-hour period was determined. The stimulation of cells due to the continued presence of mEGF-URO (○) is compared with the response of cells washed free of mEGF-URO at the indicated times (●) and the response of washed, unstimulated cells (△). The error bars, when larger than the symbols, indicate the standard deviation of values from triplicate monolayers.

tively poor source of receptor. Attention has therefore been focused on membranes from rat liver and human placenta; these preparations are readily obtained and are a comparatively rich source of receptor (O'Keefe *et al.,* 1974). As in the intact cell, binding of EGF-URO to membranes from either rat liver or human placenta is rapid, saturable, ligand-specific, and of high affinity. At 24°C the binding is readily reversible and has a dissociation half-life of about 21 minutes; little if any degradation of EGF-URO accompanies the binding process. The characteristics of EGF-URO binding by liver and placenta membranes are summarized in Table III.

In placental membranes, the receptor properties have been explored with the use of a number of enzymic and lectin probes. As with other peptide receptors, the EGF-URO receptor is quite sensitive to trypsin. More than 50% of the binding is cleaved from membranes upon incubation with 50 μg/ml trypsin for 20 minutes at 37°C; more than 95% of the receptor is cleaved by treatment with 200 μg/ml for 40 minutes (O'Keefe *et al.,* 1974). In placental membranes, neuraminidase treatment (Fig. 4) augments EGF-URO binding, with a more pronounced

TABLE III

CHARACTERISTICS OF MOUSE EPIDERMAL GROWTH FACTOR–UROGASTRONE
(mEGF-URO) BINDING BY MEMBRANES[a,b]

Tissue	Dissociation constant (mol liter^{-1})	Half-life of complex (min)	Rate constants		Binding capacity (pmol/mg protein)
			k_1 (liter mol^{-1} sec^{-1})	k_{-1} (sec^{-1})	
Rat liver	1.5×10^{-9}	21	1×10^6	5.5×10^{-4}	0.4
Human placenta	1×10^{-9}	19	2.6×10^6	6.1×10^{-4}	20

[a] Data were adapted from O'Keefe et al. (1974) and Hock and Hollenberg (1980).

[b] Membranes were prepared from tissue homogenates (Polytron) by differential centrifugation, as described (Cuatrecasas, 1972). Binding measurements were performed on the crude "microsomal fraction."

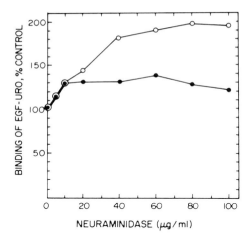

F$_{IG}$. 4. Effect of neuraminidase of the binding of mouse ● and human (○) epidermal growth factor–urogastrone (EGF-URO) to placental membranes. Membranes (200 μg) were pretreated with neuraminidase (15 minutes at 37°C, pH 5.0) at the indicated concentrations, and the binding of both hEGF-URO and mEGF-URO was then determined. Binding is expressed as a percentage of the binding to membranes similarly preincubated in the absence of enzyme. Data were taken from Hock and Hollenberg (1980).

effect on the binding of hEGF-URO (about 2-fold increase) than on mEGF-URO (about 1.2-fold increase in binding) (Hock and Hollenberg, 1980). Treatment of membranes with phospholipases A$_2$, C, and D also augments EGF-URO binding by membranes. Whereas phospholipase A$_2$ treatment causes the largest increase in binding (about 3-fold), phospholipases C (1.7-fold increase) and D (1.12-fold increase) were less effective (Hock and Hollenberg, 1980).

A variety of plant lectins compete for the binding of EGF-URO both in placental membranes (Hock and Hollenberg, 1977, 1980) and in fibroblast monolayers (Carpenter and Cohen, 1977). Lectins that compete effectively for EGF-URO binding include those that interact with mannose (Con A), N-acetylgalactosamine–N-acetylglucosamine (phytohemagglutinin), galactose (ricin, abrin), and N-acetylglucosamine (wheat germ agglutinin). It is of interest that, although both Con A and wheat germ agglutinin can interact with the EGF-URO receptor, neither of these lectins stimulates DNA synthesis in fibroblasts (M. D. Hollenberg, unpublished observations); like EGF-URO, Con A (but not wheat germ agglutinin) can, however, enhance α-aminoisobutyrate uptake in such cells (Hollenberg and Cuatrecasas, 1975). These results are in contrast to the insulin-like effects of these two lectins in fat cells (Cuatrecasas and Tell, 1973), presumably resulting from perturbation (possibly cross-linking) of the insulin receptor. The results suggest that, in contrast with the insulin receptor, the oligosaccharide portion of the EGF-URO receptor may not be involved in cellular activation.

From the studies summarized above, the membrane-bound EGF-URO receptor appears to be a glycoprotein, partially masked both by membrane lipid and by sialic acid residues, with the ligand recognition site readily accessible to agents the size of trypsin. Trypsin treatment of membranes specifically cross-linked to ^{125}I-labeled EGF-URO (see below) releases a relatively large molecular weight constituent; this suggests that only one-fifth to one-tenth of the receptor (about MW 20,000) is anchored in the membrane (Sahyoun et al., 1978).

2. Affinity Labeling and Solubilization of the EGF-URO Receptor

Unlike the insulin receptor, but like the muscarinic cholinergic receptor, the EGF-URO receptor loses its ligand recognition property upon solubilization. Thus, although detergents such as Triton X-100, Nonidet P-40, and Ammonyx-LO can solubilize most of the receptor from placental membranes, the binding activity cannot be monitored in the soluble fraction by routine procedures (summarized by Cuatrecasas and Hollenberg, 1976), such as agarose chromatography or polyethylene glycol precipitation. Therefore, it was necessary to develop new approaches for the study of the EGF-URO receptor.

In view of the sensitivity of binding toward detergent, it was decided to take advantage of the high specificity and affinity of EGF-URO binding to membranes and to cross-link the radioactively labeled peptide covalently to the receptor prior to solubilization. Two methods of "affinity cross-linking" were developed (Fig. 5). First, glutaraldehyde was employed as a bifunctional cross-linking reagent (Fig. 5); upon reduction of the Schiff base with borohydride, the receptor ^{125}I-labeled EGF-URO conjugate is sufficiently stable to permit membrane solubilization and fractionation of the specifically labeled membrane constituent(s) (Fig. 6). Just as "specific" binding in receptor studies with radioactive probes can be defined as the binding for which unlabeled parent compound does compete, so specific affinity cross-linking can be defined as that radioactivity coupled by the cross-linking reagent for which the unlabeled ligand can successfully compete. Chromatography of affinity-labeled solubilized rat liver membranes on Sepharose 6B demonstrates the presence of a major fraction

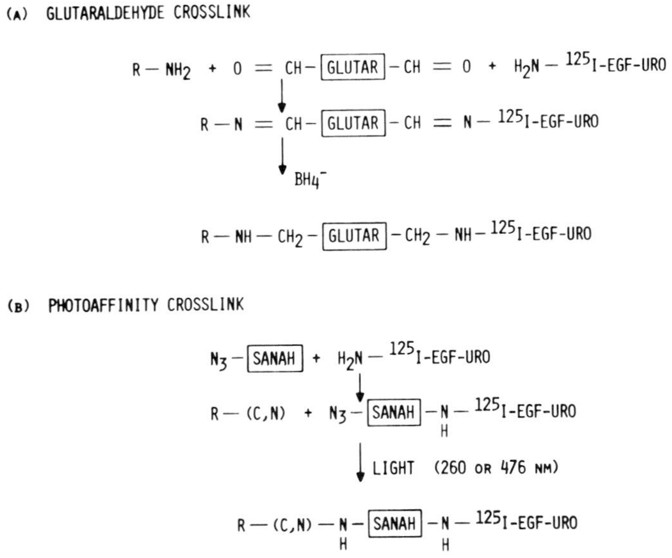

(A) GLUTARALDEHYDE CROSSLINK

$$R - NH_2 + 0 = CH - \boxed{GLUTAR} - CH = 0 + H_2N - {}^{125}I\text{-EGF-URO}$$

$$R - N = CH - \boxed{GLUTAR} - CH = N - {}^{125}I\text{-EGF-URO}$$

$$\downarrow BH_4^-$$

$$R - NH - CH_2 - \boxed{GLUTAR} - CH_2 - NH - {}^{125}I\text{-EGF-URO}$$

(B) PHOTOAFFINITY CROSSLINK

$$N_3 - \boxed{SANAH} + H_2N - {}^{125}I\text{-EGF-URO}$$

$$R - (C,N) + N_3 - \boxed{SANAH} - \underset{H}{N} - {}^{125}I\text{-EGF-URO}$$

$$\downarrow LIGHT \quad (260 \text{ OR } 476 \text{ NM})$$

$$R - (C,N) - \underset{H}{N} - \boxed{SANAH} - \underset{H}{N} - {}^{125}I\text{-EGF-URO}$$

FIG. 5. Scheme for the affinity cross-linking of epidermal growth factor–urogastrone (EGF-URO) to the receptor. (A) Cross-linking with glutaraldehyde (GLUTAR). (B) Cross-linking with the photoaffinity reagent N-succinimidyl-6(4′-azido-2′-nitrophenylamino)hexanoate (SANAH). The details of the cross-linking procedures are described elsewhere (Sahyoun et al., 1978; Hock et al., 1979); the cross-linking reactions for glutaraldehyde and arylazides have been discussed by Peters and Richards (1977).

(peak 2a, Fig. 6A) that can be cross-linked to ^{125}I-labeled EGF-URO; this material can be absorbed to and eluted from Con A–Sepharose columns with sugar (Fig. 6B), yielding a modest (about 30-fold) purification of the receptor and providing evidence independent of binding-competition data of the glycoprotein nature of the receptor. The same glutaraldehyde procedure developed for EGF-URO also works for the affinity labeling of membranes with insulin (Sahyoun et al., 1978).

The receptor for EGF-URO can also be labeled with photoaffinity reagents (Fig. 5) (Das et al., 1977; Hock et al., 1979). With this method, the photolabile EGF-URO derivative is first allowed to bind to the receptor and the reagent is then activated by light. The specificity of cross-linking can be demonstrated both by competition for labeling with native EGF-URO and by the use of cell mutants that do not possess receptors for EGF-URO (Das et al., 1977).

Both the glutaraldehyde method and the photoaffinity method have been used successfully for the specific labeling of the EGF-URO recep-

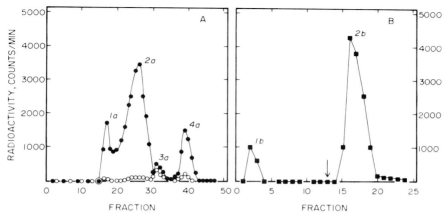

FIG. 6. Partial purification of epidermal growth factor–urogastrone (EGF-URO) bind-ing material from rat liver membranes. (A) Profile of ^{125}I-labeled EGF-URO radioactiv-ity solubilized from liver membranes after glutaraldehyde–sodium borohydride cross-linking with ^{125}I-labeled hEGF-URO in the absence (●-●) or the presence (○-○) of unlabeled EGF-URO (2 μg/ml). Identical aliquots of membrane protein were applied to a 1.2 × 60 cm Sepharose 6B column, and 1.2 ml fractions were collected. (B) Peak 2a was placed on a 0.3 × 4 cm Con A-Sepharose column, and the column was washed with 14 ml of 0.1% (v/v) Triton X-100–50 nM Tris-HCl, pH 7.7, followed by elution (arrow) with 50 mM acetate buffer, pH 6.2, containing 1 M α-methylmannopyranoside, 0.1% (v/v), Triton X-100, and 4 M urea. Data were taken from Sahyoun et al. (1978).

tor from human placental membranes (Hock et al., 1979). Elec-trophoretic analysis demonstrates the specific labeling by both pro-cedures of two prominent constituents (bands I and II, Fig. 7) having apparent molecular weights of about 160,000 and 180,000. A major constituent of about MW 200,000 is labeled in rat liver membranes (R. A. Hock, unpublished observations). The same two labeled com-ponents from placental membranes can be selectively adsorbed by a variety of lectin–agarose derivatives and can be eluted with ap-propriate lectin-specific sugars (Table IV). The amounts of bands I and II present appear to vary from one membrane preparation to another; the two constituents may be interrelated by either a biosyn-thetic or a degradative process.

When cross-linked to the receptor, EGF-URO can still be recognized by antibody (Fig. 8). Thus, it has been possible to effect considerable purification by combined affinity chromatography using lectin- and antibody–Sepharose derivatives (Hock et al., 1979) (Figs. 7 and 8). Although it was not possible to determine the protein content of the material isolated by these combined methods, the purification prob-ably approaches the theoretical maximum (about 1000-fold).

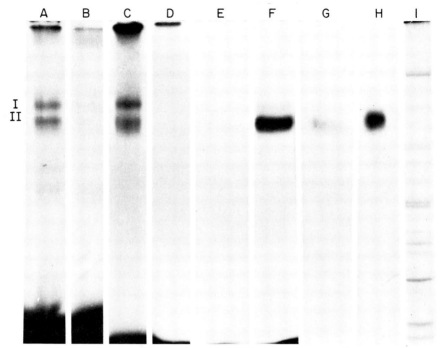

F<small>IG</small>. 7. Electrophoretic analysis and autoradiography of receptor in placental membranes affinity-cross-linked to ^{125}I-labeled mouse epidermal growth factor–urogastrone (mEGF-URO). Placental membranes were affinity cross-linked to ^{125}I-labeled mEGF-URO by either the glutaraldehyde (channels A and B) or the photoaffinity method (channels C and D). Affinity labeling was done either in the absence (A and C) or the presence (B and D) of a large excess of unlabeled EGF-URO. The photoaffinity-labeled receptor was then purified first by adsorption to wheat germ agglutinin–agarose (unadsorbed fraction, channel E; fraction eluted with N-acetylglucosamine, channel F) and then by application of the lectin-adsorbed fraction to a column of EGF-URO antibody-agarose. Channel H shows the analysis of the material that adsorbed to the antibody column. Channel G shows the unabsorbed material. Channel I shows the protein profile of the placental membranes as detected by Coomassie blue stain; channels A–H show the ^{125}I-labeled proteins detected by autoradiography of fixed, dried gels. The calibration of the gel was with the molecular weight markers β-galactosidase (130 K), phosphorylase A (94 K), bovine serum albumin (68 K), and pyruvate kinase (54 K). Data were taken from Hock *et al.* (1979).

In more recent work, methods have been devised to detect the EGF-URO receptor in solution without the need for affinity labeling (Nexø *et al.*, 1979). In brief, the soluble receptor can be "insolubilized" by adsorption to agarose–lectin beads and washed free of detergent, whereupon the specific binding of ^{125}I-labeled EGF-URO can be detected. Using this method to detect the EGF-URO receptor in col-

TABLE IV

BINDING OF AFFINITY-LABELED EPIDERMAL GROWTH FACTOR–UROGASTRONE
(EGF-URO) RECEPTOR FROM HUMAN PLACENTA BY LECTIN-AGAROSE
DERIVATIVES[a,b]

Lectin	Radioactivity (%)		Eluting sugar	Receptor detected in eluate
	Adsorbed	Unadsorbed		
Concanavalin A	6.9	93.1	α-Methylmannoside	+
Wheat germ agglutinin	5.2	94.8	N-Acetylglucosamine	+
Phytohemagglutinin	4.5	95.5	N-Acetylgalactosamine	+
Lens culinaris	4.2	95.8	α-Methylmannoside	+
Ricinus communis	0.3	99.7	Galactose	−
Peanut lectin	0.2	99.8	Galactose	−

[a] Adapted from Hock et al. (1979).

[b] The receptor in placental membranes was photoaffinity-labeled with ^{125}I-labeled mEGF-URO-SANAH and solubilized with NP-40; the extract was clarified by centrifugation. The soluble material was passed over lectin-agarose columns and the percentage of radioactivity absorbed was measured. Columns were then washed with buffer and subsequently eluted with buffer containing an appropriate lectin-specific sugar. Receptor in the eluate was detected (bands I and II, Fig. 7) by electrophoresis and autoradiography.

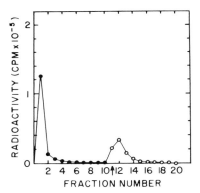

FIG. 8. Purification of affinity-cross-linked receptor from placental membranes with antibody–agarose. Soluble photoaffinity-labeled receptor was first partially purified by adsorption to wheat germ agglutinin–agarose and then applied to a mouse epidermal growth factor–urogastrone (mEGF-URO) antibody–agarose column. Electrophoretic analyses of the unadsorbed fraction (first peak) and the fraction eluted with 10% v/v formic acid (second peak) are shown in Fig. 8 (channels G and H). Data were taken from Hock *et al.* (1980).

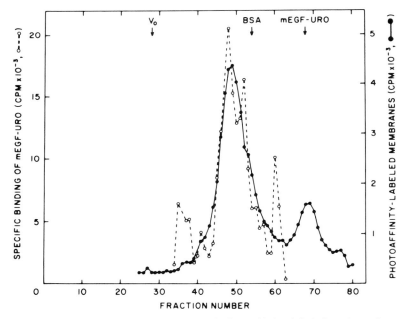

FIG. 9. Chromatography of the native and photoaffinity-labeled epidermal growth factor–urogastrone (EGF-URO) receptor on Sepharose 6B. The elution profiles of ^{125}I-labeled EGF-URO-labeled receptor (●) and of solubilized native receptor (○) are shown. The presence of native receptor in effluent fractions was detected by first ad-

umn fractions subsequent to chromatography on Sepharose 6B, it can be shown that the affinity-labeled and native soluble receptor have the same chromatographic properties (Fig. 9). The result of the work described above is to make methods available for the characterization of the receptor by a variety of standard physiochemical techniques. In principle, it should be possible to isolate sufficient pure material to determine the complete structure of this most interesting growth factor receptor.

VI. STRUCTURE–ACTIVITY RELATIONSHIPS FOR RECEPTOR BINDING AND BIOLOGICAL ACTIVITY

Remarkably, despite 16 differences between the amino acid sequences of human and mouse EGF-URO (Fig. 1), both polypeptides are equipotent, both *in vivo* (Cohen and Carpenter, 1975; Gregory, 1975) and *in vitro* (Carpenter and Cohen, 1976b; Hollenberg and Gregory, 1976). Similarly, both peptides can bind to the human fibroblast receptor with approximately equal affinity (Carpenter and Cohen, 1976a; Hollenberg and Gregory, 1976). As discussed in Section II, the differences between the amino acid residues of mouse and human EGF-URO would lead to considerable differences in the chemical microenvironment of the two peptides, particularly in the sequence comprising residues 1–28; in contrast, comparatively minor differences are evident in the third "loop" and tail portions of the two peptides, comprising residues 33–53 (Fig. 1). In terms of structure–activity relationships, it is therefore of interest to focus on the C-terminal portion of the molecule. To date, only the importance of the sequence 47–53 has been studied in detail.

Derivatives of EGF-URO lacking either the carboxy-terminal residue (hEGF-URO 1–52; also termed γ-urogastrone) or lacking two carboxy-terminal amino acids (mEGF-URO 1–51) possess the same activity as that of the intact molecule both *in vivo* and *in vitro* (Cohen *et al.*, 1975; Savage *et al.*, 1972; Gregory, 1975; Hollenberg and Gregory, 1977). In contrast, derivatives lacking either five (mEGF-

---

sorbing the receptor in such fractions to Con A–agarose and then measuring the binding of ^{125}I-labeled mEGF-URO to the immobilized receptor (data from Hock *et al.*, 1980). The column void volume and the position of elution of bovine serum albumin (BSA) and mEGF-URO are also indicated.

URO 1–48) or six (hEGF-URO 1–47 and mEGF-URO 1–47) carboxy-terminal amino acids, when compared with the intact molecule, exhibit a marked reduction in both receptor affinity and mitogenic potency *in vitro* (Figs. 10 and 11 and Table V) (Cohen *et al.*, 1975; Hollenberg and Gregory, 1980). Suprisingly, hEGF-URO 1–47 is equipotent with hEGF-URO 1–53 in the acid inhibition assay (Hollenberg and Gregory, 1980). This assay monitors a relatively rapid action of the peptides and could readily detect a 10-fold difference in potency between the two derivatives. Likewise, in the mouse eyelid opening bioassay, mEGF-URO 1–48 and the intact molecule have been observed to have similar potencies (Savage *et al.*, 1972).

The data obtained for the binding and action of derivatives in fibroblasts underscore the importance of the C-terminal portion of the molecule (especially the tripeptide 49–51: Trp Trp Glu) for both receptor affinity and mitogenic potency. Simply mixing the comparatively low-potency polypeptides (i.e., EGF-URO 1–47 or EGF-URO 1–48) with the C-terminal portion of the molecule (i.e., EGF-URO 48–53 or EGF-URO 49–53) does not simulate the potency of the intact molecule. Further, the terminal fragments themselves (e.g., hEGF-URO 48–53 or mEGF-URO 49–53) neither compete for the binding of ^{125}I-labeled EGF-URO nor exhibit mitogenic activity in human fibroblasts (Cohen *et al.*, 1975; Hollenberg and Gregory, 1980). In con-

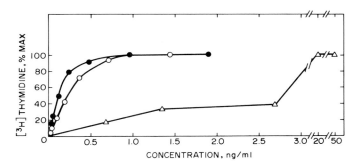

FIG. 10. Stimulation of DNA synthesis in human fibroblasts by human epidermal growth factor–urogastrone (hEGF-URO) derivatives. Confluent human fibroblast monolayers were stimulated with increasing concentrations of intact hEGF-URO (○, URO 1–53) and with derivatives lacking either one (●, URO 1–52) or six (△, URO 1–47) carboxyterminal amino acids. The incorporation of [³H]thymidine during a 3-hour period, begun 22 hours after the initial stimulus, was measured as previously described (Hollenberg and Cuatrecasas, 1975) and is expressed as the percentage of the maximum incorporation above baseline for each monolayer tray. Data were taken from Hollenberg and Gregory (1980).

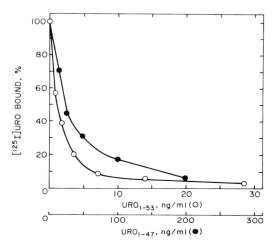

FIG. 11. Binding of human epidermal growth factor–urogastrone (hEGF-URO) and hEGF-URO 1–47 to human fibroblast monolayers. The competition for the binding of ^{125}I-labeled hEGF-URO by native hEGF-URO ($\bigcirc$, URO 1–53; $k_i = 0.5$ng/ml) and by hEGF-URO lacking the six carboxy-terminal amino acid residues ($\bullet$, URO 1–47; $k_i = 4.3$ ng/ml) was measured in replicate monolayer trays, essentially as previously described (Hollenberg and Cuatrecasas, 1975). The concentration of peptide for which the binding of labeled ligand was 50% of the amount bound in the absence of competitor (IC_{50}) was used to calculate the inhibitor dissociation constant (K_i), according to the equation: $K_i = IC_{50}/(1 + L^*/K^*)$, where L^* and K^* represent the concentration and dissociation constant of ^{125}I-labeled hEGF-URO (Cheng and Prusoff, 1973). Data were taken from Hollenberg and Gregory (1980).

trast with the importance of the C-terminal portion of the peptides for activity and receptor binding, blocking of the N terminal of mEGF-URO either with relatively small (fluorescein isothiocyanate) or comparatively large (fluorescein-labeled lactalbumin) substituents does not markedly affect receptor binding or biological activity (Shechter *et al.*, 1978a; Haigler *et al.*, 1978). Despite the reduced potency of the derivatives lacking the C-terminal hexapeptide, the sequence 1–47 is capable of causing a full biological response (Fig. 10) and thus contains the residues critical to the intrinsic activity of the molecule. Except that at least one intact disulfide bond is required for receptor binding and mitogenic activity (carboxamido-hEGF-URO is inactive) (Hollenberg and Gregory, 1980), it is not possible at present to speculate further as to the structural requirements for biological activity.

The markedly reduced potencies *in vitro* of the 1–47 or 1–48 derivatives, relative to the intact molecule, are not paralleled by the

TABLE V

COMPARISON OF RECEPTOR BINDING AND BIOLOGICAL ACTIVITIES
OF DERIVATIVES OF EPIDERMAL GROWTH FACTOR–UROGASTRONE
EGF-URO[a,b]

Compound	Binding K_D (ng/ml)	Bioactivity	
		[³H]Thymidine ED_{50}(ng/ml)	Acid inhibition ED_{50} (μg/kg)
hEGF-URO 1–53	0.57 ± 0.11 (5)	0.27 ± 0.05 (5)	0.5–0.6
hEGF-URO 1–52	0.48 ± 0.10 (3)	0.13 ± 0 (2)	0.5–0.6
hEGF-URO 1–47	6.3 ± 2.0 (4)	3.2 ± 0.7 (2)	0.5–0.6
mEGF-URO 1–53	1.6 ± 0.4 (4)	0.24 ± 0.11 (10)	0.5–0.6
mEGF-URO 1–47	7.2 ± 2.3 (6)	2.1 ± 0.5 (3)	ND

[a]Data were taken from Hollenberg and Gregory (1980).
[b]The binding and biological activities were determined for both native human and mouse EGF-URO (hEGF-URO 1–53; mEGF-URO 1–53) and for derivatives lacking either one (hEGF-URO 1–52) or six (hEGF-URO 1–47; mEGF-URO 1–47) carboxy-terminal amino acids. The dissociation constants and ED_{50}s for [³H]thymidine incorporation were determined in human fibroblast monolayers as illustrated in Figs. 10 and 11. The acid inhibitory potencies were determined *in vivo*. ND not determined. Values represent the mean ± SD for the number of estimates indicated in parentheses.

apparently equal potencies of all these derivatives *in vivo*. In the mouse eye-opening bioassay, cleavage of the intact molecule to mEGF-URO 1–48 *in vivo* over the comparatively long time period of the assay might explain the apparent discrepancy with the assay *in vitro*. However, metabolism, unless extremely rapid, is less likely to explain the equal potency of the 1–47 and 1–53 derivatives in the acid inhibition bioassay, where a rapid dose-discriminatory response to an intravenous bolus of peptide is monitored. An equally likely hypothesis to explain the different relative potencies (*in vitro* versus *in vitro*) is that the receptor involved in the mitogenic stimulus may differ from the one responsible for the inhibition of acid secretion.

VII. THE EGF-URO RECEPTOR, CELL TRANSFORMATION, AND TUMORIGENESIS

Studies of the interaction of mEGF-URO with a variety of normal and virally transformed cell lines have revealed that cells transformed by murine or feline sarcoma viruses can no longer bind EGF-URO, whereas the binding of EGF-URO is unaffected in either cells transformed by DNA tumor viruses or those infected by nontransforming RNA viruses (Todaro *et al.*, 1976, 1977). The loss in EGF-URO binding occurs *pari passu* with cell transformation. Viruses are not the only tumor-associated agents that affect EGF-URO receptors. Cells transformed by benzo[a]pyrene exhibit a reduction in EGF-URO receptors (Todaro *et al.*, 1976; Yeh and Holley, 1977; Hollenberg *et al.*, 1979), and cells treated with tumor-promoting phorbol esters also lose their ability to bind EGF-URO (Lee and Weinstein, 1978). Interestingly, nontransformed variants of mouse 3T3 cells (AD6) that display altered morphological characteristics also exhibit a reduction in EGF-URO binding (Pratt and Pastan, 1978). In the AD6 cells, which are deficient in membrane glycosylation (Pouyssegur *et al.*, 1977), the reduction in EGF binding can be partially overcome by incubating cells with *N*-acetylglucosamine, so as to bypass the enzymic defect (Pratt and Pastan, 1978).

It has been proposed that the reduction of EGF-URO binding in murine sarcoma virus-transformed cells is due to the production of a virally induced substance that occupies the receptors (Todaro *et al.*, 1976). In agreement with this hypothesis, it has been possible to isolate from such transformed mouse 3T3 cells a growth-promoting factor (SGF) that competes with EGF-URO for cellular binding in a radioreceptor assay, but does not crossreact with mEGF-URO antibodies (DeLarco and Todaro, 1978). It is as yet not known whether the reduction in EGF-URO binding caused by the SGF occurs by competition at the EGF-URO binding site or via a noncompetitive mechanism such as that exhibited by phorbol esters (Lee and Weinstein, 1978).

In view of the effects of tumorigenic virus transformation on EGF-URO binding, it was of interest to examine the receptors for EGF-URO in a number of chemically transformed tumorigenic Syrian hamster embryo (SHE) cell lines (Hollenberg *et al.*, 1979). A highly tumorigenic cell line (BP6T), derived by benzo[a]pyrene treatment, exhibits a selective reduction in the binding of EGF-URO compared to the parent SHE cell strain, whereas the binding of insulin is unaffected (Fig. 12). The reduced binding could not be attributed to receptor destruction, to cell density effects, to the production of receptor-occupying factor(s), or to an *N*-acetylglucosamine-reversible defect like the one in AD6 cells (Hollenberg *et al.*, 1979). The binding kinetics of the receptors in the transformed cells are the same as those in the parent cell strain. The reduced receptor availability in the trans-

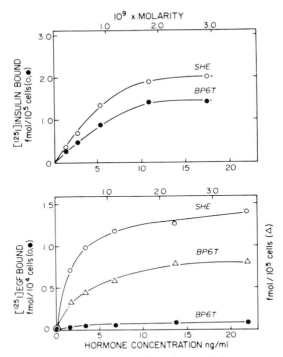

FIG. 12. Binding of insulin and mouse epidermal growth factor–urogastrone (mEGF-URO) to normal and tumorigenic Syrian hamster embryonic fibroblasts (SHE). The binding of ^{125}I-labeled insulin (upper) and mEGF-URO (lower) to both normal (SHE) and transformed, tumorigenic (BP6T) Syrian hamster embryonic fibroblast monolayers was measured by previously described methods (Hollenberg and Cuatrecasas, 1975). An expanded scale (right-hand ordinate) is used to illustrate the binding of mEGF-URO to BP6T cells. Data were taken from Hollenberg *et al.* (1979).

formed cells is most likely due to decreased receptor synthesis or increased receptor turnover or both.

Like the BP6T cell line, a number of other similarly derived tumorigenic cell lines also exhibit reduced EGF-URO binding (Table VI). It is important that in the several lines studied the level of EGF-URO binding by cells does not correlate either with the cellular growth characteristics (doubling time; growth in soft agar) or with the ability of the cells to cause tumors *in vivo* (Table VI). Thus the causal relationship(s), if any, between cell transformation, tumorigenesis, and reduced EGF-URO receptors may be difficult to establish. That there is a connection between these three cellular characteristics is, however, most provocative.

TABLE VI

BINDING OF MOUSE EPIDERMAL GROWTH FACTOR–UROGASTRONE (mEGF-URO)
BY TRANSFORMED TUMORIGENIC SYRIAN HAMSTER EMBRYONIC (SHE) CELL LINES[a,b]

Cell line	Binding (% relative to BP6T)	Tumorigenicity (TD_{50})	Generation time (hours)
BP6T	100	10	16.1
BP12A	46 ± 15	50	40.0
BP14	64 ± 21	10,000	46.1
BP12	111 ± 25	10,000	67.7
BP17	189 ± 21	1,000	37.6
BP6	221 ± 42	50	30.2

[a]Data were taken from Hollenberg et al. (1979).

[b]Tumorigenic cell lines, derived consequent to benzo[a]pyrene treatment of SHE cells
(Barrett et al., 1978), were seeded (approximately 10^4 cells/well) in replicate multidish
trays in sets that always included BP6T cells for comparison. After about 4 days'
growth, the binding of ^{125}I-labeled mEGF-URO (3.9 ng/ml) was measured (Hollenberg
and Cuatecasas, 1975), and cell counts were determined in replicate dishes. The binding per cell of each cell line, representing the average ± SD for independent
estimates, is expressed relative to the binding by BP6T cells; the parent strain SHE
cells bind about 900% of the EGF-URO bound by BP6T cells (Fig 12). The
tumorigenicity (number of cells producing palpable tumors in 50% of test animals
within one year of subcutaneous administration) and the generation times of the
various cell lines, determined independently (Barrett et al., 1979), are also recorded.

VIII. Is EGF-URO a Hormone?

In view of the many biological actions of EGF-URO that can be
observed at concentration ranges over which polypeptide hormones
are known to act, given the limited number of specific receptors that
are present on responsive cells in numbers appropriate for other peptide hormones and given the wide tissue distribution of receptors for
EGF-URO, it is tempting to propose that EGF-URO plays a hormonal role perhaps as fundamental as that of insulin. EGF-URO, like
other polypeptide hormones, also appears to be distributed among a
wide variety of species (Table VII). The presence of EGF-URO in a
given animal can be inferred on the basis of cross-reactivity in an immunoassay or radioreceptor assay of a tissue, blood, or urine extract
(the receptor apparently does not readily distinguish species differences as do the antibodies); on the basis of the binding of
^{125}I-labeled EGF-URO to tissues; or on the basis of the action of EGF-
URO on tissues or cells either in vivo or in vitro. Other evidence to

TABLE VII

OCCURRENCE OF EPIDERMAL GROWTH FACTOR–UROGASTRONE
(EGF-URO) IN VARIOUS SPECIES[a]

Animal	Evidence for Presence of EGF-URO	Reference(s)
Man	Isolation and structure determination	Gregory (1975)
Macaque	Immunoreactivity of urine with hEGF-URO	Gregory et al. (1978a)
Dog	Action in vivo	Gregory et al. (1978a)
Cat	Binding to fibroblasts action in vivo	Todaro et al. (1976)
Cow	Binding and action in cultured cells and binding to cell membranes	Vlodavsky et al. (1978); O'Keefe et al. (1974)
Sheep	Action in vivo	Sundell et al. (1975)
Mink	Action in vitro	Todaro et al. (1976)
Mouse	Isolation and structure determination	Carpenter and Cohen (1978)
Rat	Isolation and amino acid composition	Moore (1978)
	Action on tissues in vitro	Carpenter and Cohen (1978)
	Immunoreactivity of urine with mEGF-URO antibody	Gregory et al. (1978)
	Binding to cultured cells	O'Keefe et al. (1974)
	Binding to tissues in vivo	Covelli et al. (1972b)
Rabbit	Action and binding in cultured cells; reactivity of urine in a radioreceptor assay	Hollenberg (1975); E. Nexø and M. D. Hollenberg, unpublished data; Carpenter and Cohen (1978)
Guinea pig	Immunoreactivity of urine with mEGF-URO antibody	Gregory et al. (1978)
Hamster	Action and binding in cultured cells	Hollenberg et al. (1979)
Chicken	Action and binding in cultured cells	Carpenter and Cohen (1978)
Frog	Action on cells in vitro	Gregory et al. (1978)

[a] As discussed in the text, the presence of EGF-URO in the species indicated can be inferred by a variety of data other than chemical analysis. In many instances the appropriate data are found in the quoted review articles; in several instances references to specific studies are made. The references selected are representative only and are not intended to be exhaustive.

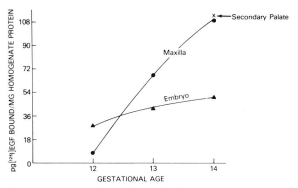

FIG. 13. Binding of mouse epidermal growth factor–urogastrone (mEGF-URO) by developing mouse embryo tissue. The binding of mEGF-URO to membranes from homogenates either of maxilla or whole embryo derived from animals of increasing gestational age (days) was measured by previously described methods (Cuatrecasas and Hollenberg, 1976). The binding by embryo tissues is compared with the binding by homogenates of the secondary palate. Data were taken from Pratt *et al.* (1978).

suggest a hormonal role for EGF-URO includes the occurrence in the mouse and in man of serum levels (about 1 ng/ml or lower; $1.7 \times 10^{-10} M$) appropriate for a polypeptide hormone and the hormonal modulation in the mouse of serum (catecholamines) and submaxillary (catecholamines, androgens) EGF-URO levels (Cohen and Taylor, 1974; Bynny *et al.*, 1974; Barthe *et al.*, 1974). Furthermore, studies of the action and binding of EGF-URO in embryonic chick tissues of different ages (results reviewed by Carpenter and Cohen, 1978), in the developing mouse palate (Hassell and Pratt, 1977), incisor and eyelid (Carpenter and Cohen, 1978), in embryonic mouse tissues (Pratt *et al.*, 1978), and in membranes from both the basal plate (O'Keefe *et al.*, 1974) and amnion* (Hock and Hollenberg, 1977) of the human placenta suggest that the EGF-URO may play a very important role in organ development. In the developing mouse embryo there may be variations not only in the amount of available EGF-URO, but also in the receptor content of a potential target tissue, such as the palate (Fig. 13) (Pratt *et al.*, 1978). Indeed, the possibility exists that the early developmental requirements for EGF-URO may be such that defects in EGF-URO function may be lethal to the embryo. This hypothesis could explain the lack to date of disease processes that can be attributed to a malfunction of EGF-URO or its receptor.

Despite the preceding evidence, it is not yet possible to ascribe to

*hEGF-URO has recently been detected in human amniotic fluid (Barka *et al.*, 1978).

EGF-URO a "traditional" hormonal[†] role with feedback regulatory controls, for instance like those for adrenocorticotropic hormone. Moreover, the lack of a single major tissue of origin (EGF-URO serum levels in the mouse remain high, even after removal of the submaxillary gland), and the existence in the circulation in man and possibly other mammals of large amounts of EGF-URO precursor (Gregory *et al.*, 1979; Hirata and Orth, 1978) may render exceedingly difficult experiments designed to study the consequences of a lack of EGF-URO on developmental or other processes. Yet, the weight of evidence cited above indicates that EGF-URO can, and probably normally does, influence a variety of vital processes *in vivo* and may be representative of a new class of polypeptide modulating factors that exhibit multiple actions and are not adequately described as "hormones" in the classical sense of the term. In future work it will thus be of great interest to determine the factor(s) that control the levels and action of EGF-URO *in vivo*. One can anticipate many exciting developments concerning the physiology and pathophysiology of this most interesting polypeptide.

REFERENCES

Acher, R., Manoussos, G., and Olivry, G. (1955). *Biochim. Biophys. Acta* **16**, 155.

Aharonov, A., Pruss, R. M., and Herschman, H. R. (1978a). *J. Biol. Chem.* **253**, 3970.

Aharonov, A., Vlodavsky, I., Pruss, R. M., Fox, C. F., and Herschman, H. L. (1978b). *J. Cell. Physiol.* **95**, 195.

Anderson, R. G. W., Goldstein, J. L., and Brown, M. S. (1977). *Nature (London)* **270**, 695.

Armelin, H. A. (1973). *Proc. Natl. Acad. Sci. U.S.A.* **70**, 2702.

Baker, J. B., Barsh, G. S., Carney, D. H., and Cunningham, D. D. (1978). *Proc. Natl. Acad. Sci. U.S.A.* **75**, 1882.

Baker, J. B., Simmer, R. L., Glenn, K. C., and Cunningham, D. D. (1979). *Nature (London)* **278**, 743.

Barka, T., Vandernoen, H., Gresik, E. W., and Kerenyi, T. (1978). *J. Cell Biol.* **79**, 186a.

Barrett, J. C., Crawford, B. D., Mixter, L. O., Schechtman, L. M., Ts'o, P. O. P., and Pollack, R. (1979). *Cancer Res.* **39**, 1504.

Barthe, P. L., Bullock, L. P., Mowszowicz, I., Bardin, C. W., and Orth, D. N. (1974). *Endocrinology* **95**, 1019.

Baseman, J. B., and Hayes, N. S. (1975). *J. Cell Biol.* **67**, 492.

Bennett, G. V., O'Keefe, E., and Cuatrecasas, P. (1975). *Proc. Natl. Acad. Sci. U.S.A.* **72**, 33.

Benveniste, R., Speeg, K. V., Carpenter, G., Cohen, S., Lindner, J., and Rabinowitz, D. (1978). *J. Clin. Endocrinol. Metab.* **46**, 169.

Bertsch, S., and Marks, F. (1974). *Nature (London)* **251**, 517.

Blosse, P. T., Fenton, E. L., Henningsson, S., Kahlson, G., and Rosengren, E. (1974). *Experientia* **30**, 22.

[†]It is rather interesting that EGF-URO, like the peptides for which the term hormone was coined (secretin and gastrin), is a gastrointestinal polypeptide.

Boeynaems, J. M., and Dumont, J. E. (1977). *Mol. Cell Endocrinol.* **7**, 33.
Brunk, U., Schellens, J., and Westermark, B. (1976). *Exp. Cell Res.* **103**, 295
Bynny, R. L., Orth, D. N., and Cohen, S. (1972). *Endocrinology* **90**, 1261.
Bynny, R. L., Orth, D. N., Cohen, S., and Doyne, E. S. (1974). *Endocrinology* **95**, 776.
Carpenter, G. (1978). *J. Invest. Dermatol.* **71**, 283.
Carpenter, G., and Cohen, S. (1976a). *J. Cell Biol.* **71**, 159.
Carpenter, G., and Cohen, S. (1976b). *J. Cell. Physiol.* **88**, 227.
Carpenter, G., and Cohen, S. (1977). *Biochem. Biophys. Res. Commun.* **79**, 545.
Carpenter, G., and Cohen, S. (1978). *Biochem. Actions Horm.* **5**, 203.
Carpenter, G., Lembach, K. J., Morrison, M., and Cohen, S. (1975). *J. Biol. Chem.* **250**, 4297.
Carpenter, G., King, L., Jr., and Cohen, S. (1978). *Nature (London)* **276**, 409.
Chen, L. B., Gudor, R. C., Sun, T. T., Chen, A. B., and Mosesson, M.W. (1977). Science **197**, 776.
Cheng, R.-C., and Prusoff, W. H. (1973). *Biochem. Pharmacol.* **22**, 3099.
Cohen, S. (1960). *Proc. Natl. Acad. Sci. U.S.A.* **46**, 302.
Cohen, S. (1962). *J. Biol. Chem.* **237**, 1555.
Cohen, S. (1965). *Dev. Biol.* **12**, 394.
Cohen, S. (1972). *J. Invest. Dermatol.* **59**, 13.
Cohen, S., and Carpenter, G. (1975). *Proc. Natl. Acad. Sci. U.S.A.* **72**, 1317.
Cohen, S., and Savage, C. R., Jr. (1974). *Recent Prog. Horm. Res.* **30**, 551.
Cohen, S., and Stastny, M. (1968). *Biochim. Biophys. Acta* **166**, 427.
Cohen, S., and Taylor, J. M. (1974). *Recent Prog. Horm. Res.* **30**, 533.
Cohen, S., Carpenter, G., and Lembach, K. J. (1975). *Adv. Metab. Disorders* **8**, 265.
Covelli, I., Mozzi, R., Rossi, R., and Frati, L. (1972a). *Hormones* **3**, 183.
Covelli, I., Rossi, R., Mozzi, R., and Frati, L. (1972b). *Eur. J. Biochem.* **27**, 225.
Cuatrecasas, P. (1972). *Proc. Natl. Acad. Sci. U.S.A.* **69**, 1277.
Cuatrecasas, P. (1974). *Annu. Rev. Biochem.* **43**, 169.
Cuatrecasas, P., and Hollenberg, M. D. (1976). *Adv. Prot. Chem.* **30**, 251.
Cuatrecasas, P., and Tell, G. P. E. (1973). *Proc. Natl. Acad. Sci. U.S.A.* **70**, 485.
Das, M., and Fox, C. F. (1978). *Proc. Natl. Acad. Sci. U.S.A.* **75**, 2644.
Das, M., Miyakawa, T., Fox, C. F., Pruss, R., Aharonov, A., and Herschmann, H. R. (1977). *Proc. Natl. Acad. Sci. U.S.A.* **74**, 2790.
Dean, C. R., Hollenberg, M. D., and Hope, D. B. (1967). *Biochem. J.* **104**, 8C.
DeHaen, C. (1976). *J. Theor. Biol.* **58**, 383.
DeLarco, J. E., and Todaro, G. J. (1978). *Proc. Natl. Acad. Sci. U.S.A.* **75**, 4001.
Elder, J. B., Williams, G., Lacey, E., and Gregory, H. (1978). *Nature (London)* **271**, 466. **16**, 887.
Elder, J. B., Williams, G., Lacey, E., and Gregory, H. (1978). *Nature (London)* **271**, 466.
Farebrother, D. A., and Mann, C. B. (1970). *Biochem. J.* **118**, 33P.
Feldman, E. J., Aures, D., and Grossman, M. I. (1978). *Proc. Soc. Exp. Biol. Med.* **159**, 400.
Frati, L., Daniels, S., Delogu, A., and Covelli, I. (1972). *Exp. Eye Res.* **14**, 135.
Frati, L., Cenci, G., Sbaraglia, G., Teti, D. V., and Covelli, I. (1976). *Life Sci.* **18**, 905.
Gerring, E. L., Bower, J. M., and Gregory, H. (1974). *In* "Chronic Duodenal Ulcer" (C. Wastell, ed.), p. 171. Butterworth, London.
Gordon, A. S., Davis, C. G., Milfay, D., and Diamond, I. (1977). *Nature (London)* **267**, 539.
Gospodarowicz, D., Ill, C. R., and Birdwell, C. R. (1977a). *Endocrinology* **100**, 1108.
Gospodarowicz, D., Moran, J. S., and Owashi, N. D. (1977b). *J. Clin. Endocrinol. Metab.* **44**, 651.

Gray, J. S., Wieczorowski, E., and Ivy, A. C. (1939). *Science* **89**, 489.

Gregory, H. (1975). *Nature (London)* **257**, 325.

Gregory, H., and Preston, B. M. (1977). *Int. J. Peptide Protein Res.* **9**, 107.

Gregory, H., and Willshire, I. R. (1975). *Hoppe-Seyler's Z. Physiol. Chem.* **356**, 1765.

Gregory, H., Holmes, J. E., and Willshire, I. R. (1977). *J. Clin. Endocrinol. Metab.* **45**, 668.

Gregory, H., Bower, J. M., and Willshire, I. R. (1978). *In* "Growth Factors" (K. W. Kastrup and J. H. Nielsen, eds.), p. 75 Pergamon, (FEBS Colloq, B3, Vol. 48). Oxford.

Gregory, H., Walsh, S., and Hopkins, C. R. (1979). *Gastroenterology* **77**, 313.

Haigler, H., Ash, J. F., Singer, S. J., and Cohen, S. (1978). *Proc. Natl. Acad. Sci. U.S.A.* **75**, 3317.

Hassell, J. R. (1975). *Dev. Biol.* **45**, 90.

Hassell, J. R., and Pratt, R. M. (1977). *Exp. Cell Res.* **106**, 55.

Heimberg, M., Weinstein, I., LeQuire, V. S., and Cohen, S. (1965). *Life Sci.* **4**, 1625.

Hershko, A., Mamont, P., Shields, R., and Tomkins, G. M. (1971). *Nature (London) New Biol.* **232**, 206.

Hirata, Y., and Orth, D. N. (1978). *Endocrinology* (*Proc. 60th Annu. Endocrinol. Meeting* Abst. No. 409), p. 279.

Ho, P. C., Davis, W. H., Elliot, J. H., and Cohen, S. (1974). *Invest. Ophthalmol.* **13**, 804.

Hock, R. A., and Hollenberg, M. D. (1977). *Clin. Res.* **25**, 665A.

Hock, R. A., and Hollenberg, M. D. (1980). *J. Biol. Chem.* Submitted.

Hock, R. A., Nexφ, E., and Hollenberg, M. D. (1979). *Nature (London)* **277**, 403.

Hock, R. A., Nexφ, E., and Hollenberg, M. D. (1980). *J. Biol. Chem.* Submitted.

Holladay, L. A., Savage, C. R., Jr., When, S., and Puett, D. (1976). *Biochemistry* **15**, 2624.

Hollenberg, M. D. (1975). *Arch. Biochem. Biophys.* **171**, 371.

Hollenberg, M. D. (1976). *Pan Am. Assoc. Biochem. Soc. Rev.* **5**, 265.

Hollenberg, M. D. (1978). *In* "Neurotransmitter Receptor Binding" (H. I. Yamamura, S. J. Enna, and M. J. Kuhar, eds.), p. 13 Raven New York.

Hollenberg, M. D., and Cuatrecasas, P. (1973). *Proc. Natl. Acad. Sci. U.S.A.* **70**, 2964.

Hollenberg, M. D., and Cuatrecasas, P. (1975). *J. Biol. Chem.* 250, 3845.

Hollenberg, M. D., and Cuatrecasas, P. (1978). *Prog. Neuropsychopharm.* **2**, 287.

Hollenberg, M. D., and Gregory, H. (1976). *Life Sci.* **20**, 267.

Hollenberg, M. D., and Gregory, H. (1977). *Clin. Res.* **25**, 312A.

Hollenberg, M. D., and Gregory, H. (1980). *Molec. Pharmacol.* **17**, in press.

Hollenberg, M. D., and Hope, D. B. (1968). *Biochem. J.* **106**, 557.

Hollenberg, M. D., and Schneider, E. L. (1979). *Mech. Ageing Dev.* **11**, 37.

Hollenberg, M. D., Barrett, J. C., Ts'o, P. O. P., and Berhanu, P. (1979). *Cancer Res.* **39**, 4166.

Holley, R. W., Armour, R., Baldwin, J. H., Brown, K. D., and Yeh, Y.-C. (1977). *Proc. Natl. Acad. Sci. U.S.A.* **74**, 5046.

Hoober, J. K., and Cohen, S. (1967a). *Biochim. Biophys. Acta* **138**, 347.

Hoober, J. K., and Cohen, S. (1967b). *Biochim. Biophys. Acta* **138**, 357.

Hosam, A., Horowitz, S. G., Hollenberg, M. D., and Makman, M. H. (1976). *Fed. Proc. Fed. Am. Soc. Exp. Biol.* **35**, 1731.

Jacobs, S., and Cuatrecasas, P. (1976). *Biochim. Biophys. Acta* **433**, 482.

Jacobs, S., and Cuatrecasas, P. (1978). *Science* **200**, 1283.

Kahn, C. R., Baird, K. L., Jarrett, D. B., and Flier, J. S. (1978). *Proc. Natl. Acad. Sci. U.S.A.* **75**, 4209.

Knox, E., Reynolds D. W., Cohen, S., and Alford, C. A. (1978). *J. Clin. Invest.* **61**, 1635.
Koffman, C. G., Elder, J. B., Ganguli, P. C., Gillespie, I. E., Gregory, H., and Geary, C. (1977). *Gastroenterology* **72**, 1082.
Krieger, D. T., Hauser, H., Liotta, A., and Zelenetz, A. (1976). *Endocrinology* **99**, 1589.
Lee, L.-S., and Weinstein, I. B. (1978). *Science* **202**, 313.
Leffert, H. L. (1974). *J. Cell Biol.* **62**, 767.
Lembach, K. J. (1976). *J. Cell. Physiol.* **89**, 277.
Lindgren, A., and Westermark, B. (1976). *Exp. Cell Res.* **99**, 357.
Linsley, P. S., Blifeld, C., Wrann, M., and Fox, C. F. (1979). *Nature (London)* **278**, 743.
Mann, C. B., and Fenton, E. L. (1970). *Biochem. J.* **118**, 33P.
Maxfield, F. R., Schlessinger, J., Shechter, Y., Pastan, I., and Willingham, M. C. (1978). *Cell* **14**, 805.
Moore, J. B., Jr. (1978). *Arch. Biochem. Biophys.* **189**, 1.
Nexø, E., Nelson, J., Lamberg, S. I., and Hollenberg, M. D. (1977). *Clin. Res.* **25**, 657A.
Nexø, E., Hock, R. A., and Hollenberg, M. D. (1979). *J. Biol-Chem.* **254**, 8740.
O'Keefe, E., Hollenberg, M. D., and Cuatrecasas, P. (1974). *Arch. Biochem. Biophys.* **164**, 518.
Pasquini, F., Petris, A., Sbaraglia, G., Scopelliti, R., Cenci, G., and Frati, L. (1974). *Exp. Cell Res.* **86**, 233.
Peters, K., and Richards, F. M. (1977). *Annu. Rev. Biochem.* **46**, 523.
Pouyssegur, J., Willingham, M., and Pastan, I. (1977). *J. Biol. Chem.* **252**, 1639.
Pratt, R. M., and Pastan, I. (1978). *Nature (London)* **272**, 68.
Pratt, R. M., Figueroa, A. A., Nexø, E., and Hollenberg, M. D. (1978). *J. Cell Biol.* **79**, 24a.
Raff, M. (1976). *Nature (London)* **259**, 265.
Reynolds, V. H., Boehm, F., and Cohen, S. (1965). *Surg. Forum* **16**, 108.
Rheinwald, J. G., and Green, H. (1977). *Nature (London)* **265**, 421.
Richman, R. A., Claus, T. H., Pilkus, S. J., and Friedman, D. L. (1976). *Proc. Natl. Acad. Sci. U.S.A.* **73**, 3593.
Roberts, M. L. (1974). *Biochem. Pharmacol.* **23**, 3308.
Roberts, M. L. (1977). *Naunyn-Schmeideberg's Arch. Pharmacol.* **296**, 301.
Rose, S. P., Pruss, R. M., and Herschman, H. R. (1976a). *J. Cell. Physiol.* **86**, 593.
Rose, S. P., Stan, R., Passovoy, D. S., and Herschman, H. R. (1976b). *Experientia* **32**, 913.
Sahyoun, N., Hock, R. A., and Hollenberg, M. D. (1978). *Proc. Natl. Acad. Sci. U.S.A.* **75**, 1675.
Sandweiss, D. J., Sugarman, M. H., Friedman, M. H. F., Salzstein, H. C., and Farbman A. A. (1941). *Am. J. Dig. Dis.* **8**, 371.
Savage, C. R., and Cohen, S. (1972). *J. Biol. Chem.* **247**, 7609.
Savage, C. R., and Cohen, S. (1973). *Exp. Eye Res.* **15**, 361.
Savage, C. R., Jr., Inagami, T., and Cohen, S. (1972). *J. Biol. Chem.* **247**, 7612.
Savage, C. R., Jr., Hash, J. H., and Cohen, S. (1973). *J. Biol. Chem.* **248**, 7669.
Schlessinger J., Shechter, Y., Willingham, M. C., and Pastan, I. (1978a). *Proc. Natl. Acad. Sci. U.S.A.* **75**, 2659.
Schlessinger, J., Shechter, Y., Cuatrecasas, P., Willingham, M. C., and Pastan, I. (1978b). *Proc. Natl. Acad. Sci. U.S.A.* **75**, 5353.
Shechter, Y., Schlessinger J., Jacobs, S., Chang, K.-J., and Cuatrecasas, P. (1978a). *Proc. Natl. Acad. Sci. U.S.A.* **75**, 2135.
Shechter, Y., Hernaez, L., and Cuatrecasas, P. (1978b). *Proc. Natl. Acad. Sci. U.S.A.* **75**, 5788.

Shodell, M. (1972). *Proc. Natl. Acad. Sci. U.S.A.* **69**, 1455.

Smith, L. F. (1966). *Am. J. Med.* **40**, 662.

Starkey, R. H., Cohen, S., and Orth, D. N. (1974). *Science* **189**, 800.

Stastny, M., and Cohen, S. (1970). *Biochim. Biophys. Acta* **204**, 578.

Stoker, M. G. P., Pigott, D., and Taylor-Papadimitriou, J. (1976). *Nature (London)* **264**, 764.

Sun, T. T., and Green, H. (1976). *Cell* **9**, 511.

Sun, T. T., and Green, H. (1977). *Nature (London)* **269**, 489.

Sundell, H., Serenius, F. S., Barthe, P., Friedman, Z., Kanarek, K. S., Escobedo, M. B., Orth, D. N., and Stahlman, M. T. (1975). *Pediatr. Res.* **9**, 371.

Taylor, J. M., Mitchell, W. M., and Cohen, S. (1972). *J. Biol. Chem.* **247**, 5928.

Taylor, J. M., Mitchell, W. M., and Cohen, S. (1974). *J. Biol. Chem.* **249**, 2188.

Teichberg, V. I., Sobel, A., and Changeux, J.-P. (1977). *Nature (London)* **267**, 540.

Todaro, G. J., DeLarco, J. E., and Cohen, S. (1976). *Nature (London)* **264**, 26.

Todaro, G. J., DeLarco, J. E., Nissley, S. P., and Rechler, M. M. (1977). *Nature (London)* **267**, 526.

Turkington, R. W. (1969a). *Exp. Cell Res.* **57**, 79.

Turkington, R. W. (1969b). *Cancer Res.* **29**, 1459.

Turkington, R. W., Males, J. L., and Cohen, S. (1971). *Cancer Res.* **31**, 253.

Van Noorden, S., Heitz, P., Kasper, M., and Pearse, A. G. E. (1977). *Histochemistry* **52**, 329.

Varon, S., Nomura, J., and Shooter, E. M. (1967). *Biochemistry* **6**, 2202.

Vlodavsky, I., Brown, K. D., and Gospodarowicz, D. (1978). *J. Biol. Chem.* **253**, 3744.

Westermark, B. (1976). *Biochem. Biophys. Res. Commun.* **69**, 304.

Westermark, B. (1977). *Proc. Natl. Acad. Sci. U.S.A.* **74**, 1619.

Wolf, L., Kohler, N., Boehm, C., and Lipton, A. (1975). *Exp. Cell Res.* **92**, 63.

Yeh, Y.-C., and Holley, R. W. (1977). *Fed. Proc.* **36**, 711.

Control of ACTH Secretion by Corticotropin-Releasing Factor(s)

ALVIN BRODISH

Department of Physiology and Pharmacology,
Bowman Gray School of Medicine of Wake Forest University,
Winston-Salem, North Carolina

I.	Introduction	111
II.	Central Nervous System Activation of Corticotropin-Releasing Factor (CRF)	112
III.	Nature of Hypothalamic CRF	113
IV.	Dynamic Changes in ACTH Secretion	115
	A. The Impact of Radioimmunoassays of ACTH and Cortisol	118
	B. Circadian Rhythm and Feedback Regulation	121
V.	CRF in Peripheral Blood	123
VI.	Hypothalamic Control Center for ACTH Release	125
VII.	Nature of the Functional Deficit in Rats with Hypothalamic Lesions	128
	A. Delayed Response to Stress	129
	B. Sensitization to Stress	131
VIII.	Assays for CRF	132
	A. *In Vivo* CRF Assays	132
	B. *In Vitro* CRF Assays	135
IX.	Hypothalamic and Extrahypothalamic CRF in Peripheral Blood	138
	A. Time Course of Response to Hypothalamic CRF	139
	B. Hypothalamic CRF in Blood	140
	C. ACTH Release by Extrahypothalamic CRF	141
X.	Tissue CRF	143
	A. Time Course of Median Eminence CRF and Tissue CRF	143
	B. Regulation of Tissue CRF Activity	145
	C. Suppression of Tissue CRF	146
	D. Significance of Tissue CRF	147
	References	150

I. Introduction

This review of the control of ACTH secretion by corticotropin-releasing factor is not intended to be complete or necessarily authoritative with respect to current dogma. Instead, the review reflects a personal assessment and involvement by the author that selectively presents his bias and emphasis on research efforts and contributions from his laboratory.

Neuroendocrinology has earned a respectable place in endocrinology. It is now firmly established that the synthesis and release of the hormones of the adenohypophysis are controlled by substances released from nerve endings in the hypothalamus and conveyed to the anterior pituitary gland by the portal vessels. The evidence that demonstrated the fundamental importance of the hypothalamus and the hypothalamo-hypophysial portal vessels came primarily from experiments that involved pituitary stalk transection, transplantation of the pituitary gland to a site remote from the sella turcica, and selective destruction or stimulation of the hypothalamus.

In 1948, Geoffrey Harris concluded that there was presumptive evidence to favor neural control of the adenohypophysis and that nervous stimuli activate the anterior pituitary gland by means of humoral transmission through the hypophysial portal vessels (Harris, 1948).

The realization that the hypothalamus contains substances capable of affecting pituitary activity naturally led to attempts to isolate and identify these neurohormones. The traditional transmitters of the autonomic nervous system were quickly ruled out as possible candidates; therefore, several laboratories embarked on extensive programs to extract and separate the hypothalamic hormones or "releasing hormones." Several hypothalamic releasing hormones have been isolated and their structures determined. It was originally postulated that each pituitary hormone is controlled by a single hypothalamic hormone, but it now appears that the system is much more complex.

II. Central Nervous System Activation of Corticotropin-Releasing Factor (CRF)

It is generally accepted that many aspects of ACTH release are modulated by the central nervous system (CNS). Such regulation is mediated by a corticotropin-releasing factor. The sites of production of such a factor within the CNS and its chemical nature still remain to be elucidated. Current thought holds that production of CRF occurs within neurosecretory cells that in addition to their secretory properties, share with other nerve cells the property of synaptic activation by neurotransmitter substances. It is presumed that some of these neurotransmitters are similar to those whose functions have been described in the peripheral nervous system. Chemical and fluorescence techniques have demonstrated the presence of acetylcholine, norepinephrine, serotonin, and dopamine within the CNS. Regional and circadian variation of levels of these substances within areas of the hypothalamic–limbic system have also been demonstrated. These are neural areas that have been shown through lesion and stimulation experiments to have significant effects on ACTH secretion (Mangili *et al.*, 1966) and to be sites of corticosteroid concentration (McEwen *et al.*, 1970). It is likely that these transmitter substances, by acting on the neurosecretory cells involved in the production of CRF, could affect its release in response to the varied stimuli that are known to influence ACTH levels. There is no definitive evidence that neurotransmitter substances modify ACTH release by direct action on the pituitary gland itself (Guillemin and Rosenberg, 1955).

III. Nature of Hypothalamic CRF

Although CRF was the first hypothalamic releasing factor to be demonstrated in hypothalamic tissue (Saffran and Schally, 1955), it remains the least well characterized of the releasing hormones. The lack of understanding of the nature of CRF might be attributed to difficulty in effectively assaying this substance in hypothalamic tissue, not to mention the difficulties in measuring ACTH itself. Other problems have surfaced in the attempts at purification of CRF. It has been reported that CRF activity is lost as purification proceeds until little or no activity remains (Chan *et al.*, 1970). Thus, much of the knowledge concerning CRF structure and function has necessarily been obtained through indirect methods.

Some clues concerning the nature of CRF have been obtained by studying the action of substances with known structure that can stimulate ACTH secretion in a manner similar to that described for hypothalamic extract (HSME). Many early studies showed that CRF was present in the posterior lobe of the pituitary and may therefore involve neurohypophysial function. Some investigators proposed that vasopressin itself was the physiological CRF (Sobel *et al.*, 1955; Martini and Morpurgo, 1955; McCann, 1957). Guillemin *et al.* (1957) isolated a neurohypophysial CRF that he called β-CRF. Schally and Bowers (1964) subsequently proposed a structure for β-CRF of posterior pituitary origin. The proposed structure consisted of a polypeptide of 12 amino acids that shared a common sequence with lysine vasopressin for 10 of the amino acids. Previously, Schally *et al.* (1960) postulated that there were several CRF-like substances in the posterior pituitary: vasopressin itself, melanocyte-stimulating hormone (αMSH), and β-CRF. However, there is convincing evidence that in addition to the aforementioned compounds some other substance from the hypothalamus could additionally release ACTH from the anterior pituitary (Saffran and Schally, 1955; McDonald *et al.*, 1957; Guillemin *et al.*, 1957; Royce and Sayers, 1958.)

Corticotropin-releasing factor of hypothalamic origin may or may not be identical with or related to neurohypophysial CRF, but the similarities between the CRF activity of vasopressin and hypothalamic CRF have stimulated additional studies to determine whether a vasopressin-like compound may be a physiological CRF. Data reported by Andersson *et al.* (1972) indicate that the ability of vasopressin to release ACTH and cortisol does not depend upon its antidiuretic or pressor activity. Analogs of vasopressin, which exert significant pressor and maximal antidiuretic action in human subjects, did not change cortisol levels whereas 1–10 ng of lysine vasopressin given intravenously to similar subjects did cause significant adrenal steroid release.

The CRF-like activity of vasopressin has also been observed in rat anterior pituitary cell preparations (Portanova and Sayers, 1973a,b). In contrast to the findings of Arimura *et al.*, (1969) and Chan *et al.* (1969), who have reported similarities in dose-response relationships of hypothalamic extracts and vasopressin preparations in several *in vivo* and *in vitro* assay systems, the *in vitro* cell suspension procedures of Portanova and Sayers demonstrated unique dose-response relationships, thereby permitting distinction between these preparations.

More recent evidence from Miller *et al.* (1974) indicates that vasopressin and/or other CRF-like substances from the posterior pituitary are not necessarily involved in the control of ACTH release from the anterior pituitary. These investigators examined the anterior pituitary–adrenal axis in the absence of the posterior pituitary. They found that the axis functioned essentially normally in the absence of the posterior pituitary gland. Although vasopressin or vasopressin-like compounds may stimulate ACTH release, it appears that vasopressin is probably not essential for the stress-induced release of ACTH.

If hypothalamic CRF is not identical to vasopressin of posterior pituitary origin, what then is its nature? Chan *et al.* (1969) reviewed some of the chemical properties of CRF of hypothalamic origin; subsequent reports have been sparse since that time. Observations by Chan *et al.* (1969) indicated that there may be two CRFs in hypothalamic tissue. Acetone precipitation, thin-layer chromatography, and gel filtration produced two areas of CRF activity. The fact that thioglycolate produced only partial inactivation suggested that one of the factors contained sulfide bonds, whereas the second did not.

The conclusion that there are two components of hypothalamic CRF activity has recently been substantiated by Pearlmutter *et al.* (1975). Data from these investigators show that there are high and low molecular weight fractions from rat and bovine hypothalamic stalk median eminence tissue that exhibit CRF activity when assayed *in vitro*. Separation of the two fractions, using a Sephadex–gel column, resulted in the loss of considerable CRF activity. The larger molecular weight fraction alone showed moderate activity, whereas the smaller weight fraction exhibited little activity. Recombination of the two fractions restored the full ACTH-releasing activity. Such findings can help explain previous reports of loss of activity associated with purification and the numerous inconsistencies in reports from different laboratories concerning the characteristics of CRF. There is now hope that the purification necessary for further chemical analysis can proceed, and elucidation of the chemical identity of CRF may be forthcoming.

Recently, a new approach to the study of the chemical nature of CRF has been devised by Jones *et al.* (1976). These investigators found that serotonin selectively stimulated release of CRF from hypothalamic tissue *in vitro* whereas vasopressin was ineffective. These investigators isolated two peptide fractions with CRF activity from the incubation medium of the hypothalamus; one fraction of approximate molecular weight 1000 resembled vasopressin in size, and the other fraction was considerably larger. These authors reported that the fractions were relatively unstable, thereby making identification difficult.

Currently, the most widely held view is that CRF is probably peptidic in nature, as are other well characterized hypothalamic hormones, but that it is distinct from vasopressin. As Saffran and Schally (1977) concluded recently, the majority of observations support the idea that vasopressin does release ACTH. Although the characteristics of the release of ACTH may not be the same as the release caused by other agents, vasopressin may be involved in the acute response to stress. Saffran and Schally (1977) continue to remind us that the original concept of stress, proposed by Hans Selye (1936) and C. N. H. Long (1952), emphasized that multiple mechanisms and agents could bring about the discharge of ACTH in response to stress.

IV. Dynamic Changes in ACTH Secretion

When I first became involved in endocrine research in 1952, ACTH in blood could not easily be measured. It was therefore difficult to study the dynamic changes in ACTH secretion. Before studies on

ACTH regulation could be undertaken, it was necessary to develop a means of quantitating ACTH in the blood.

Since a direct method was not available for determination of ACTH, previous investigators had to resort to indirect indices of ACTH secretion such as adrenal ascorbic acid depletion. However, the depletion of ascorbic acid in the adrenal of intact rats could only indicate that ACTH secretion had occurred, but could not be used to infer the pattern of ACTH secretion, i.e., magnitude or duration of ACTH release. On the other hand, hypophysectomized animals could be used as assay recipients to quantitate ACTH. One method of blood ACTH assay, employed by Sayers and his colleagues, was to inject a quantity of blood (usually limited to 4 ml taken from donor animals at intervals after an experimental stimulus) directly into hypophysectomized rats and then to determine the changes in the adrenal ascorbic acid of the recipient preparation in the absence of an endogenous source of ACTH. This method was limited by the small amounts of ACTH normally present in the blood and the small volume of blood that could be infused into bioassay recipients as a single injection. In fact, the direct injection of blood could detect the elevated blood ACTH levels of adrenalectomized rats, but the level of sensitivity was inadequate to measure ACTH routinely in the blood of intact rats. Other investigators pooled large quantities of blood from groups of rats subjected to the same procedure, then extracted and concentrated the ACTH prior to injection into the hypophysectomized recipient for assay. However, loss, inactivation, or fragmentation into greater units of hormone activity was possible as a consequence of applied chemical procedures. It soon became apparent that investigators who employed different extraction procedures reported results that were not in agreement.

Before I began to investigate the regulation of ACTH secretion , I felt it necessary to develop a method to assay ACTH in blood that would avoid the problems of extraction yet provide for the assay of large volumes of blood in order to detect the minute ACTH concentration in the blood of intact animals. A cross-circulation technique was developed in the rat whereby the blood level of ACTH in its natural state in the circulation could be measured. This method of cross-circulation in the rat permitted accurate control of blood volume transfers between two animals, and the apparatus was designed so that the blood volumes of two rats could be kept in balance while volumes as large as 100 ml were exchanged without detriment to the partners (Brodish and Long, 1956a). By this method, large volumes of blood were assayed for ACTH activity (Fig. 1) (Brodish and Long,

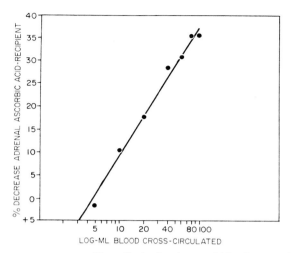

FIG. 1. Dose-response curve. The effect of volume of blood cross-circulated from normal donors on percentage change in adrenal ascorbic acid of hypophysectomized recipients.

1956b). Usually, 20-ml transfers were employed for most physiological studies.

Development of the cross-circulation procedure for the assay of ACTH in blood made it possible to study the dynamics of ACTH secretion in response to stress. The magnitude of the change as well as the duration of the change in ACTH secretion was determined by uniting the stressed animal with a hypophysectomized assay partner at various times after the application of the stress. Variations in the secretion of ACTH by the intact donor rat were reflected by proportional changes in the adrenal ascorbic acid of the hypophysectomized partner. The results of these studies (Fig. 2) demonstrated a transient high rate of ACTH secretion after application of stress, followed by reduced levels of ACTH 3–6 hours later. The decline in ACTH secretion was observed even after the stress of bilateral adrenalectomy, which suggested that elevated adrenocortical hormone levels were not solely responsible for the decline in ACTH release. Additional stress could release additional ACTH during the period of reduced ACTH secretion, which implied that the capacity for release of ACTH was intact but that there was reduced sensitivity. Control ACTH levels were reestablished 24 hours after the stress, whereas hypersecretion of ACTH was evident 2 weeks after removal of both adrenals. We interpreted these results to suggest that there are two phases of ACTH

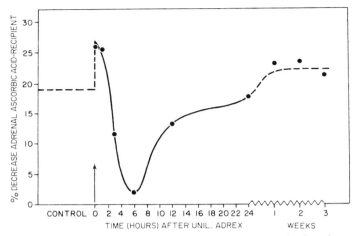

FIG. 2. Blood levels of ACTH at various times after unilateral adrenalectomy (unil. adrex) of normal donor rats. Levels were estimated by the percentage of depletion in the adrenal ascorbic acid of its hypophysectomized recipient partner.

secretion in response to stress—an initial phase of rapid but short-lasting ACTH hypersecretion, probably under neural control, followed by a second phase that develops somewhat more slowly and possibly involves humoral regulation (Brodish and Long, 1956c).

A. The Impact of Radioimmunoassays of ACTH and Cortisol

Prior to the development of radioimmunoassays by Berson and Yalow, investigation into pituitary–adrenal physiology was hampered by lack of suitable methods for measuring most of the hormones of the hypothalamic–pituitary–adrenal system. Only cortisol and its metabolites could be measured easily and reliably. Methods for other hypothalamic–pituitary–adrenal hormones were either nonexistent or too impractical for extensive use. The situation improved greatly with the advent of radioimmunoassay into the field in 1964 when Berson and Yalow published their first paper on a radioimmunoassay for plasma ACTH (Yalow et al., 1964).

Radioimmunoassays have contributed much new and important information that has improved our understanding of pituitary–adrenal physiology. One of the most important contributions of radioimmunoassays has been a better definition of the complexity of circadian rhythms. New information on when cortisol and ACTH are secreted has led to important revisions of formerly accepted concepts of the hypothalamic-pituitary-adrenal circadian rhythm.

Before development of radioimmunoassays for plasma ACTH and cortisol, assays required large volumes of blood, so that measurements had to be carried out at infrequent intervals of 4–6 hours. These infrequent measurements led to the conclusion that cortisol and ACTH blood levels in the resting state changed slowly but continuously in a smooth diurnal pattern that, in man, peaked in the early morning and reached minimal levels at about midnight.

With the increased sensitivity of the radioimmunoassay, much smaller volumes of blood were required and measurements could be made as frequently as every 10 minutes throughout the day. More frequent measurements revealed that past concepts had been oversimplified; instead of a sustained secretory pattern, the adrenal secreted cortisol intermittently in short bursts that lasted for only a few minutes (Berson and Yalow, 1968; Weitzman et al., 1971).

Secretory episodes were observed most frequently during the 6–8 hours of sleep, whereas the fewest secretory episodes occurred in the period 2–4 hours prior to the onset of sleep. Plasma ACTH levels usually paralleled the cortisol levels except that as expected, ACTH preceded cortisol by a few minutes (Graber et al., 1965). This type of secretion has been designated "episodic secretion" to distinguish it from previous measurements of smooth diurnal variation. It is now known that other hormones, in addition to hypothalamic- pituitary-adrenal hormones, are secreted episodically. It has been suggested that a control center or "biological clock" in the hypothalamus or higher brain centers initiates or terminates cortisol secretion by stimulating or suppressing the secretion of CRF by the hypothalamus, which is in turn followed by modification of pituitary ACTH release. The critical question is: What tells the CNS control center when to initiate this process (teleologically because the body needs more cortisol) and what tells it when to stop to avoid overproduction? For years, it was felt that blood cortisol levels served this regulatory function. However, the following observations, notable from studies of episodic secretion, have led to serious doubts that blood cortisol levels alone are involved in the regulation of ACTH secretion.

1. Plasma cortisol levels may fall to extremely low levels for several hours without increase in ACTH release (Berson and Yallow, 1968).
2. ACTH secretion may occur at a time when cortisol levels are in the high normal range (Berson and Yalow, 1968).

3. An essentially normal circadian rhythm for plasma ACTH, at higher than normal levels, persists in adrenal insufficiency despite undetectable cortisol levels (Besser et al., 1970; Smelik, 1970).

4. After adrenalectomy in rats, there is a considerable time lag between the fall in corticosterone and the rise in ACTH (Kendall et al., 1972).

If episodic secretion is independent of blood cortisol concentration, it is possible that cortisol concentration in the central nervous system control center itself might regulate pituitary–adrenal activity. The observation that hypothalamic–pituitary–adrenal activity was inhibited by implantation of corticosteroids in the hypothalamus and that radioactive corticosteroids localized in the hypothalamus and higher brain centers after systemic administration lend some support to this concept (Jubiz et al., 1970).

The possibility that blood cortisol concentration might influence the CNS control center has not been completely ruled out. If the maximum cortisol levels (i.e., peak values for each secretory episode throughout the day) are plotted against time, a reasonably smooth curve is obtained with a maximum during the early morning hours and a minimum at midnight. This curve is somewhat reminiscent of those drawn to illustrate cortisol diurnal variation before the discovery of episodic secretion; it appears to represent the cortisol level that will terminate ACTH secretion at any given time. Since this threshold level is continuously changing along a smooth gradient, this theory has been called the variable setpoint theory.

A similar plot of the minimum cortisol levels for each secretory episode appears to represent the threshold level at which ACTH secretion is initiated. It appears to operate only during the early morning hours, whereas throughout the rest of the day other factors must initiate ACTH release.

When blood cortisol levels were maintained at a level over 7.5 μg/100 ml throughout the day by means of a constant intravenous infusion, ACTH secretion was completely abolished in normal subjects (Krieger, 1970). When plasma cortisol levels were maintained at lower levels, ACTH was secreted in the usual pattern, but in smaller amounts. These findings suggest that there is a threshold blood cortisol level that turns ACTH secretion off. It can also be argued that it is not the level of cortisol in the blood but the level in the CNS control center that is regulating hormone release. In studies of episodic secretion, blood cortisol levels frequently rose to levels much higher than 7.5 μg/100 ml before ACTH secretion was terminated. This observation led to the suggestion that the level of cortisol in the control center must build up to a critical level before ACTH secretion is turned off and that the blood levels may not be the same as the hormone levels in the control center.

There are objections to the "variable setpoint theory":

1. In most normal subjects, the cortisol threshold curves for inhibition and stimulation are fairly continuous and smooth, but the basic pattern is interrupted sporadically by large bursts of secretion for no apparent reason.
2. In some normal subjects, the secretory episodes seem to occur erratically throughout the day with no basic underlying pattern.
3. Within a brief period of time, the levels of cortisol associated with either ACTH suppression or stimulation may fluctuate widely.

To explain these objections, it has been suggested that a variable set point operates to establish a baseline pattern of secretion, but that this baseline pattern can be modified by intervention of the hypothalamus and higher brain centers in response to a variety of stimuli (Krieger, 1970; Krieger et al., 1971).

B. Circadian Rhythm and Feedback Regulation

Rhythmicity in the daily secretory activity of the pituitary gland and the adrenal cortex has been well documented by many investigators. A diurnal rhythm of ACTH in the blood and in the pituitary gland persisted even in adrenalectomized animals (Cheifetz et al., 1969; Hiroshige and Sakakura, 1971). Our laboratory was one of the first to detect CRF activity in the hypothalamus of nonstressed rats and to show a diurnal rhythm in the level of this activity (David-Nelson and Brodish, 1969). As seen in Fig. 3, the CRF activity of the rat hypothalamus gradually increased from the early morning hours to late afternoon and peaked at 3 PM. The peak level of CRF was followed by a precipitous drop of hypothalamic CRF activity at 6 PM, followed by a return to a higher level several hours later. The hypothalamic CRF activity preceded the rise and fall of peripheral corticosterone levels and presumably was responsible for the diurnal rhythms of ACTH and corticosterone.

The rhythms of CRF in the hypothalamus, although not necessarily influenced by negative feedback of corticosterone, could conceivably be modulated by cyclic changes in circulating ACTH levels. Further

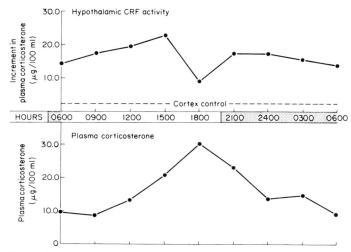

FIG. 3. Diurnal rhythm of hypothalamic corticotropin-releasing factor (CRF) activity (upper curve) and plasma corticosterone (lower curve) in nonstressed male rats during a controlled 24-hour light–dark cycle. The level of stimulation of extracts of cerebral cortex in lesioned recipients is indicated by the dashed line.

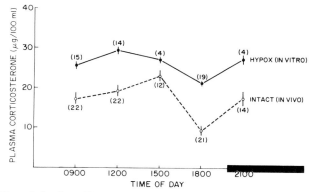

FIG. 4. Diurnal rhythm of hypothalamic corticotropin-releasing factor (CRF) activity in hypophysectomized rats. Each point represents the hypothalamic CRF activity of hypophysectomized donor rats sacrificed at the specified time of day. CRF activity was determined by incubating pituitaries from intact male rats with hypothalamic extract and assaying the ACTH content of the incubation medium by injection into hypophysectomized assay rats. Brackets at each point denote the standard error of the mean; the numbers in parentheses represent the number of hypophysectomized recipients at each point (upper curve). The lower curve shows the rhythm of intact rats that were tested *in vivo* (from Fig. 3).

experiments were therefore carried out in chronically hypophysec-tomized rats to determine whether the rhythm of hypothalamic CRF activity persisted in the virtual absence of feedback from ACTH or adrenal steroids. The results of these experiments, shown in Fig. 4, demonstrate that the previously reported rhythm of hypothalamic CRF activity found in intact and adrenalectomized rats persisted in the absence of hormone feedback from the pituitary gland or the adrenal cortex. The rhythm seen in hypophysectomized rats was similar to that observed in intact rats, which suggests that the rhythm of hypothalamic CRF activity is not caused by the feedback of peripheral hormones, but is an inherent property of the nervous system (Seiden and Brodish, 1972).

V. CRF in Peripheral Blood

Interpretations based upon CRF content of the hypothalamus must be tempered with caution, since the content represents the net effects of synthesis and release. Since hypothalamo-hypophysial portal blood was inaccessible, direct evidence for secretion of releasing factors from the hypothalamus to regulate pituitary hormone release was generally not available. During the course of our experiments on ACTH in blood, we inadvertently obtained evidence for CRF in peripheral blood.

In the cross-circulation technique for ACTH assay, rapid changes in ACTH could not be detected since the cross-circulation itself required at least 10–30 minutes for completion. In order to assess the more rapid changes in ACTH secretion, we developed a modification of a procedure employed by Sayers and his colleagues (Sayers, 1957) in which blood was withdrawn from an intact donor rat and then infused into a hypophysectomized recipient animal. When the two methods of ACTH assay (cross-circulation vs infusion-withdrawal) were compared (Fig. 5), it was found that the cross-circulated animals consistently ex-hibited higher levels of blood ACTH than animals assayed by the infusion-withdrawal technique but otherwise subjected to the same experimental procedure. In the cross-circulation technique, an ex-change of blood occurred between the normal rat and the hypophysec-tomized rat during the assay for blood ACTH, whereas in the infusion-withdrawal method, the normal rat was not exposed to the blood of the hypophysectomized rat. It seemed entirely possible that the

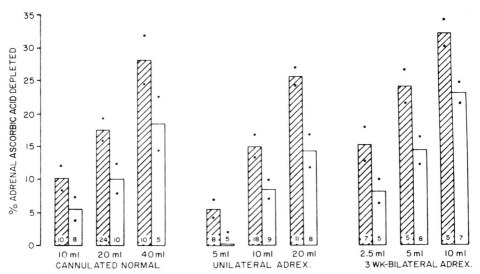

FIG. 5. Blood level of ACTH as indicated by the percentage of depletion of adrenal ascorbic acid in hypophysectomized recipient rats. A cross-circulation method ▨ of ACTH assay is compared with an infusion-withdrawal method ☐ after (a) cannulation of femoral blood vessels 15 minutes earlier; (b) removal of an adrenal 1 hour earlier; (c) removal of both adrenals for 3 weeks. The number of experiments is indicated by numeral at base of each bar; the standard error by dots above each bar. Adrex., adrenalectomized.

elevated blood ACTH levels observed during the cross-circulation might be caused by circulatory transfer of CRF from the hypophysectomized animal to the normal animal. Indeed, an ACTH-releasing substance (CRF) was subsequently demonstrated in the peripheral circulation of rats, and a technique was devised for its detection and quantitation under various experimental conditions (Brodish and Long, 1962).

Previous investigators (Porter and Jones, 1956; Porter and Rumsfeld, 1956, 1959; Schapiro et al., 1956) had reported the presence of ACTH-releasing substances in hypophysial portal blood or in blood draining the brain, but they did not conclusively show that the substance(s) originated in the hypothalamus. Others, particularly Hume and Wittenstein (1950), suggested that a hypothalamic humoral agent could enter the systemic circulation and be carried to the anterior pituitary to release ACTH, but they did not establish the neural origin (i.e., hypothalamus) of this substance. In our studies, the hypothalamic origin of the CRF in the peripheral blood of hypophysectomized rats was clearly indicated when it was shown that the CRF activity disappeared after placement of lesions in the hypothalamus of these animals. Hence, our findings raised serious questions concerning those reports that attempted to "isolate" the pituitary gland from the central nervous system by transplantation to distant sites. It is possible that some of the controversial findings reported by a number of investigators could be explained by the transfer of hypothalamic releasing hormones via the systemic circulation to influence a pituitary transplant at a remote site (Brodish and Long, 1962).

We provided the first definitive experimental evidence of hypothalamic releasing factor activity in the peripheral circulation by demonstration of CRF in the systemic blood of hypophysectomized animals. Since that time other investigators have reported the existence of several other hypothalamic releasing factors in the peripheral circulation of hypophysectomized rats, i.e., luteinizing hormone-releasing factor (LRF) (Nallar and McCann, 1965); follicle hormone-releasing factor (FRF) (Saito *et al.*, 1967; Negro-Vilar *et al.*, 1968); growth hormone-releasing factor (GRF) (Falconi 1966; Müller *et al.*, 1967). The relative inaccessibility of the hypothalamic–hypophysial portal circulation made it difficult to study hypothalamic CRF secretion. Since changes in CRF content of the hypothalamus (commonly employed) were difficult to interpret, we reasoned that studies of CRF in peripheral blood might provide insight into the dynamic responses of hypothalamic neurons as regulators of ACTH secretion.

VI. HYPOTHALAMIC CONTROL CENTER FOR
ACTH RELEASE

Before comprehensive studies of CRF release could be carried out, a suitable test system had to be devised for CRF assay. *In vitro* pituitary incubation assays for CRF were being criticized incessantly for lack of specificity; therefore we were interested in developing an *in vivo* preparation for CRF assay in which relatively large volumes of blood could be assayed. Although a suitable test animal for the study of hypothalamic releasing factors would be an animal with an appropriate hypothalamic lesion that presumably destroyed the nuclei concerned with the synthesis and release of specific releasing factors, neither the extent nor the precise location of these essential hypothalamic structures had been defined, at least for CRF. For ACTH secretion, there was no agreement as to the location of hypothalamic structures essential for ACTH release. Certain investigators reported that lesions in the posterior hypothalamus effectively blocked a stress response, whereas equally prominent investigators reported that lesions placed in the anterior hypothalamus produced the same result. In order to reconcile these controversial reports, and to provide a reliable test animal for CRF assay, we attempted to define precisely the region of the hypothalamus that controls ACTH release from the anterior pituitary gland. To determine the extent of a hypothalamic area that regulates ACTH release, the hypothalamus of the rat was systematically divided into four zones between the optic chiasm and the mammillary bodies (Fig. 6), and the effects on ACTH release of bilateral lesions of the individual zones, as well as on several combinations thereof, were determined. In addition to varying the location of the lesions, the degree of hypothalamic damage was also varied so that the effects of small and large lesions in the same area could be compared. By using a standard animal population and by standardization of the stereotaxic placement techniques in the same laboratory, it was possible to control lesion size and location and therefore make reliable comparisons. Furthermore, the nature of the stress imposed on these animals was essentially the same, so that the stress-induced test for ACTH release was also standardized (Brodish, 1963).

Certain investigators (McCann, 1953; Bouman et al., 1957) had reported that lesions in the anterior or posterior region of the hypothalamus did not impair a pituitary–adrenal response to unilateral adrenalectomy stress until at least 80% of the median eminence was destroyed, whereupon the response to stress was blocked and no adrenal ascorbic acid depletion occurred. In our studies, by using ether as the stimulating agent and plasma corticosterone levels as the

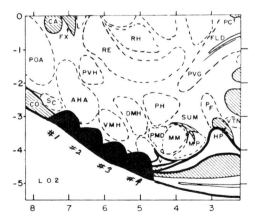

FIG. 6. Sagittal section of rat brain taken from the DeGroot atlas showing four black peaks at the base of the hypothalamus that correspond to lesioned zones 1, 2, 3, and 4, as described in the text.

index of pituitary–adrenal activation, we were able to grade the
response to a given stressful agent. Therefore, the effectiveness of a
particular lesion was evaluated in terms of the percentage of normal
response that remained rather than whether or not a response to
stress was possible. Consequently, as a result of the ability to grade
the response, it was shown (Fig. 7) that a small lesion, placed in any of

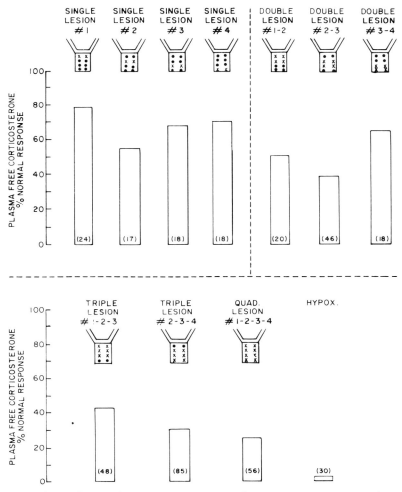

FIG. 7. Plasma free corticosterone response to ether stress, as percentage of normal
controls, in rats with various hypothalamic lesions. The type of lesion is designated by
symbol above each bar, and the number of experiments is indicated by a numeral at
base of each bar. Hypox., hypophysectomy.

the four zones of the hypothalamus, significantly impaired the full expression of a stress-induced response. These findings implied that the entire region of the ventral hypothalamus, extending from the optic chiasm to the mammillary bodies, was involved in ACTH release, albeit the median eminence–tuberal region seemed particularly important. Graded hypothalamic destruction resulted in graded pituitary ACTH response. A small lesion permitted an attenuated corticosterone release in response to stress, whereas a larger lesion resulted in greater attenuation of response. A lesion encompassing the entire ventral hypothalmus produced the greatest deficit with respect to ACTH release and resulted in corticosterone levels that remained essentially at basal control values.

The results of these investigations established that a small, discretely localized, hypothalamic nucleus did not exist for the control of ACTH release. To the contrary, there appears to be a diffuse area at the base of the hypothalamus, extending from the optic chiasm to the mammillary bodies, that influences the secretion of ACTH in response to a variety of stimuli (Brodish, 1963). This study unequivocally resolved the question of precise localization of the control of ACTH secretion in a circumscribed hypothalamic nucleus and was instrumental in dispelling the prevailing concept of compartmentalization of hypothalamic control of anterior pituitary activity. Currently, it is held that there are overlapping areas in the hypothalamus for the regulation of anterior pituitary secretions. These conclusions were affirmed by other investigators who employed stimulation techniques (D'Angelo *et al.*, 1964, for TSH; Redgate *et al.*, 1973, for ACTH).

VII. NATURE OF THE FUNCTIONAL DEFICIT IN RATS WITH HYPOTHALAMIC LESIONS

Further studies on lesioned rats led us to a series of unexpected, but extremely significant, observations. In general, previous studies by other investigators on lesioned or chemically blocked animals, consisted of examinations of stress-induced responses within a 1-hour period. An experimental design, confined to observations within the first hour after application of stress, could detect failure only of rapid responses in effectively lesioned animals but obviously gave no opportunity to detect delayed hormone secretion. In our laboratory, we carried out studies that were intended to evaluate the nature of the impairment in ACTH secretion that followed placement of hypothalamic lesions in rats. The effects of small and large lesions in various regions of the hypothalamus were investigated with respect to the rapidity of stress-induced ACTH release.

A. DELAYED RESPONSE TO STRESS

One of the consequences of a hypothalamic lesion was to delay, rather than to prevent entirely, the ACTH secretory response to stress. The duration of the delay was proportional to size of lesion; small lesions delayed for 1 hour, whereas larger lesions delayed for 2 hours, the increased secretion of ACTH following an appropriate stimulus. As shown in Fig. 8, rats with single bilateral hypothalamic lesions did not show evidence of increased ACTH release in response to unilateral adrenalectomy (i.e., insignificant adrenal ascorbic acid

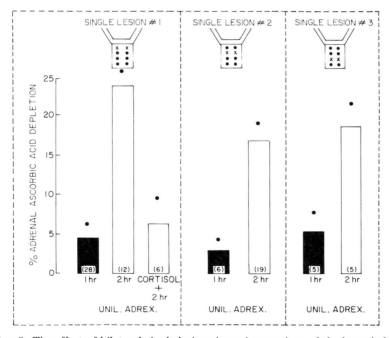

FIG. 8. The effect of bilateral single lesions in various regions of the hypothalamus on ACTH release as judged by adrenal ascorbic acid depletion. The number of experiments is indicated by a numeral at the base of each bar; the standard error of the mean by a dot above each bar. Unit Adrex., unilateral adrenalectomy.

depletion) in the first hour after stress, whereas significant ACTH secretion was evident in the second hour. Similarly, in Fig. 9, multiple bilateral hypothalamic lesions uniformly blocked ACTH release during the first hour after stress and in most instances also during the second hour, but ACTH release nonetheless did occur sometime between the second and fourth hours after onset of the stress. These studies showed that "effective" hypothalamic lesions prevented the usual rapid stress-induced release of ACTH, but they did not prevent a substantial delayed response in which plasma corticosterone concentrations reached levels comparable to those observed in control rats exposed to the same stress (Brodish, 1964a,b).

The delayed response of lesioned animals was unexpected and did not fit the dogma of the time, which assumed that "effective" lesions prevented increased secretion of ACTH in response to stress. Our studies contradicted the prevailing assumption that animals bearing hypothalamic lesions could not further increase ACTH secretion. Although lesioned rats did not release ACTH immediately after

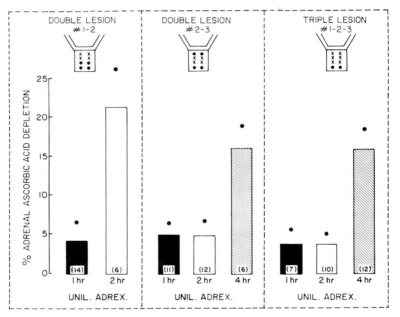

Fig. 9. The effect of multiple lesions in various parts of the hypothalamus on secretion of ACTH after unilateral adrenalectomy (Unil. Adrex.). Adrenal ascorbic acid depletion was determined 1 hour, 2 hours, and 4 hours after onset of the surgical procedure. The number of experiments is indicated by a numeral at the base of each bar; the standard error of the mean by a dot above each bar.

stress, under certain conditions they did show delayed hypersecretion of ACTH and elevated plasma corticosterone concentrations similar to those of intact animals. The delayed hypersecretion of ACTH and corticosterone were not sustained and returned to initial levels 24 hours later (Brodish, 1969). Thus a delayed transient elevation of ACTH was possible despite considerable hypothalamic destruction. It was not until several years later that an explanation was forthcoming to clarify these findings.

B. SENSITIZATION TO STRESS

In the course of experiments in which lesioned rats were used as recipients for CRF bioassay, it became apparent that extracts of either hypothalamic or nonhypothalamic tissue could, under certain conditions, induce ACTH release whereas ether stress alone was without effect. The mechanism of this "breakthrough" was not known. However, the responses to nonhypothalamic tissue extracts were eventually eliminated by avoiding "prior sensitization" of the recipient without at the same time impairing the responses to hypothalamic material. Conditions were therefore developed so that lesioned rats could be used reliably for the assay of CRF in tissue extracts (Witorsch and Brodish, 1972a).

When conditions were established for the reliable use of lesioned rats to assay CRF, it was shown that hypothalamic extracts evoked rapid release of ACTH in rats bearing hypothalamic lesions. ACTH release was elicited from extracts of nonhypothalamic tissue only after lesioned recipients has been stressed ("sensitized") before the injection of the extract. Neither the previous stress itself nor injection of nonhypothalamic extract, when applied separately, were effective in releasing ACTH. On the other hand, hypothalamic extract evoked the release of ACTH in lesioned rats even in the absence of prior stress. Since the recipient animals had extensive hypothalamic lesions that consistently blocked stress-induced ACTH release and the response to nonhypothalamic tissue extract depended upon prior manipulation of the recipient, further experiments investigated whether hypothalamic or extrahypothalamic pathways were involved. Expanded hypothalamic lesions were made that destroyed virtually all the hypothalamus; the response nevertheless persisted, although it was somewhat attenuated. Moreover, removal of all brain tissue anterior to the mesencephalon (pituitary isolation) did not entirely eliminate an evoked increase in plasma corticosterone. The observations of rapid stress-induced increases in plasma corticosterone in rats bearing ventral hypothalamic lesions, expanded hypothalamic lesions, and pituitary islands led us to propose that extrahypothalamic pathways were perhaps responsible for acute ACTH release in these rats (Witorsch and Brodish, 1972b).

VIII. Assays for CRF

At the present time CRF activity is detected and quantitated by means of bioassay. *In vivo* or *in vitro* methods have been used that essentially measure the amount of ACTH released into the peripheral circulation or into the medium, respectively, after administration of extracts containing CRF (Brodish, 1973a).

The ideal *in vivo* CRF assay requires a physiological preparation in which the response to stress has been abolished without altering the functional integrity of the anterior pituitary. Although no single *in vivo* CRF assay is available that fulfills these criteria completely, several attempts have been made to approximate these requirements. Stereotaxic lesions (Brodish, 1963) have been employed, adrenocortical suppression (Vernikos-Danellis, 1964) has been used, and central depressants (Arimura *et al.*, 1967) have been administered for purposes of assaying CRF. Each of these preparations has its merits and limitations in regard to ease of preparation, specificity, sensitivity, and successful utilization.

A. *In Vivo* CRF Assays

Hedge *et al.* (1966) developed an assay for CRF by stereotaxically injecting material directly into the pituitary gland in pharmacologically blocked rats (dexamethasone, pentobarbital, and morphine sulfate). Because of the difficulty in localizing intrapituitary injections by stereotaxic methods, Hiroshige *et al.* (1968) developed a direct intrapituitary microinjection technique in which tissue extracts were administered in 0.5 μl volumes directly into the adenohypophysis, which was exposed parapharyngeally, in a pharmacologically blocked (dexamethasone, chlorpromazine, pentobarbital) rat. These investigators have successfully demonstrated quantitative physiological changes in hypothalamic CRF with this technique (Hiroshige *et al.*, 1969; Hiroshige and Sato, 1970).

Witorsch and Brodish (1972a) systematically analyzed and established the conditions that must be met in order to use the lesioned rat reliably for the assay of CRF in tissue extracts. As shown in Table I, when large ventral hypothalamic lesions were employed, 95% of lesioned rats failed to show a significant elevation in plasma corticosterone after ether stress and thus, by the criteria established previously, were considered to be effectively blocked. It is of interest to note that corticosterone levels after ether stress were not significantly different from prestress levels, but that prestress (resting) corticosterone levels were significantly greater than those observed in hypophysectomized rats.

Most efforts to improve assays for CRF have been designed to enhance sensitivity without appreciable change in specificity and without a means to examine the dose responsiveness of a particular extract preparation. Lymangrover and Brodish (1973a) described a procedure for the multiple use of a lesioned assay preparation that makes it possible for an investigator to evaluate the animal's sensitivity to a standard CRF preparation, its blockade effectiveness or specificity, and its dose responsiveness (slope) after administration of two different doses of an unknown CRF preparation. Lesioned rats are reliable for CRF assays when they are prepared and used appropriately. Twenty-four hours after placement of the lesion, the animals were uniformly unresponsive to a variety of test stimuli, as shown in Fig. 10. Effectively lesioned animals showed a corticosterone response

TABLE I

PLASMA CORTICOSTERONE CONCENTRATIONS IN
SHAM-LESIONED, LESIONED, AND HYPOPHYSECTOMIZED RATS

Type of rat	No. of rats	Procedure	Plasma corticosterone ($\mu g/100$ ml)
Sham-lesioned	15	Ether stress	36.5 ± 1.1[a]
Lesioned			
Unblocked	26	Ether stress	26.6 ± 1.2
Blocked	552	Ether stress	9.8 ± 0.2
Blocked	27	Prestress	8.7 ± 0.8
Hypophysectomized	38	Ether stress	4.3 ± 0.3

[a] Mean $\pm$ standard error.

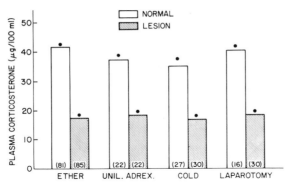

FIG. 10. Plasma corticosterone levels of normal rats and lesioned rats 20 minutes after ether stress, unilateral adrenalectomy (unil. adrex.) stress, cold stress, or laparotomy stress. In this and in Figs. 11–13, the number in parentheses at the base of each bar refers to the number of animals sampled, and the dot above each bar represents the standard error of the mean.

to stress that was generally less that 20 μg per 100 ml of plasma compared to levels of 40 μg or more for normal male rats. Multiple use of the lesioned animals for CRF assay was validated in a study that showed effective maintenance of blockade to ether stress when lesioned animals were tested at 2-hour intervals (Fig. 11). Moreover, the response to median eminence extract was essentially the same when the same dose was administered intravenously at 2-hour intervals (Fig. 12). Finally, randomized sequential injections of median eminence or cerebral cortex or exposure to ether stress (Fig. 13) clearly demonstrated the reliability of the lesioned rat as an assay preparation for CRF when used in the prescribed manner. A linear log-dose response to varying amounts of median eminence extract administration was also demonstrated (Fig. 14) that allowed for CRF quantitation and made it possible to use this preparation to detect changes in CRF levels.

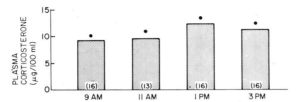

FIG. 11. Plasma corticosterone levels of lesioned rats subjected to ether stress or control intravenous injections of 0.1 N HCl at 2-hour intervals throughout the day. Values are essentially prestress values and indicate persistence of blockade to stress.

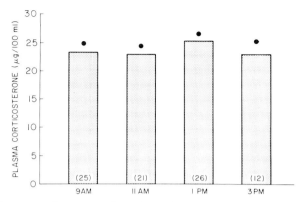

Fig. 12. Plasma corticosterone elevations of lesioned rats to intravenous injections of a pool of median eminence extract at 2-hour intervals throughout the day. Similar responses were obtained at each test period.

B. *In Vitro* CRF Assays

Sayers and his colleagues have employed dispersed pituitary cells for CRF assays and for elucidation of CRF effects on pituitary cells. By use of suspensions of trypsin-dispersed anterior pituitary cells, Portanova *et al.* (1970) showed that extracts of hypothalamic median eminence added to these cells produced increased release of ACTH into the medium in a log-dose relationship to the amount of extract.

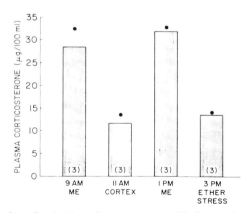

Fig. 13. Effect of randomization of test sequence. Median eminence (ME) extract at 9 A.M. and at 1 P.M. elicited similar corticosterone responses, whereas administration of cerebral cortex extracts at 11 A.M. or exposure to ether stress at 3 P.M. did not produce significant changes in plasma corticosterone.

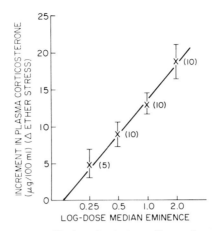

FIG. 14. Log-dose response of lesioned rats to median eminence (ME) extract. On the abscissa is plotted the log-dose of a pool of ME extract, and on the ordinate is plotted the increment in plasma corticosterone (postinjection plasma corticosterone value minus the ether stress plasma corticosterone value obtained 2 hours previously). The numbers in parentheses indicate the number of experiments, and vertical bars represent standard errors of the mean.

Energy dependence (Portanova, 1972; Portanova and Sayers, 1972) was demonstrated, and vasopressin and other neurohypophysial-type peptides stimulated ACTH release in a manner that suggested that they are partial agonists for ACTH secretion (Portanova and Sayers, 1973b). Portanova and Sayers (1972, 1973a) have developed the isolated pituitary cell suspension into a sensitive assay for CRF.

Lowry (1974) subsequently developed the technique of cell-column perfusion so that isolated cells, packed in an inert matrix and continuously perfused with incubation medium, were allowed to recover from the trauma of isolation before any stimulation was started, thereby leading to lower background levels and greater sensitivity. A 4-minute pulse of hypothalamic extract followed by a 4-minute wash was sufficient to obtain adequate stimulation and relaxation profiles when fractions of the effluent were collected and assayed for ACTH. Mulder and Smelik (1975) applied Lowry's column perfusion system to study the dynamics of ACTH release from isolated cells. Short pulses of CRF-containing extract caused bursts of ACTH release from the cells; these bursts were diminished by prior inclusion of corticosterone in the superfusion medium. Similarly, prior treatment of the pituitary donor animals with corticoids *in vivo* also had a profound inhibitory effect on ACTH release *in vitro*.

A further modification of the dispersed cell technique for CRF assay is the use of monolayer cultures of pituitary cells. Fleischer and Rawls (1970) prepared pituitary cell monolayer cultures to quantitate ACTH synthesis, storage, and release and to measure effects of the glucocorticoids dexamethasone and corticosterone on these parameters. They showed that new synthesis of ACTH occurred in monolayer pituitary cell culture and that ACTH secretion can decrease without apparent change in ACTH synthesis, thus dissociation between ACTH synthesis and secretion was demonstrated. Other investigators (Watanabe *et al.*, 1973) have used the cloned mouse pituitary tumor cell line as a model system to study the effects of glucocorticoids on ACTH production. Their results suggest that the response of the neoplastic cells resembles that of normal pituitary cells and support the localization of negative feedback inhibition of ACTH secretion, at least in part, at the level of the pituitary.

Availability of pituitary cells that synthesize and secrete hormones in culture provides a system that allows for long-term studies of hormone regulation and synthesis, in contrast to other *in vitro* models that are hampered by limited viability. By use of monolayer cultures, it is possible to view the cells during the experiments and to correlate the biochemical with the morphological findings. Lang *et al.* (1975) used cyclic AMP and theophylline to stimulate ACTH release in rat pituitary monolayer cultures. Both substances promoted the secretion of ACTH in a dose-dependent fashion, and the authors conclusively demonstrated the synthesis of new hormone by incorporation of labeled amino acids into the hormone during culture. These results presented direct evidence for the ability of rat anterior pituitary cells growing in culture to synthesize ACTH and may become a model system for future studies of the metabolism of ACTH.

Takebe *et al.* (1975) developed a reliable and relatively simple technique for CRF assay that uses cultured rat anterior pituitary cells according to the method of Vale *et al.* (1972) and Tang and Spies (1974). The authors believe that the combined use of pooled cultured anterior pituitary cells and ACTH measurement by radioimmunoassay provides a convenient method for CRF assay that is more accurate and sensitive than most of those previously described, while possessing the general advantages of *in vitro* assays. Graded doses of rat hypothalamic extract were added to dishes that contained dispersed, pooled rat adenohypophysial cells cultured for several days. ACTH secretion into the medium gave a linear log-dose response curve over a 100-fold range between 0.01 and 1 mg of NIH-HE (0.0125–1.25 rat hypothalamus). Forty percent of the maximal ACTH secretion in response to a given dose of hypothalamic extract occurred within 3 minutes of administration. No decrease in intracellular ACTH was observed at any time with any dose of extract, which suggested that secretion was always balanced by production. The same cultured cells could be used in repetitive assays performed on the same or different days. Yasuda *et al.* (1976) applied their technique to study basal and CRF-induced ACTH secretion and intracellular ACTH content in cultured adenohypophysial cells derived from adrenalectomized, dexamethasone-treated, or intact rats. They found that even after 4 days of culture, pituitary cells obtained after adrenalectomy or dexamethasone administration *in vivo* preserved characteristic supra- or infranormal secretion of ACTH.

IX. Hypothalamic and Extrahypothalamic CRF in Peripheral Blood

Although it is well accepted that CRF from the hypothalamus regulates ACTH release, Egdahl in 1960 jolted the neuroendocrine community by demonstrating pituitary–adrenal function in dogs after removal of the entire nervous system rostral to the hindbrain. Egdahl (1960, 1961, 1962) observed elevated levels of adrenal corticosteroids in dogs with "pituitary islands" and also showed that these animals responded to additional stresses, such as inferior vena cava constriction or hemorrhage. Explanations of Egdahl's findings ranged from "pituitary leakage" to removal of an "inhibitory input" from the central nervous system. In any event, Egdahl's findings were unexpected and provocative and did not fit the established concepts of the era.

In our laboratory our research efforts have often challenged the current dogma, and results from our laboratory were, at times, instrumental in revising certain concepts of endocrine control. Appropriate methodology had to be developed to improve existing methods so that valid results could be obtained. For example, by development of a cross-circulation technique, quantitative measurements of changing ACTH levels in individual rats became possible without need for artifact-producing extraction procedures. Demonstration of a diffuse ventral hypothalamic system for ACTH release dispelled the concept of discrete compartmentalization that was in vogue at the time and resolved much of the controversy regarding the effectiveness of lesions placed in different parts of the hypothalamus. Application of the concept of diffuseness permitted the development of a reproducible and effective assay for CRF in lesioned rats. The studies that demonstrated a delayed secretion of ACTH in lesioned rats raised questions concerning the universality of hypothalamic control of ACTH secretion. Questions concerning the "absoluteness" of blockade had to be reconciled and therefore directed attention to other pathways for pituitary ACTH release. Our findings of delayed stress-induced responses in lesioned animals suggested the possible involvement of an extrahypothalamic humoral CRF.

A. Time Course of Response to Hypothalamic CRF

When crude extracts of the median eminence (ME) were injected intravenously into ether-anesthetized lesioned rats, peak elevations of plasma corticosterone were observed 20 minutes later, followed by declining levels thereafter. In Fig. 15, the ordinate is the *increase* in corticosterone levels 20 minutes after injection of extract compared to the preinjection levels after ether stress alone. Extracts of the equivalent of 0.5 ME produced significant increments at 20 minutes with return to control levels at 40 minutes. One ME equivalent produced an even greater elevation in corticosterone at 20 minutes than did 0.5 ME-equivalent and was followed by declining levels that approached control levels at 1 hour. After 2 ME-equivalents, elevations were again observed at 20 minutes and the return to baseline values was slower than with the lower doses. An obvious dose-response relationship was obtained, characterized by peak levels of corticosterone at 20 minutes, irrespective of the dose of ME administered, followed

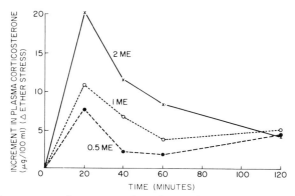

Fig. 15. Time course of response of median eminence (ME) lesioned animals to injection of 0.5, 1, or 2 ME-equivalent extracts.

by more gradual declines to control values with greater amounts of ME extract. Two hours after injection of ME extract, corticosterone levels had essentially returned to control values. It should be emphasized that, after administration of ME extracts that produced considerable elevations in plasma corticosterone, the peak response was always at 20 minutes whereas lower levels of corticosterone were always observed at 60 minutes or later—a characteristic pattern of the response to ME CRF (Lymangrover and Brodish, 1973b; Brodish, 1973b).

B. HYPOTHALAMIC CRF IN BLOOD

Detectable levels of CRF in the peripheral blood of hypophysectomized rats had been reported previously from our laboratory (Brodish and Long, 1962), but quantitation and time-course studies had not been carried out. In an attempt to study the dynamics of CRF secretion from the median eminence, we initiated a series of investigations on ME CRF in peripheral blood.

By means of an infusion–withdrawal procedure (Brodish and Long, 1962), 1 ml of donor blood was infused per minute into a jugular vein of a lesioned recipient rat while an equal volume of recipient blood was withdrawn at a rate of 1 ml per minute from the opposite jugular vein. Blood from various donor types was assayed for CRF in this manner.

When the infusion-withdrawal procedure was used, 8 ml of blood from hypophysectomized donor rats were shown to produce significant increments in plasma corticosterone 20 minutes and 1 hour after infusion into lesioned recipients (Fig. 16), whereas an equivalent volume of blood from lesioned donor animals produced no significant change in the plasma corticosterone of the lesioned recipients. Four milliliters of blood from hypophysectomized donors produced smaller increments, whereas when blood from hypophysectomized rats that had been lesioned was infused, the CRF in the blood was reduced. Presumably then, the CRF in the blood was of hypothalamic origin, and its effect was relatively transient since baseline levels of corticosterone were reestablished at 3 hours.

We have thus characterized the time course of response of lesioned rats to CRF in the blood that presumably originated in the median eminence of the hypothalamus.

At the present time, purified CRF is not available to us. In fact, it is not known what CRF is, since its chemical nature or structure remains uncharacterized. Therefore, we have taken the position that a

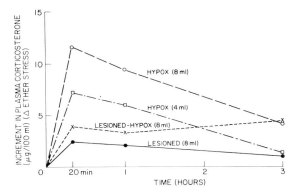

Fɪɢ. 16. Response of lesioned rats to corticotropin-releasing factor (CRF) in blood. Effect of infusion-withdrawal of blood from various donors on the time course of corticosterone responses of lesioned recipients. Failure of blood from lesioned or lesioned and hypophysectomized (Hypox) donors to stimulate ACTH and corticosterone secretion while 4 and 8 ml of blood from hypophysectomized donors elicited significant elevations of plasma corticosterone. Each point represents the mean value of at least six animals.

reasonable approach at this time is to attempt to provide a description of CRF in terms of "what CRF does" by characterization of the time course of the pituitary–adrenal response of lesioned rats to extracts that contain CRF activity. By characterization of the elicited response, we may be in a better position to determine whether one or more physiological CRFs exist.

Encouraged by the similarity of the time course of response to ME CRF in hypothalamic extracts and in blood, and convinced that dose-response quantitation was possible, we were prepared to embark on an intensive study of the dynamics of CRF release. However, we chanced upon a series of unexpected observations that looked both promising and exciting and may indeed prove to be highly significant for our understanding of the regulation of the pituitary–adrenal system.

C. ACTH Release by Extrahypothalamic CRF

It became increasingly apparent to us that, under certain conditions, lesioned rats (with the ventral hypothalamus destroyed) released ACTH in response to stress (Brodish, 1964b; Witorsch and Brodish, 1972b). The stress response of lesioned animals was usually observed several hours after the onset of the stress, but not all stresses elicited a response. Figure 17 shows the response of lesioned

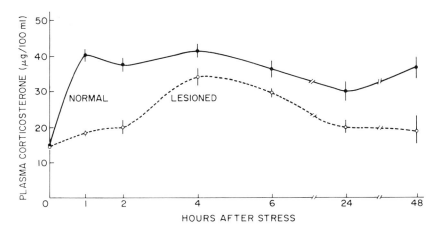

F<small>IG</small>. 17. Plasma corticosterone concentration of normal and lesioned rats after surgical laparotomy. The upper curve shows the rapid and sustained elevation of plasma corticosterone levels in intact animals. The lower curve shows the delay of the stress-induced elevation in lesioned rats, which approached normal levels 4 and 6 hours later. Vertical bars represent standard errors of the mean, and each point is the mean value of 7–31 animals.

rats to the stress of surgical laparotomy. No response was detected at 1 or at 2 hours after the stress, but at 4 and at 6 hours, elevated plasma corticosterone levels were observed. Similar results were obtained following cold stress or unilateral adrenalectomy (Brodish, 1964a).

A delayed response was characterized by the expected absence of an immediate response of lesioned rats to stress, whereas a later (delayed) elevation of plasma corticosterone occurred that approached levels attained in intact rats. We subsequently showed that this phenomenon was pituitary dependent, since it was not observed when the lesioned rat was hypophysectomized shortly after the onset of the stress (Brodish, 1969). Furthermore, the steroid elevation apparently did not represent a change in steroid metabolism, since Porter (1963) also observed a delayed elevation of plasma corticosterone in blood collected directly from the adrenal venous effluent of lesioned rats.

Do all stresses produce a delayed response in rats?

Surgical laparotomy, cold, or unilateral adrenalectomy all have the common characteristic of a prolonged stimulus to the animal. Is this a characteristic that is responsible for a delayed response?

We have investigated this question by subjecting lesioned rats to other types of stress, some of which presumably produce a prolonged stimulation.

The withdrawal and reinfusion of 8 ml of blood at a rate of 1 ml per minute did not result in an elevated plasma corticosterone level in the lesioned recipient 2 or 4 hours later. Therefore the recirculation of blood did not in itself produce a delayed response. Lesioned rats subjected to physical restraint by immobilization on their backs for 1 or 2 hours did not show elevated corticosterone levels 2 or 4 hours after onset of restraint. Therefore, prolonged restraint did not produce a delayed pituitary–adrenal response in lesioned rats. On the other hand, the stress of laparotomy consistently produced considerable corticosterone elevations at 4 or 6 hours after the onset of the stimulus. These results suggested that prolonged stress in itself was not the essential condition for eliciting a delayed response.

X. Tissue CRF

To determine whether a blood-borne factor was involved in the delayed stress response of lesioned rats, the following experiments were carried out.

Lesioned rats that were hypophysectomized and also subjected to the stress of laparotomy served as donor animals 5 hours later. Hypophysectomy was carried out by the transauricular approach (Tanaka, 1955), and laparotomy was performed immediately thereafter. Five hours after the combined stress of hypophysectomy and laparotomy, blood was withdrawn and assayed for CRF activity in recipient lesioned rats. Figure 18 shows the large increments in plasma corticosterone elicited in the lesioned recipients after administration of 2 or 4 ml of blood from laparotomy-stressed lesioned and hypophysectomized donor rats whereas blood from lesioned and hypophysectomized animals not subjected to laparotomy stress had little effect.

A. Time Course of Median Eminence and Tissue CRF

When a comparison was made of the responses of lesioned recipients to CRF of median eminence (ME) origin and to CRF in the blood 5 hours after hypophysectomy and laparotomy stress, several distinguishing features became apparent. In Fig. 19, the solid line shows a typical pattern of response to a large dose of ME extract in which the

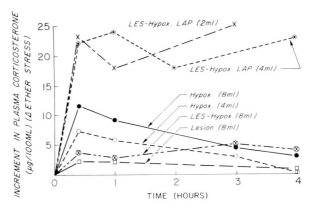

FIG. 18. Time course of response of lesioned recipients to blood from various types of donor animals. Blood from lesioned (LES) or lesioned and hypophysectomized (LES-Hypox.) donors had no detectable corticotropin-releasing factor (CRF) activity, whereas 4 ml or 8 ml of blood from hypophysectomized animals showed dose-related CRF activity that produced peak corticosterone levels at 20 minutes followed by delining levels to preinjection values within 3 hours. Blood, 2 or 4 ml, from lesioned and hypophysectomized rats subjected to laparotomy stress 5 hours earlier had considerable CRF activity that produced maximal peak corticosterone responses at 20 minutes and sustained levels for at least 3–4 hours (at least 6 animals per point). LAP, laparotomy.

maximal corticosterone levels produced at 20 minutes declined to preinjection levels 2 hours later. A similar pattern of response was observed after administration of 8 ml of blood from hypophysectomized donors that presumably contained CRF from the ME (shown by the broken line of the lower curve in Fig. 19). Contrast these curves with those produced by the blood of lesioned rats subjected to hypophysectomy and laparotomy stress 5 hours previously. Relatively small volumes (0.5, 2, and 4 ml) produced significant immediate and prolonged elevations in plasma corticosterone. The high potency of this CRF suggested to us that it was not of hypothalamic origin, and the term "tissue CRF" was coined to distinguish it from ME CRF of the hypothalamus (Lymangrover and Brodish, 1973b).

The action of tissue CRF was pituitary dependent since it had no effect on hypophysectomized recipients (Lymangrover and Brodish, 1973b). By means of direct pituitary microinjection, it was shown that tissue CRF acted directly on the pituitary gland to release ACTH. Therefore, tissue CRF seemed to have all the characteristics that we usually attribute to a releasing factor or hormone (Lymangrover and Brodish, 1973b).

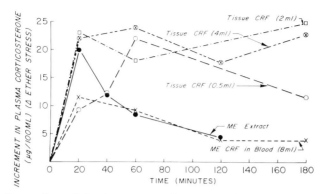

FIG. 19. Comparison of the time courses of response of lesioned recipients to median eminence (ME) extract, ME CRF in blood, and to varying volumes of blood containing tissue CRF. ME extract and ME CRF in blood produced the same time course of response illustrated by peak increments of plasma corticosterone at 20 minutes followed by declines to previous basal levels at 2 hours. In contrast, 2 or 4 ml of blood containing tissue CRF produced comparable peak corticosterone responses at 20 minutes that were sustained for at least a 3-hour period. With 0.5 ml of blood containing tissue CRF, submaximal corticosterone levels were elicited at 20 minutes, whereas maximal levels were attained at 1 hour and appeared to be declining at 3 hours, although they were still significantly elevated.

B. REGULATION OF TISSUE CRF ACTIVITY

Is the delayed response brought about by tissue CRF a physiological phenomenon of some utility to the organism? We have investigated this question by determining whether the delayed response was subject to modification or regulation (Lymangrover and Brodish, 1974).

When lesioned rats were subjected to laparotomy stress, an immediate release of ACTH was not induced and plasma corticosterone levels had not changed significantly in the blood samples obtained 20 minutes after the stress (Fig. 20). However, the lesioned animals did show the characteristic steroid elevations 4 and 6 hours later (solid line, Fig. 20). When 20 mU of ACTH were administered subcutaneously in divided doses 30 minutes apart (10 mU immediately after laparotomy and 10 mU 30 minutes later), plasma corticosterone levels were increased in the physiological range at 20 minutes whereas at 2 hours the values had returned to preinjection levels. Significantly, however, suppression of the delayed response to the laparotomy stress was observed 4 and 6 hours later (shown by the dashed line in Fig. 20).

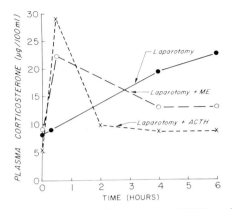

F IG. 20. Effect of median eminence (ME) extract or ACTH on the delayed response of lesioned rats to laparotomy stress. Laparotomy alone (●) did not elicit a rapid 20-minute corticosterone response but did produce a delayed response 4–6 hours later. Administration of ME extract (○) or ACTH (X) immediately after laparotomy stress suppressed the delayed corticosterone elevation 4–6 hours later (5–7 animals per point).

These results demonstrated that the delayed response was suppressed by prior pituitary–adrenal activation; hence it is not unreasonable to speculate that the appearance or absence of a delayed response may depend upon prior activity of the pituitary–adrenal system in response to certain kinds of stress.

C. SUPPRESSION OF TISSUE CRF

Suppression of the delayed response by ME extract or ACTH could have been brought about by direct suppression of the pituitary gland itself (making it unresponsive to tissue CRF) or by inhibition of the release of the tissue CRF.

To determine the manner of suppression, lesioned and hypophysectomized donor rats were subjected to laparotomy stress, and 5 hours later 4-ml blood samples were withdrawn rapidly from the abdominal aorta and assayed for CRF activity in lesioned recipient rats by means of the infusion-withdrawal procedure. As shown by the solid line in Fig. 21, a rapid increase in corticosterone was observed in the lesioned animal after it had received the 4 ml of donor blood, a characteristic CRF effect. A significant elevation in plasma corticosterone was elicited 20 minutes after the infusion, and, of interest, there was a sustained steroid elevation 1 hour later. Other lesioned and hypophysectomized donor rats were subjected to laparotomy stress, but in

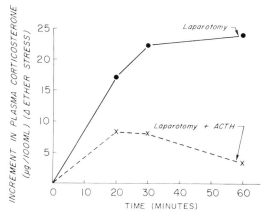

FIG. 21. Suppression of tissue corticotropin-releasing factor (CRF) by ACTH. Time course of response of lesioned recipients to 4 ml of blood from lesioned and hypophysectomized donor rats subjected to laparotomy stress 5 hours earlier. Blood from donor rats subjected to laparotomy stress (●—●) had considerable tissue CRF activity, whereas blood from donor rats subjected to laparotomy stress and also injected with ACTH (X—X) showed significantly reduced levels of tissue CRF (at least 6 animals per point).

addition were also injected with 30 mU of ACTH subcutaneously (in three divided doses of 10 mU each, given 30 minutes apart). Five hours after laparotomy, they were likewise sampled for CRF activity. As shown by the dashed line in Fig. 21, blood from the ACTH-treated donors had relatively little CRF activity in comparison to the untreated group, which suggests significant reduction of tissue CRF by prior administration of ACTH. The ACTH injections decreased the amount of tissue CRF in the blood. These results therefore suggest that the suppression of the delayed response with ME extract or ACTH was caused by reduction of tissue CRF release rather than by an impairment of its action on the pituitary gland itself.

The demonstration that tissue CRF in blood was significantly decreased by prior ACTH administration suggests that increased pituitary–adrenal activity may suppress tissue CRF, and, conversely, increased tissue CRF release may result when pituitary–adrenal activity is inadequate.

D. SIGNIFICANCE OF TISSUE CRF

Corticotropin-releasing factor in the blood of hypophysectomized rats showed a time course of response (i.e., corticosterone elevation) similar to that observed after administration of hypothalamic extract

(ME CRF). Therefore, it was reasonable to conclude that the CRF in the blood of hypophysectomized rats represented CRF released from the median eminence of the hypothalamus. On the other hand, when lesioned animals were subjected to laparotomy stress and hypophysectomy, and 5 hours later had blood withdrawn for CRF assay, it was found that the delayed response (i.e., elevated corticosterone levels) was caused by a potent CRF that produced an action that was distinctive compared to the effects normally observed with median eminence CRF (ME CRF). On the basis of its extreme potency and unique time course of action, it is probable that "tissue CRF" is different from ME CRF of hypothalamic origin.

Tissue CRF has been distinguished from CRF of median eminence origin on the basis of its relative instability (compared to ME CRF), its extreme potency, its prolonged action on the pituitary–adrenal system, and its persistence even after the entire hypothalamus has been removed. Recent reports from our laboratory clearly demonstrate a humoral factor in the peripheral blood of stressed rats that can activate the pituitary–adrenal axis and result in a massive and prolonged secretion of corticosterone. Because the substance appeared in animals with extensive ventral hypothalamic lesions that were also hypophysectomized 5 hours earlier, it seems unlikely that this potent pituitary–adrenal activation was evoked by ME CRF.

Nonhypothalamic CRF (tissue CRF) seems to stimulate the pituitary–adrenal system in a sufficiently unique manner to suggest that it is not identical to hypothalamic ME CRF. "Tissue CRF" characterizes the nonhypothalamic humoral substance that can directly stimulate the secretion of ACTH. There are a number of reasons why such terminology is suggested. This substance is probably not of hypothalamic origin; therefore it is not unreasonable to assume that it is released from a more peripheral site in response to stress. Our studies as well as those of other investigators suggest that the types of stress that presumably activate an extrahypothalamic mechanism are extensive surgery, caval constriction, laparotomy, prolonged cold exposure, and high altitude; all seem to produce, in common, tissue anoxia or tissue destruction, or both. We have postulated that intense and prolonged stress, which results in tissue damage, may evoke the release of tissue CRF to supplement the rapid ME CRF mechanism and thereby produce a prolonged output of adrenal cortical steroids in time of need.

What is the possible physiological role of tissue CRF? Transient secretion of ACTH, presumably by hypothalamic activation, may be an appropriately rapid response to acute stress. The subsequent feedback suppression of the hypothalamic–pituitary system by the secreted hormones may be a means of preventing overstimulation and excessive secretion of the system.

In cases of severe trauma associated with extensive tissue damage, hypothalamic–pituitary suppression by the secreted hormones may be premature and inappropriate. Therefore a mechanism may exist whereby the affected tissues themselves can sustain adrenocortical activation by releasing tissue CRF as a signal to the pituitary for continued need. Tissue CRF release would represent a valuable mechanism for damaged tissues to sustain the signals for the hormones or metabolites that are needed. When the tissue damage has been repaired or stabilized, then tissue CRF release would cease.

One can further speculate that the mechanism whereby corticosterone suppresses tissue CRF secretion is similar to the membrane stabilization theory proposed by Weissman and Thomas (1964). If tissue CRF is a common factor that is found in all tissues and is released as a result of tissue destruction, then the suppression could be mediated through corticosterone acting at the cell membrane of lysosomes to stabilize the cellular lysosomes and prevent the release of enzymes that could disrupt the cell and release tissue CRF. Further clarification must await purification of tissue CRF and studies of its secretory process.

The significance of this new finding is that it suggests that tissue CRF is under physiological regulation and thus may play a role in the ability of an organism to adapt to its environment. The tissue CRF system may be related to a fundamental mechanism for the control of ACTH secretion. Normally, a transient response to stress is observed, which, if sufficient, may be terminated by neural adaptive mechanisms that prevent overstimulation and oversecretion of the pituitary–adrenal system. During continued stress of relatively high intensity, the needs of the organism may not be met by the hypothalmic (ME CRF) mechanism and another system (tissue CRF) may be brought into play to sustain pituitary–adrenal secretions. Although the tissue CRF hypothesis may be viewed as somewhat radical with respect to previous concepts, it is of such potential significance in our understanding of pituitary–adrenal regulation that confirmation in other laboratories is eagerly awaited. CRF production at extraneural sites may indeed be a mechanism for proper adjustments to prolonged or chronic alterations that are generally referred to as adaptations to stress.

REFERENCES

Andersson, K. E., Arner, B., Hedner, P., and Mulder, J. L. (1972). *Acta Endocrinol. (Copenhagen)* **69**, 640.

Arimura, A., Saito, T., and Schally, A. V. (1967). *Endocrinology* **81**, 235.

Arimura, A., Schally, A. V., and Bowers, C. Y. (1969). *Endocrinology* **84**, 579.

Berson, S. A., and Yalow, R. S. (1968). *J. Clin. Invest.* **47**, 2725.

Besser, G. M., Cullen, D. R., Irvine, W. J., Ratcliffe, J. G., and Landon, J. (1970). *Br. Med. J.* **1**, 374.

Bouman, P. R., Gaarenstroom, J. H., Smelik, P. G., and De Wied, D. (1957). *Acta Physiol. Pharmacol. Neer.* **6**, 368.

Brodish, A. (1963). *Endocrinology* **73**, 727.

Brodish, A. (1964a). *Endocrinology* **74**, 28.

Brodish, A. (1964b). *In* "Major Problems in Neuroendocrinology" (E. Bajusz and G. Jasmin, eds.), p. 177. Karger, Basel.

Brodish, A. (1969). *Neuroendocrinology* **5**, 33.

Brodish, A. (1973a). *In* "Methods in Investigative and Diagnostic Endocrinology" (S. A. Berson and R. S. Yalow, eds.), p. 391. North Holland Publ., Amsterdam.

Brodish, A. (1973b). *In* "Brain-Pituitary-Adrenal Interrelationship (A. Brodish and E. S. Redgate, eds.), p. 177. Karger, Basel.

Brodish, A., and Long, C. N. H. (1956a). *Yale J. Biol. Med.* **28**, 644.

Brodish, A., and Long, C. N. H. (1956b). *Yale J. Biol. Med.* **28**, 650.

Brodish, A., and Long, C. N. H. (1956c). *Endocrinology* **59**, 666.

Brodish, A., and Long, C. N. H. (1962). *Endocrinology* **71**, 298.

Chan, L. J., De Wied, D., and Saffran, M. (1969). *Endocrinology* **84**, 967.

Chan, L. T., Schaal, S. M., and Saffran, M. (1970). *In* "Hypophysiotropic Hormones of the Hypothalamus" (J. Meites, ed.), p. 253. Williams & Wilkins, Baltimore, Maryland.

Cheifetz, P. N., Gaffud, N. T., and Dingman, J. F. (1969). *J. Endocrinol.* **43**, 521.

D'Angelo, S. A., Snyder, J., and Grodin, J. M. (1964). *Endocrinology* **75**, 417.

David-Nelson, M. A., and Brodish, A. (1969). *Endocrinology* **85**, 861.

Egdahl, R. H. (1960). *Endocrinology* **66**, 200.

Egdahl, R. H. (1961). *Endocrinology* **68**, 226.

Egdahl, R. H. (1962). *Endocrinology* **71**, 926.

Falconi, G. (1966). *Experientia* **22**, 333.

Fleischer, N., and Rawls, W. E. (1970). *Am. J. Physiol.* **219**, 445.

Graber, A. L., Givens, J. R., Nicholson, W. E., Island, D. P., and Liddle, G. W. (1965). *J. Clin. Endocrinol. Metab.* **25**, 804.

Guillemin, R., and Rosenberg, B. (1955). *Endocrinology* **57**, 599.

Guillemin, R., Hearn, W. R., Cheek, W. R, and Householder, D. F. (1957). *Endocrinology* **60**, 488.

Harris, G. W. (1948). *Physiol. Rev.* **28**, 139.

Hedge, G. A., Yates, M. B., Marcus, R., and Yates, F. E. (1966). *Endocrinology* **70**, 328.

Hiroshige, T., and Sakakura, M. (1971). *Neuroendocrinology* **7**, 25.

Hiroshige, T., and Sato, T. (1970). *Endocrinol. Jpn.* **17**, 1.

Hiroshige, T., Kunita, H., Yoshimura, K., and Itoh, S. (1968). *Jpn. J. Physiol.* **18**, 179.

Hiroshige, T., Sato, T., Ohta, R., and Itoh, S. (1969). *Jpn. J. Physiol.* **19**, 866.

Hume, D. M., and Wittenstein, G. J. (1950). *In* "Proceedings of the First Clinical ACTH Conference" (J. R. Mote, ed.), p. 134. McGraw-Hill (Blakiston), New York.

Jones, M. T., Hillhouse, E. W., and Burden, J. (1976). *In* "Frontiers in Neuroendocrinology" (W. F. Ganong and L. Martini, eds.), p. 195. Raven, New York.

Jubiz, W., Matsukura, S., Meikle, A. W., Harada, G., West, C. D., and Tyler, F. H. (1970). *Arch. Intern. Med.* **125**, 468.

Kendall, J. W., Jacobs, J. J., and Kramer, R. M. (1972). In "Brain-Endocrine Interaction. Median Eminence Structure and Function" *(Int. Symp. Munich, 1971)*, p. 342. Karger, Basel.

Krieger, D. T. (1970). *Trans. N. Y. Acad. Sci.* **32**, 316.

Krieger, D. T., Allen, W., Rizzo, F., and Krieger, H. P. (1971). *J. Clin. Endocrinol.* **32**, 266.

Lang, R. E., Hilwig, I., Voigt, K. H., Fehm, H. L., and Pfeiffer, E. F. (1975). *Acta Endocrinol.* **79**, 421.

Long, C. N. H. (1952). *Recent Prog. Horm. Res.* **7**, 75.

Lowry, P. J. (1974). *J. Endocrinol.* **62**, 163.

Lymangrover, J. R., and Brodish, A. (1973a). *Neuroendocrinology* **12**, 98.

Lymangrover, J. R., and Brodish, A. (1973b). *Neuroendocrinology* **12**, 225.

Lymangrover, J. R., and Brodish, A. (1974). *Neuroendocrinology* **13**, 234.

McCann, S. M. (1953). *Am. J. Physiol.* **175**, 13.

McCann, S. M. (1957). *Endocrinology* **60**, 664.

McDonald, R. K., Wagner, E. N., and Weise, V. K. (1957). *Proc. Soc. Exp. Biol. Med.* **96**, 652.

McEwen, B. S., Weiss, J. M., and Schwartz, L. S. (1970). *Brain Res.* **17**, 471.

Mangili, G., Motta, M., and Martini, L. (1966). In "Neuroendocrinology" (L. Martini and W. F. Ganong, eds.), Vol. 1, p. 297. Academic Press, New York.

Martini, L., and Morpurgo, C. (1955). *Nature (London)* **175**, 1127.

Miller, R. E., Yueh-Chien, H., Wiley, M., and Hewitt, R. (1974). *Neuroendocrinology* **14**, 233.

Mulder, G. H., and Smelik, P. G. (1975). *Acta Endocrinol. (Copenhagen) Suppl.* **199**, 207.

Müller, E. E., Arimura, A., Saito, T., and Schally, A. V. (1967). *Endocrinology* **80**, 77.

Nallar, R., and McCann, S. M. (1965). *Endocrinology* **76**, 27.

Negro-Vilar, A., Dickerman, E., and Meites, J. (1968). *Endocrinology* **82**, 939.

Pearlmutter, A. F., Rapino, E., and Saffran, M. (1975). *Endocrinology* **97**, 1336.

Portanova, R. (1972). *Proc. Soc. Exp. Biol. Med.* **140**, 825.

Portanova, R., and Sayers, G. (1972). In "Brain–Pituitary–Adrenal Interrelationships" (A. Brodish and E. S. Redgate, eds.), p. 319. Karger, Basel.

Portanova, R., and Sayers, G. (1973a). *Neuroendocrinology* **12**, 236.

Portanova, R., and Sayers, G. (1973b). *Proc. Soc. Exp. Biol. Med.* **143**, 661.

Portanova, R., Smith, K. K., and Sayers, G. (1970). *Proc. Soc. Exp. Biol. Med.* **133**, 573.

Porter, J. C. (1963). *Am. J. Physiol.* **204**, 715.

Porter, J. C., and Jones, J. C. (1956). *Endocrinology* **58**, 62.

Porter, J. C., and Rumsfeld, H. W., Jr. (1956). *Endocrinology* **58**, 359.

Porter, J. C., and Rumsfeld, H. W., Jr. (1959). *Endocrinology* **64**, 948.

Redgate, E. S., Fahringer, E. E., and Szechtman, H. (1973). In Brain–Pituitary–Adrenal Interrelationships" (A. Brodish and E. S. Redgate, eds.), p. 152. Karger, Basel.

Royce, P. C., and Sayers, G. (1958). *Proc. Soc. Exp. Biol. Med.* **98**, 677.

Saffran, M., and Schally, A. V. (1955). *Can. J. Biochem.* **33**, 408.

Saffran, M., and Schally, A. V. (1977). *Neuroendocrinology* **24**, 359.

Saito, T., Sawano, S., Arimura, A., and Schally, A. V. (1967). *Endocrinology* **81**, 1226.

Sayers, G. (1957). *Ciba Found. Colloq. Endocrinol. (Proc.)* **11**, 138.

Schally, A. V., and Bowers, C. Y. (1964). *Metabolism* **13**, 1190.

Schally, A. V., Anderson, R. N., Lipscomb, H. S., Long, J. M., and Guillemin, R. (1960). *Nature (London)* **188**, 1192.

Schapiro, S., Marmorston, J., and Sobel, H. (1956). *Proc. Soc. Exp. Biol. Med.* **91**, 382.

Seiden, G., and Brodish, A. (1972). *Endocrinology,* **90**, 1401.

Selye, H. (1936). *Nature (London)* **138**, 32.

Smelik, P. G. (1970). *Prog. Brain Res.* **32**, 20.

Sobel, H., Levy, R. S., Marmorston, J., Schapiro, S., and Rosenfield, S. (1955). *Proc. Soc. Exp. Biol. Med.* **89**, 10.

Takebe, K., Yasuda, N., and Greer, M. A. (1975). *Endocrinology* **97**, 1248.

Tanaka, A. (1955). *Shionogi Kenkyusho Nempo* **5**, 678.

Tang, L. K. L., and Spies, H. G. (1974). *Endocrinology* **94**, 1016.

Vale, W., Grant, G., Amoss, M., Blackwell, R., and Guillemin, R. (1972). *Endocrinology* **91**, 562.

Vernikos-Danellis, J. (1964). *Endocrinology* **75**, 514.

Watanabe, H., Nicholson, W. E., and Orth, D. N. (1973). *Endocrinology* **93**, 411.

Weissman, G., and Thomas, L. (1964). *Recent Prog. Horm. Res.* **20**, 215.

Weitzman, E. D., Fukushima, D., Nogeire, C., Roffwarg, H., Gallagher, T. F., and Hellman, L. (1971). *J. Clin. Endocrinol. Metab.* **33**, 14.

Witorsch, R. J., and Brodish, A. (1972a). *Endocrinology* **90**, 552.

Witorsch, R. J., and Brodish, A. (1972b). *Endocrinology* **90**, 1160.

Yalow, R. S., Glick, S. M., Roth, J., and Berson, S. A. (1964). *J. Clin. Endocrinol. Metab.* **24**, 1219.

Yasuda, N., Takebe, K., and Greer, M. A. (1976). *Endocrinology* **98**, 717.

Modulation of Memory by Pituitary Hormones and Related Peptides

HENK RIGTER AND JOHN C. CRABBE

CNS Pharmacology Department, Scientific Development Group, Organon, Oss, The Netherlands

I. General Introduction	154
II. Memory Processes	154
A. Aspects of Processing	154
B. Some Paradigms for Assessment of Memory	158
III. Effects of Peptides on Memory—Introduction	162
IV. Amelioration of Behavioral Deficits	165
A. Hypophysectomy	165
B. Selective Ablation of the Anterior and Posterior Lobes of the Pituitary	170
C. Hereditary Diabetes Insipidus	176
D. Old Animals	179
E. Experimental Amnesia	181
F. Summary	181
V. Effects in Normal Animals	182
A. Treatments Administered after Training	182
B. Treatments Administered before Testing for Retention	190
C. Summary of Effects in Normal Animals	196
VI. Effects on Experimental Amnesia	196
A. Introduction	196
B. Prevention of Amnesia	197
C. Reversal of Amnesia	200
D. Summary of Effects on Amnesia	202
VII. The Endorphins: A New Field of Research	202
A. Introduction	202
B. Interactions between Endorphins and ACTH and Vasopressin	203
C. Possible Effects of Opioids on Memory	207
VIII. Peptides and Memory Processes: Human Data	210
A. Introduction	210
B. Studies in Normal Subjects	211
C. Studies in Cognitively Impaired Subjects	215
D. Summary of Peptide Effects in Humans	218
IX. Possible Sites and Mechanisms of Actions	219
A. Neuroanatomy	219
B. Neurophysiology	225
C. Neurochemistry	227
X. Concluding Comments	231
References	233

153

I. General Introduction

To state that the endocrine system is intimately involved in adaptive processes is tautological: indeed, the principal function of the endocrine system would seem to be to maintain important homeostases. For the most part, the early history of endocrinological research examined peripheral physiological functions. More recently, greater recognition of the interrelationships between endocrine responses and behavioral systems has led to interesting research, some of which is reviewed in this chapter. The interest in hormonal involvement in memory processes may, in one sense, be traced to the work of Selye on analysis of the stress response. The recognition that endocrine mechanisms are involved in the ability of an organism to adapt to a stressful change in its environment, and that experimental manipulation of endocrine balance could prevent it from so doing, led to the hypothesis that related adaptational mechanisms might come into play during learning. Certainly, for a laboratory animal, stress is an inevitable concomitant of most assessments of learning.

We do not, in this review, discuss in detail the seminal lines of research. One such line has provided ample evidence that, during the course of learning and memory, changes in pituitary–adrenal activity occur (Lissák and Endröczi, 1965; Brush and Levine, 1966; Wertheim et al., 1969; Levine and Levin, 1970; Van Delft, 1970). Other studies have demonstrated that an intact pituitary–adrenal system may aid the performance of animals in a variety of behavioral tests and that manipulations of pituitary–adrenal activity may interfere with behavioral performance (Mirsky et al., 1953; Levine, 1968; De Wied, 1969; Levine and Levin, 1970; Brush and Froelich, 1975). From these studies, the idea arose that hormones may have a role in memory processes. Experiments designed specifically to test this hypothesis are the main subject of the present review.

II. Memory Processes

A. Aspects of Processing

1. Analysis of Memory

The phenomenon of memory can be differentiated into a number of conceptual classifications according to various schemata (Klatzky, 1975; Gold and McGaugh, 1975). To provide a basis for discussion of the relation between hormones and memory, we may assume that memory processing involves at least four steps: (a) selection of some stimuli from the perceptual environment; (b) consolidation or storage into memory by some little-understood neurobiological mechanisms; (c) decay, or the eventual forgetting of information; and (d) retrieval (or recall) of stored information by an equally ill-understood neurobiological mechanism. A key assumption in this conceptual scheme is that a burgeoning memory "trace" is labile.

There are essentially two theoretical schools regarding the neurobiological basis for memory storage relevant for this review. Classical "consolidation theory" suggests that there are two independent sequentially organized storage mechanisms—short-term and long-term memory. Entry of information into short-term memory is followed by consolidation, or transfer, into long-term memory (Hebb, 1949; Glickman, 1961; McGaugh and Dawson, 1971). The lability of memory from this viewpoint means that interference with or facilitation of either short-term memory or consolidation can alter the strength of the memory trace stored in long-term memory. A recently proposed alternative theory holds that the initiation of a memory activates a single process that will decay rapidly (like short-term memory) unless some other process, not strictly memorial, arrests decay of the memory trace (Gold and McGaugh, 1975). The influence of treatments given at about the time of learning on eventual memory strength is assumed to be mediated through effects on the modulatory process. In the absence of externally applied treatments, such a modulatory process must be activated quickly after an experience in order to strengthen the initiated memory trace. The rapid action of hormones and their intimate association with central nervous system arousal make them clear candidates for such a modulatory role.

For our purposes here, the validation of one or the other of these theories is not essential. The experimental literature can generally be explained by either theory. Rather, we will analyze memory processing by describing essentially two aspects, storage and retrieval. Such a distinction is sound logically; practically, it is impossible to assess the strength of a stored memory without first retrieving it from storage. However, experimental designs may be employed that allow specific inferences about the adequacy of storage or retrieval. These designs exploit a corollary feature of memory lability, that it is time-dependent. To demonstrate how time-dependent features may be exploited, we turn to some specific samples.

2. Effects of Treatments on Memory Storage

Until 1961, most studies of the effects of a treatment on memory processes followed the paradigm of applying the treatment each day before training the animal. Thus, for example, Karl Lashley demonstrated (in 1917) that daily administration of low doses of strychnine or caffeine to rats could enhance the acquisition of a complex maze. However, as McGaugh pointed out in 1961, the effects of such a schedule of drug administration cannot be specifically ascribed to an effect on memory. Strychnine might, for example, have simply aroused Lashley's rats, made them more attentive to the relevant cues of the problem or more highly motivated.

A methodological improvement introduced by McGaugh (1961) was to administer treatments *after* training but still long before testing for retention. A drug given after training cannot logically be affecting such processes as attention, arousal, and motivation and must be assumed to be acting directly on some aspect of memory storage. A variety of treatments applied after training have been shown to facilitate memory storage (McGaugh and Petrinovich, 1965; McGaugh and Herz, 1972).

Duncan (1949) placed rats in a box and trained them to run to an adjoining chamber to avoid shock. In such a one-way avoidance problem, an animal's retention is measured by the latency of its run into the "safe" compartment on subsequent trials. Long entrance latencies on subsequent trials are assumed to reflect good memory for the shock. They may also reflect nonspecific fear, or general over- or underarousal. Appropriate control groups can be employed to strengthen the interpretation of latency differences as being owed to memory. At different intervals after the daily training trial, an electroconvulsive shock (ECS) was administered. If the ECS followed the trial within 1 hour, a graded loss of the avoidance response was exhibited, presumed to represent amnesia for the response. The strength of amnesia was dependent upon the training-ECS interval. ECS administered more then 1 hour after trial produced no retrograde amnesia and, therefore, presumably it no longer impaired memory storage. A variety of agents can similarly produce retrograde amnesia when administered shortly after training.

Both retrograde amnesia and posttraining facilitation of memory exhibit time-dependence. That is, the longer after training a treatment is given, the less effective it becomes (Duncan, 1949; Cherkin, 1969; McGaugh and Herz, 1972). The demonstration of such a posttrial time gradient strengthens in two ways the interpretation that there has been an effect on memory storage processes. First, the lability of memory storage, whether caused by consolidation of short-term to long-term memory or by the tonic modulation of a single storage mechanism, would logically be expected to decline the further in time from the initiation of the memory trace. Second, if treatment is effective when given immediately but not, for example, 4 hours after treatment, it is difficult to ascribe its efficacy to nonspecific effects that are carried over to later retention tests.

3. *Isolation of Effects on Storage and Retrieval*

Similar procedural manipulations may be employed to differentiate the effects of a drug on storage and retrieval. For example, when mice are given intracerebral puromycin shortly after training, their later performance is impaired (Flexner and Flexner, 1968). Such impairment could represent amnesia for the response. It could also, however, be caused by a failure to retrieve an adequately stored memory. Such an amnesia may be reversed at a later time by intracerebral injections of saline (Flexner and Flexner, 1968). Since one action of puromycin is to form abnormal peptides that are hypothesized to interfere with synaptic transmission by physically clogging the synaptic cleft, saline injection could simply have "flushed" the synapse and restored memory by restoring the retrieval process (Roberts *et al.*, 1970). If memory storage were blocked, such a block by definition should be irreversible. Puromycin, therefore, would seem to block the retrieval of information stored in memory.

On the other hand, cycloheximide, acetoxycycloheximide, actinomycin D, and anisomycin are protein synthesis inhibitors that may block the storage of memory entirely. While high doses of *d*-amphetamine, if not unduly delayed, can protect the forming memory trace against the amnesic effect of cycloheximide, if administration of the amphetamine is delayed more than 6 hours after training it cannot reverse amnesia previously induced by a protein synthesis inhibitor (Barondes and Cohen, 1968). The effect of cycloheximide, then, may be blockade of memory storage rather than blockade of retrieval.

4. *Human and Nonhuman Memory*

The most significant difficulty in comparing human and animal memory is the difference in type of problems amenable to experimentation in humans and in animals. Studies of human memory largely deal with the retention of verbal material. This is natural, since we appear to code lexically even nonverbal material to a great extent (Deutsch and Deutsch, 1975; Klatzky, 1975). Having no direct experience of how an animal perceives its experimental environment, we are forced to make many assumptions regarding its motivational state, arousal level, and presumed memory strength. Thus, the specific response measured in animal tests is presumably influenced by but cannot be equated with memory. Specifically, as we shall discuss in more detail in the following section, it is virtually impossible in animals to distinguish effects of treatments on motivation, attention, or perception from effects on memory retrieval. Consequently, in discussing animal studies we will employ the term retrieval to include such processes as motivation, attention, and perception, all of which influence retrieval per se but are not easily differentiated from it. In research on human subjects, however, some paradigms permit discrimination among these alternatives.

It should come as no surprise, then, that it is frequently difficult to obtain comparable results with treatments that affect memory processing in humans and animals. Nonetheless, for both ethical and practical reasons, it is obviously necessary that we continue to attempt to model human memory with animal research, while keeping in mind the limits of interpretation of such research.

B. Some Paradigms for Assessment of Memory

Let us consider at this point a few technical terms and experimental paradigms regarding memory and learning processes, since we will discuss in following sections research that is largely derived from such paradigms. We have already mentioned the distinction between the strength of retention of a memory and the ability to retrieve the information.

1. *Active Avoidance Learning*

In rodents, the simplest paradigm we will consider is an active avoidance problem. One such problem is the pole-jump task (Fig. 1). A rat is placed in a chamber on a grid floor, in the center of which there is a pole. After a period of familiarization, a light is turned on in the box. Five seconds later, the floor is electrified and the rat receives shock to the feet until it discovers (within a few seconds) that it is possible to climb the pole and so escape the footshock. As soon as the rat jumps onto the pole, the light and shock are turned off. The rat is then placed on the grid floor once again, and after a variable interval averaging 60 seconds, the light–shock sequence is repeated. The animal is given 10 such trials per day. Accomplishment of the task is reflected in the ability of the rat to avoid the shock entirely by jumping onto the pole during the 5-second interval between light and shock. An animal in this task will generally quickly begin to jump onto the pole, even during the intertrial interval. Clear evidence of learning is seen when the animal responds as soon as the warning

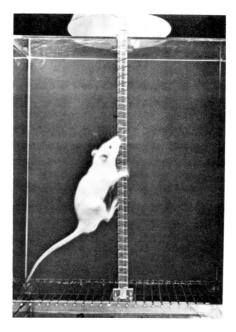

FIG. 1. Pole-jump test apparatus (with acknowledgment to Organon Nederland).

signal (the light) appears, thus always avoiding shock, but does not respond during the intertrial interval.

After several learning acquisition sessions, generally of 10 trials each, extinction of the response may be studied. In this phase of the task, the conditional stimulus is no longer followed by the footshock. Nonetheless, the rat continues to climb the pole when the light is turned on. Over several trials, the number of responses the rat makes will gradually decline until extinction is complete and it no longer climbs the pole.

The nature of responding during extinction is entirely unclear. In early stages of extinction, it is logical to assume that the level of responding is a direct measure of the strength of retention of the originally conditioned response. Until the rat fails to respond for the first time and discovers that such failure is not punished with footshock, its situation is exactly the same as during the later stages of acquisition of the problem, when it rarely received shock. However, as responding begins to extinguish and the subject begins to experience the light as no longer followed by shock, interpretation of the response rate becomes very difficult. Responding during extinction, although generally asserted to be a direct measure of retention of the original response, is without doubt a very complicated behavioral index. It measures both retention of the original response and the acquisition of the new response (that of ignoring the light). Moreover, one often sees an increase in behaviors, such as grooming and exploration, that compete with the conditioned response of climbing the pole.

A second problem frequently used is a shuttlebox (Fig. 2). In this case, the rat is placed in one compartment of a box with a grid floor, separated from another identical compartment by a small hurdle in the center of the floor. Once again, a light or a tone is presented as a conditional warning stimulus, and the rat must learn to cross the hurdle to the other compartment before shock is applied to the grid floor. After an intertrial interval, the warning signal is again presented. The rat must then shuttle back to the original compartment, in which it previously experienced shock, in order to avoid shock in the second compartment. Learning is assessed in analogous fashion to the pole jump. The rat must exhibit efficient avoidance of the footshock, at the

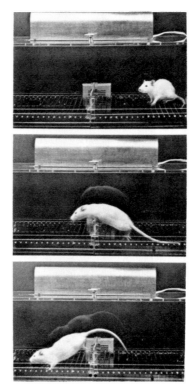

FIG. 2. Shuttlebox (with acknowledgment to Organon Nederland).

same time withholding responding during the intertrial interval. Extinction may also be assessed in a similar fashion, and the same interpretational caveats apply.

2. *Passive Avoidance Learning*

Finally, it is useful to study the ability of an animal to withhold responding, rather than actively to perform responses, in order to be certain that the conditioned responses are not confounded with changes in general arousal and/or activity. A passive avoidance problem, such as the step-through task (Fig. 3), can provide such an alternative. A rat placed beneath a light on a small ledge hanging over empty space finds the situation aversive. At the end of the platform is a darkened box with a hole. Within a very few seconds a normal rat, innately preferring the dark, will run into the hole. The rat is, however, given a footshock immediately upon entering the dark compartment. After this training experience (usually after 24 hours) the rat's retention may be tested by placing it on the platform and measuring the latency to step through the hole. Latency on the retention trial will be elevated; the rat may, indeed, never enter the dark compartment.

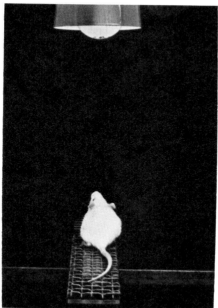

FIG. 3. Passive avoidance step-through test apparatus (with acknowledgment to Organon Nederland).

This task has the advantage of providing the ability to assess retention for a single training trial. Further, the degree of training and the presumed strength of memory may easily be titrated. By administration of a low level of footshock on the training day, a moderately increased latency on the retention trial may be induced. If the rat is immediately given a memory-enhancing treatment (for example, a low dosage of a peptide), it will subsequently display enhanced retention by exhibiting a greatly increased latency on the retention trial. The specificity of the treatment may be demonstrated by giving control animals the drug treatment after they have entered the compartment during training without footshock. If they show no similar increase in latency during retention testing, a nonmemorial effect of the drug may be eliminated. This task is sometimes employed with repeated (nonshocked) retention trials. The interpretation of latencies observed during subsequent retention trials is again complicated. Such repeated trials certainly involve learning the new problem (without shock) in addition to assessing retention of the originally trained passive avoidance problem.

We have used the passive avoidance test for studies of amnesia. A rat given carbon dioxide (CO_2) anesthesia immediately after the training trial in the step-through apparatus will enter the retention trial with as low a latency as it did during training, thus displaying amnesia for the training experience. Without additional evidence, one cannot equate amnesia with loss of memory. The fact that CO_2 is able to produce amnesia for different experiences and that this amnesia can be measured by means of different responses (Rigter and van Riezen, 1979) indicates that CO_2-induced amnesia does not result from a nonspecific disturbance of behavior, but rather may be based on a disturbance of memory. The existence of a retrograde amnesia gradient, the presence of other time-dependent features, and the lack of spontaneous recovery of memory after treatment with CO_2 (Rigter and van Riezen, 1979) all lend support to the view that CO_2-induced amnesia results from an interference with memory. Therefore, we have used with confidence our passive avoidance-amnesia test as a model for the assessment of peptide effects on memory.

III. Effects of Peptides on Memory—Introduction

We now turn our attention to the possible involvement of pituitary peptides in memory processes. The effects of two general classes of peptides, ACTH-like and vasopressin-like, will be reviewed. These peptides have been selected for the present review because sufficient data are available to enable a critical analysis of their potential effects on memory. For a number of other peptides there is also suggestive evidence for a role in memory processing, but in view of the paucity of relevant data we will refrain from a discussion of these peptides in this review. We will make one exception: pertinent effects of endorphins will briefly be discussed to outline an important direction in which the field is moving and to illustrate physiological interactions between peptides that may be relevant for an understanding of their possible effect on memory.

We will offer evidence that ACTH- and vasopressin-like peptides may act differentially on memory. Specifically, ACTH-like peptides appear to affect memory retrieval processes. Vasopressin-like peptides may exert effects not only on retrieval but also on storage processes. We will not exhaustively review the massive literature on all behavioral effects of these neuropeptides. This literature has usually been examined from a point of view not specifically intended to differentiate between effects on retrieval and on memory storage; rather the intention has generally been to attribute behavioral differences to attentional or motivational effects, which themselves clearly influence memory. We will consider in detail those critical experiments that allow further specification of peptide effects. We will at the same time consider many older studies and studies that methodologically do not permit unequivocal interpretation but have yielded results that are consistent with data derived from studies that were specifically designed to assess effects on memory.

Table I summarizes the criteria we will apply to distinguish hormone effects on memory storage, memory retrieval, and not strictly memorial factors, such as motivation and attention. We mention motivation and attention in particular, because a number of views on the mode of action of neuropeptides have been formulated around these key words. Thus, it has been proposed that ACTH-like peptides increase the motivational significance of relevant cues (De Wied, 1976a), or, in similar words, enhance selective attention (Sandman and Kastin, 1977). On methodological grounds it is difficult to distinguish in animals between effects on "cognitive" aspects of memory retrieval and the prerequisite sustaining processes, motivation and attention. Consequently, the fact that we will discuss peptide effects on memory retrieval processes should not be taken to imply that we find this conceptual framework to exclude an adequate description of peptide effects in motivational or attentional terms. Rather, we distinguish storage from retrieval and consider retrieval, motivation, and atten-

TABLE I
INTERPRETATION OF TREATMENT EFFECTS IN ANIMALS

Time of treatment	Response pattern	Interpretation as memory effect	Alternative interpretations
	A. Active Avoidance		
Before acquisition sessions[a]	↑Avoidance; no↑ITI[b]	↑Memory storage or memory retrieval	↑Motivation, perception or attention
	↑Avoidance; ↑ITI	↑Memory storage or memory retrieval	↑Motivation, perception or attention; or ↑Motility
After acquisition sessions	↑Avoidance	↑Memory storage[c]	
	B. One-Trial Passive Avoidance		
Before acquisition	↑Avoidance[d]	↑Memory storage	↑Motivation, perception or attention at the time of acquisition; or ↓Motility
After acquisition	↑Avoidance[d]	↑Memory storage[c]	
Before retention testing	↑Avoidance[d]	↑Memory retrieval[e]	↓Motility

[a] Since most studies employ more than one trial per (daily) acquisition session, preacquisition administration is usually equivalent to administration before retention testing in this paradigm.

[b] ITI = intertrial responses. Only a few of the studies to be discussed reported intertrial responses, and it is evident from the table that knowledge about intertrial responses may aid the interpretation of effects of treatments.

[c] Alternative interpretations can be excluded on the basis of time-dependence studies.

[d] As assessed at retention test.

[e] By definition: the compound of processes determining "retrieval performance" (including ancillary processes like attention, motivation, or arousal).

tion to be functionally indistinguishable in the animal literature. Thus, the issue is not the theoretical independence of motivation, attention, and memory retrieval, but the inability of existing animal research paradigms to discriminate between them. A potentially confounding factor such as change in locomotor activity, however, may be discarded as an explanation by some experimental paradigms although such possibilities have not been fully realized (cf. Table I). As a further aid to organization of the review, we will consider effects seen in hypophysectomized, aged, and genetically deficient animals apart from those in normal animals. The virtual orthogonality of the human and animal data leads us to consider the human data in a separate section.

IV. AMELIORATION OF BEHAVIORAL DEFICITS

A. HYPOPHYSECTOMY

1. *Effects of ACTH-like Peptides*

As an initial step in an attempt to assess the influence of pituitary hormones on memory processes, one might ablate the pituitary gland and examine the resulting behavioral syndromes. Accordingly, De Wied undertook an extensive series of investigations to examine the ability of hypophysectomized Wistar rats to learn and remember a shuttlebox avoidance task. Two types of behavioral impairment seen in hypophysectomized animals have been examined. In accordance with earlier reports (Applezweig and Baudry, 1955; Applezweig and Moeller, 1959), De Wied (1969) found that ablation of the pituitary seriously impaired shuttlebox avoidance acquisition. In addition, when performance during extinction was studied, a deficit was seen in this measure as well; hypophysectomized rats displayed accelerated extinction.

Since one of the principal products of the adenopypophysis is ACTH, the effects of ACTH replacement after hypophysectomy were assessed. Adrenal maintenance doses of ACTH restored avoidance acquisition in the shuttlebox to a considerable extent. Further, the extinction deficit in hypophysectomized rats could also be reversed by administration of a related peptide, melanocyte-stimulating hormone (α-MSH), during the extinction period (De Wied, 1969). The ameliorative action of ACTH was independent of the adrenocorticotropic properties of the hormone, since treatment with the synthetic glucocorticosteroid dexamethasone failed to improve deficient acquisition (De Wied, 1976a). Moreover, the fragments ACTH 4–10 and ACTH 1–10, neither of which possesses significant adrenocorticotropic activity, both returned shuttlebox acquisition to normal (De Wied, 1969).

2. *Possible Mechanisms of ACTH Action*

a. Factors Other Than Memory. Several "nonmemory" hypotheses may be invoked to explain the effects of ACTH-like peptides. One such hypothesis is that the deficient shuttlebox acquisition of hypophysectomized rats is caused by altered pain perception. ACTH-like peptides could be assumed to exert their ameliorative action through a normalization of pain sensitivity. De Wied (1968) trained rats in a runway to escape an electric shock and then hypophysectomized them. Removal of the pituitary gland interfered with rapid escape responding. Treatment with ACTH 4–10 increased the escape speed of hypophysectomized rats, although not to normal levels. De Wied (1968) argued that the escape test cannot be considered as a pure test of changes in pain perception since locomotor capacities and motivational variables, for example, also influence responding in this task. It is assumed that these latter phenomena play a lesser role in tests that assess pain sensitivity thresholds by recording flinching and a variety of other responses across a series of shock intensities. In such a test, hypophysectomy also enhanced responsiveness of rats to electric shock, but ACTH 1–10 or ACTH 1–24 did not reverse this change in responsiveness (Gispen et al., 1970, 1973). It is therefore unlikely that the efficacy of these peptides in ameliorating and conditioned behavior in hypophysectomized rats is due to their effect on pain perception.

Another possibility is that ACTH and related peptides may increase the motility of hypophysectomized rats, thereby increasing the chance that a treated animal will "shuttle" over the hurdle in the shuttlebox. Enhanced motility may be reflected in an increase in the number of crossings over the hurdle in the absence of the warning signal. However, the converse is not true. An increase in such intertrial interval (ITI) responses does not necessarily indicate an enhanced motility. Increases in levels of motivation or arousal might also be expected to increase ITI responding. Whatever the significance of changes in ITI responses, the effect of ACTH 4–10 on such responses has not been consistent. In one study, ACTH 4–10 increased ITI responses in hypophysectomized animals even over the level of sham-operated rats (De Wied, 1968), but in another study ACTH 4–10 ameliorated shuttlebox training without affecting the number of ITI responses in hypophysectomized rats (Bohus et al., 1973). Other measures of locomotor activity have also failed to detect clear effects of ACTH-like peptides on motility. ACTH 1–10 did not alter ambulation of hypophysectomized rats in an open field (De Wied, 1968) and ACTH 1–10 and ACTH 4–10 affected neither ambulation nor shock-induced suppression of ambulation in normal rats (Weijnen and Slangen, 1970; Wolthuis and De Wied, 1976).

Finally, removal of the anterior lobe of the pituitary interferes with a number of metabolic processes and thus results in physical malaise

(De Wied, 1964). It could therefore be argued that physical disability prevents hypophysectomized rats from adequately performing such a strenuous task as the shuttlebox test. De Wied (1969) has shown that hormone-replacement therapy consisting of cortisone, testosterone, and thyroxine also had a restorative action on the acquisition of a shuttlebox response in hypophysectomized animals. One obvious explanation is that the beneficial effect on shuttlebox responding of the hormone-replacement therapy was secondary to a general improvement of physical well-being, but a more specific action cannot be excluded. In any event, although the physical malaise experienced by hypophysectomized animals may have contributed to their difficulty in mastering the avoidance response, the physical condition of the subjects was not the sole cause of the behavioral deficit displayed by these animals. ACTH 1–10 and ACTH 4–10 do not alleviate the physical malaise that occurs after removal of the pituitary, but they restore impaired shuttlebox acquisition (De Wied, 1969). The lack of demonstrated peripheral effects of these ACTH fragments provides strong evidence that the specific behavioral action of these peptides is through an effect on the central nervous system.

   b. *Effects on memory.* Within the present context, we will consider the possibility that hypophysectomy interferes with memory storage and that this memory deficit is reversed by ACTH-like peptides. Data bearing on this hypothesis seem to be conflicting. It is clear that pituitary ACTH has no indispensable role in memory storage. As mentioned above, hypophysectomized rats maintained on hormone-replacement therapy were able to learn a shuttlebox avoidance response in the absence of pituitary ACTH (De Wied, 1969). However, before excluding any role for ACTH in memory storage, two further possibilities should be considered. First, future studies should address the possibility that a hypophysectomized animal may be able to master a task by utilizing extrapituitary sources of ACTH. Second, at the behavioral level, the possibility remains that ACTH and related peptides, although not essential for memory storage, may *modulate* this process (Gold and McGaugh, 1975). According to this theory, the storage of recent information may be promoted or impaired by the operation of adaptive processes generated, along with the memory trace, by the learning experience. Gold and McGaugh (1977) considered ACTH as an activator of one such memory-modulatory system. To test this view, they studied a passive avoidance response impaired by pituitary ablation. A single immediate posttrial injection of 0.3 IU per rat of ACTH normalized this deficit (Gold and McGaugh, 1977) (Fig. 4). The fact that the hormone was administered posttrial,

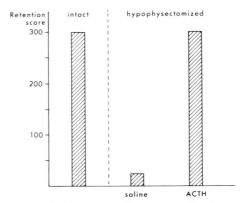

FIG. 4. Posttrial ACTH (0.3 IU per rat) restores retention of passive avoidance response. Retention score: avoidance latency in seconds. Adapted from Gold and McGaugh (1977) with permission. By courtesy of Raven Press, New York.

i.e., on termination of the training trial, precluded an ACTH effect on attentional, perceptual, motivational, or motor processes during training. The effectiveness of posttrial administration of ACTH is consistent with the view that hormonal responses to training have a modulatory effect on the storage of information generated by the training experience.

On the other hand, some findings indicate that it is improbable that the ACTH-induced amelioration of acquisition in hypophysectomized animals is exclusively due to a modulation of memory storage. An experiment by Bohus et al. (1973) may serve to illustrate this point. Hypophysectomized rats were trained in a shuttlebox for 14 days. Placebo-treated animals showed impaired acquisition; this group never scored more than an average of 50% avoidance responses. Rats treated with ACTH 4–10 during the first week attained a performance level of 80% avoidances, which suggests that relevant information had been stored in memory. In the second week of the experiment ACTH 4–10 was no longer administered and performance declined gradually to the level of the placebo-treated group (Fig. 5). If the sole effect of ACTH 4–10 had been a modulation of memory storage, there is no apparent reason why cessation of treatment after formation of memory had taken place would have led to a progressive deterioration of performance. One possible explanation is that ACTH produced a transient facilitation of retrieval processes, sufficient to maintain responding during the period of treatment but without consequence for the permanent storage of the information. The efficacy of ACTH administered before extinction in the restoration of responding in

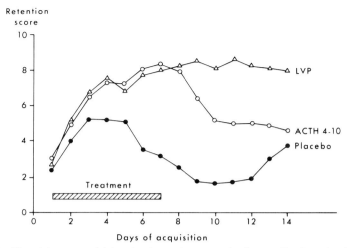

FIG. 5. Shuttlebox acquisition by hypophysectomized rats. During the indicated period of treatment, animals received daily subcutaneous injections of placebo, ACTH 4–10 (20 μg/day) or lysine vasopressin (LVP; 1 μg/day). Retention score: number of avoidance responses. From Bohus *et al.* (1973), with permission. By courtesy of S. Karger, Basel, Switzerland.

hypophysectomized rats to normal levels is consistent with such a postulated effect on retrieval processes (De Wied, 1969).

It is noteworthy in this regard that Bélanger (1958) found that hypophysectomized rats responded more slowly than control rats to a cue that signaled impending shock. The operated rats still exhibited nearly normal acquisition of the avoidance response, perhaps because Bélanger used quite a long interval (10 seconds) between the appearance of the warning cue and onset of shock. The slow response of hypophysectomized animals could not be attributed to possible sluggishness, for hypophysectomized rats are, if anything, more lively than control animals (Gispen *et al.*, 1973). Moreover, hypophysectomized animals are also deficient in the acquisition of passive avoidance responses, i.e. in paradigms in which sluggish animals would be expected to perform better than normal rats (Anderson *et al.*, 1968; Weiss *et al.*, 1970). Bélanger's results (1958), therefore, suggest that his rats had difficulty in retrieving the appropriate information in response to the warning cue, perhaps because of a motivational or attentional impairment.

Melanocyte-stimulating hormones (α-MSH and β-MSH) can also ameliorate deficient shuttlebox acquisition in operated rats (De Wied, 1969; Bohus *et al.*, 1973; Greven and De Wied, 1973). The effects of

MSH are not surprising, since it shares the amino acid sequence 4–10 with ACTH. This sequence contains sufficient information to specify the ameliorative behavioral effects (Fig. 6).

In summary, it is improbable that pituitary ACTH has an indispensable role in memory storage in rats. In certain experimental situations, however, it seems possible that ACTH may exert a modulatory effect on storage processes. In addition, there is evidence that ACTH may promote memory retrieval.

3. *Effects of Vasopressin-like Peptides*

In the experiment of Bohus *et al.* (1973) cited in the preceding section, the effects of lysine vasopressin (LVP) were also investigated. LVP given to hypophysectomized rats during the first week of acquisition of the shuttlebox problem ameliorated the acquisition deficit. However, when treatment was discontinued an interesting result was obtained (Fig. 5). The enhancement induced by LVP persisted long after treatment was discontinued, in clear contrast to the effects of ACTH described above. The effect was probably not caused by a peripheral action of LVP. The fragment deglycinamide LVP (DGLVP), which is virtually devoid of pressor, antidiuretic, oxytocin-, and corticotropin-releasing activities (De Wied *et al.*, 1972), is nonetheless able to restore shuttlebox acquisition (De Wied *et al.*, 1974). Corroboration of the lack of peripheral activity of DGLVP is provided by the absence of DGLVP effects on adrenal, testis, thymus, or body weight (Lande *et al.*, 1971).

The long-lasting consequences of administration of LVP afford indications that LVP may act on memory storage processes. Alternative explanations that invoke less specific mechanisms are possible. For example, in the study of Bohus *et al.* (1973), LVP also tended to increase ITI responding, so effects on activity or motivation cannot be excluded (see Table I). Results from studies that employed posttrial treatment with peptide (see Section V,A) support a specific effect on memory storage.

B. Selective Ablation of the Anterior and Posterior Lobes of the Pituitary

1. *Differential Roles of the Anterior and Posterior Lobes*

There is evidence that selective ablation of the pituitary lobes differentially affects the behavior of rats in the shuttlebox avoidance test. Adenohypophysectomy results in the acquisition deficit seen in

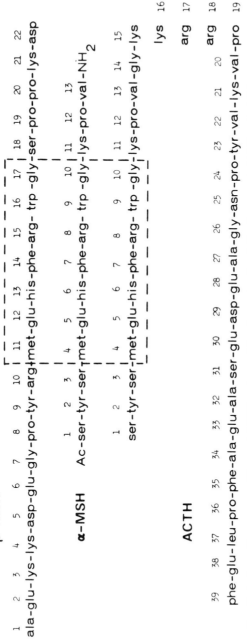

Fig. 6. Amino acid sequence of (human) ACTH and α- and β-melanocyte-stimulating hormone (α-MSH and β-MSH). The sequence ACTH 4–10 is common to all three hormones.

completely hypophysectomized subjects, whereas removal of the posterior, including the intermediate, lobes produces no such deficit (De Wied, 1964, 1965, 1969). Since the anterior lobe is the source of ACTH, the efficacy of ACTH and fragments of the hormone in restoring acquisition to normal seems logical. However, if adenohypophysectomized rats are not treated with ACTH, but rather with a hormone-replacement therapy consisting of cortisone, testosterone, and thyroxine, acquisition is also amended (De Wied, 1969). Vasopressin is also able to correct deficient acquisition of the shuttlebox response in adenohypophysectomized rats (De Wied, 1969). Thus, it would appear that this principle of the neural lobe may nonetheless reverse the deficits induced by adenohypophysectomy. This observation proves that this behavioral activity of LVP need not be mediated through a release of anterior pituitary ACTH.

Removal of the posterior pituitary lobe, including the intermediate lobe, is responsible for the extinction deficit displayed by completely hypophysectomized rats (De Wied, 1969). Neurohypophysectomy does not affect acquisition, but an acceleration of extinction ensues. This extinction deficit may be ameliorated by LVP given during either acquisition or extinction. In contrast to the LVP effect, treatment with ACTH during acquisition was not as effective as treatment during the extinction period (De Wied, 1969). The various interactions between pituitary manipulation and hormonal treatment are summarized in Tables II and III.

2. Implications for Interpreting Effects of Peptide

a. ACTH-like Peptides. Our survey of data from studies on hypophysectomized rats has shown that removal of the anterior lobe interferes with acquisition of new responses. Acquisition can be restored by ACTH, but also by a hormonal replacement therapy that does not include ACTH. Adenohyphysectomy does not affect extinction of responses, but ACTH is able to restore otherwise accelerated extinction in neurohypophysectomized rats. Apparently, pituitary ACTH is not crucial in either acquisition or extinction. Exogenous ACTH influences both processes.

The efficacy of ACTH in restoring acquisition in adenohypophysectomized animals does not necessarily imply that the sole effect of this hormone was to reverse a specific deficit that resulted from removal of the anterior lobe of the pituitary gland. It is also possible that the low baseline levels of acquisition performance displayed by adenohypophysectomized rats provide a background against which a general

TABLE II

EFFECTS OF PEPTIDES ON ACQUISITION AND EXTINCTION OF
A SHUTTLEBOX AVOIDANCE RESPONSE IN RATS [a,b]

Pituitary status	Hormone treatment during		Performance	
	Acquisition	Extinction	Acquisition	Extinction
Intact	None	None	Normal	Normal
	ACTH	None	Normal	Normal or slightly delayed
	None	ACTH	Normal	Delayed
	Vasopressin	None	Normal or improved	Delayed
	None	Vasopressin	Normal	Delayed
Hypophysectomized	None	None	Disrupted	Accelerated
	ACTH	—	Normalized	Not tested
	None[c]	None	Normalized	Accelerated
	None[c]	ACTH	Normalized	Normalized
	Vasopressin	—	Normalized	Not tested
	None[c]	Vasopressin	Normalized	Normalized

[a] Data from De Wied (1969, 1976a).
[b] Results of hypophysectomy and response to peptides given at the indicated times are shown. ACTH indicates ACTH-like peptides; vasopressin indicates vasopressin-like peptides.
[c] These animals received hormone-replacement therapy, consisting of cortisone, testosterone, and thyroxine, during the period of acquisition.

ameliorative action of ACTH can more easily be displayed. This latter view implies that ACTH-like peptides exert behavioral actions that are independent not only of the adrenal gland, but also, at least in part, of the pituitary. In accordance with this suggestion is the recent finding that material with ACTH-like activity has been extracted from brain of normal as well as hypophysectomized rats (Krieger *et al.*, 1977a). However, there is strong evidence in favor of the hypothesis that exogenous ACTH restores acquisition performance by correcting a specific deficit associated with the removal of the adenohypophysis. Verhoef *et al.* (1977) reported that in rats an intracerebroventricularly injected potent ACTH 4–9 analog (Org 2766) was preferentially taken up in the septum, a brain area implicated in the behavioral effects of ACTH-like peptides (see Section IX,A,1). Hypophysectomy enhanced septal uptake, which suggests that the uptake capacity of this brain structure was elevated because of depletion of an endogenous pituitary-related source of peptide(s). This

TABLE III
RESULTS OF SELECTIVE ADENO- AND NEUROHYPOPHYSECTOMY[a,b]

Pituitary status	Hormone treatment during		Performance	
	Acquisition	Extinction	Acquisition	Extinction
Adenohypophy-	None		Disrupted	Not tested
sectomy	ACTH		Normalized	Not tested
	Vasopressin		Normalized	Not tested
Neurophypophy-	None	None	Normal	Accelerated
sectomy	ACTH	None	Normal	Accelerated or slightly normalized
	None	ACTH	Normal	Normalized
	Vasopressin	None	Normal	Normalized
	None	Vasopressin	Normal	Normalized

[a] Data from De Wied (1964, 1965, 1969, 1976a).
[b] The subjects were rats. The test used was shuttlebox, ACTH indicates ACTH-like peptides; vasopressin indicates vasopressin-like peptides.

possibility was further supported by the finding that systemic pretreatment with structurally related peptides, ACTH 1–24 and ACTH 4–10, decreased the accumulation of Org 2766 in the septum of hypophysectomized animals, whereas pretreatments with ACTH 11–24 (a behaviorally rather inactive peptide) or DGLVP were ineffective.

Given that the behavioral activity of ACTH-like peptides is exerted at a site or sites within the brain, how it reaches these active sites must be considered. If the pituitary is a source of ACTH-like neuropeptides active in the brain, routes of transport between pituitary and brain must be assumed to exist. The general circulation may be one such route. Studies with systemically administered Org 2766 have revealed that this peptide may reach the brain, although in minute quantities (Verhoef and Witter, 1976). Additional routes of transport, bypassing the blood-brain barrier, have been suggested: retrograde transport along the pituitary stalk, transport via a microcirculation from the anterior hypophysial artery to the nucleus paraventricularis, retrograde transport via the portal vessels, or direct leakage of peptides from the pituitary into adjacent basilar cisterns (for references see De Wied, 1977; Bergland and Page, 1978).

The potential significance of some of these hypophysial–cerebral routes has been elegantly illustrated by a recent study. Labeled Org 2766 was injected into rats intravenously or into the pituitary. Much higher brain levels of radioactivity were seen after intrapituitary administration than after intravenous injection. Uptake of radioactivity into the brain was also high when the ACTH-analog was injected into the extracellular space surrounding the pituitary gland, a finding that underscores the importance of the cerebrospinal fluid as one route of transport from the pituitary to the brain (Mezey et al., 1978). There is inferential support for the view that transport of peptides within the brain may also be effected through the cerebrospinal fluid. Allen et al. (1974) found immunoreactive ACTH in cerebrospinal fluid of man; they suggested that at least part of the immunoreactivity might be attributable to ACTH fragments. Further, intracerebroventricular injection of nanogram quantities of ACTH 4–10 produced a delay of pole-jump extinction similar to that following the systemic administration of doses in the microgram range (Van Wimersma Greidanus and De Wied, 1971).

It is probable that the pituitary is not the only source of ACTH-like neuropeptides active in the brain (Krieger et al., 1977a; Watson et al., 1978a). If there exist such extrapituitary neural sources of ACTH-related peptides, their function may well be related to the behavioral activities we have discussed. For example, Pacold et al. (1978) have identified growth hormone and ACTH in the amygdala of rats. Bush et al. (1973) showed that amygdalectomized rats were deficient in shuttlebox avoidance learning and extinguished rapidly. Both deficits were reversed by ACTH administered before the single, combined acquisition and extinction session. We noted that the efficacy of hormonal replacement therapy in restoring acquisition in hypophysectomized rats argues that pituitary ACTH is not indispensable in learning. Apparently, compensatory mechanisms allow an adenohypophysectomized rat to learn. We suggest that one such mechanism may be mediated by brain-borne ACTH. A further implication is that there may be a physiological interplay between neuropeptides that arise from neural and pituitary sources in the determination of acquisition and retention responding.

b. Vasopressin-like Peptides. The persistent action of vasopressin on acquired behavior suggests that this hormone influences memory storage. It is therefore surprising that neurohypophysectomy did not result in an impairment of acquisition. Neurohypophysectomized rats exhibited an extinction deficit, but this impairment could be normalized also by agents other than vasopressin. Accordingly, one might conclude that vasopressin is important, but not crucial, for acquisition and extinction. There are alternatives to this conclusion. First, in the shuttlebox studies reviewed, training continued for a long time; in that period of time, regeneration of the neural lobe might have occurred (Moll and De Wied, 1962). Second, extrapituitary sources of vasopressin (George and Jacobowitz, 1975; Buys, 1978; Dogterom *et al.*, 1977, 1978) might have compensated for a possible effect of neurohypophysectomy. However, data obtained with another animal model, diabetes insipidus rats, tend to rule out these possibilities.

C. HEREDITARY DIABETES INSIPIDUS

In rats of the Brattleboro strain, severe hypothalamic diabetes insipidus is determined by a single autosomal locus. Homozygous diabetes insipidus (HO-DI) animals lack the ability to produce vasopressin and its associated neurophysin (Valtin *et al.*, 1962; Morris *et al.*, 1977). As revealed by radioimmunoassay, the posterior pituitary of homozygous diabetes insipidus animals contains virtually no vasopressin compared with heterozygous (HE-DI) and homozygous normal Brattleboro rats. The posterior pituitary vasopressin content of HE-DI rats is approximately 40% of that of normal Brattleboro rats (Van Wimersma Greidanus and De Wied, 1977). HO-DI rats also lack cerebral vasopressin (Dogterom *et al.*, 1978) and therefore seem to be a more suitable animal model for the study of the behavioral effects of vasopressin than neurohypophysectomized rats.

Behavioral differences between HO-DI rats and their relatively normal littermates cannot be attributed simply to the difference in availability of vasopressin, since HO-DI rats have other endocrine abnormalities in addition to a lack of vasopressin. HO-DI rats also completely lack arginine-8-vasotocin (Rosenbloom and Fisher, 1975). In addition, less oxytocin is stored in the posterior pituitaries of HO-DI rats than in HE-DI and normal Brattleboro rats (Van Wimersma Greidanus and De Wied, 1977); on the other hand, plasma levels of oxytocin are elevated in HO-DI animals (Dogterom *et al.*, 1977). The relatively depleted neurohypophysial oxytocin store of HO-DI rats probably results from periodic hyperosmolar stimulation of the hypothalamoneurohypophysial system caused by excessive water loss, since normalization of the fluid balance in HO-DI rats after treatment with exogenous vasopressin also normalizes oxytocin content of the neural lobe (Valtin *et al.*, 1975). As we shall discuss later, vasotocin and oxytocin are peptides with behavioral activity distinct from that of vasopressin. Finally, HO-DI rats have diminished pituitary–adrenal responsiveness (De Wied *et al.*, 1976) and growth hormone levels are reduced (Arimura *et al.*, 1968). This multitude of endocrine differences between HO-DI rats and HE-DI or normal rats might seem to limit the utility of HO-DI animals in studies of memory. We shall see that in some studies this objection was met by the demonstration that a memory deficiency in diabetes insipidus rats could be normalized with centrally active vasopressin-like peptides.

Compared to HE-DI animals, HO-DI rats were extremely impaired in the retention of a step-through one-trial passive avoidance response (Bohus *et al.*, 1975a). When tested immediately after termination of the acquisition trial, HO-DI rats displayed normal avoidance behavior. Three hours after the acquisition trial, however, HO-DI rats showed poor retention of the avoidance response, and the test performance of these animals was even worse when retention was assessed 24 hours after acquisition (Fig. 7). Strengthening acquisition by increasing shock level or shock duration failed to improve retention in HO-DI animals, while a single subcutaneous posttrial injection of 1 μg of arginine vasopressin (AVP) or 1 μg of DGLVP restored avoidance behavior to values indistinguishable from those of HE-DI rats. The dosage of DGLVP employed did not affect step-through latencies in nonshocked HO-DI rats (De Wied *et al.*, 1975a). Diabetes insipidus and HE-DI rats behaved similarly in the open field ambulation test (Bohus *et al.*, 1975a) and also did not differ on measures of pain sensitivity (Bohus *et al.*, 1975a; Celestian *et al.*, 1975; De Wied *et al.*,

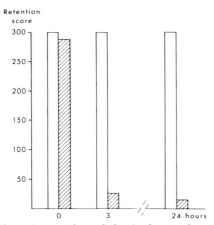

FIG. 7. Retention of passive avoidance behavior by rats homozygous (□, HO-DI) or heterozygous (▨, HE-DI) for hereditary diabetes insipidus. Retention score: avoidance latency in seconds. Adapted from Van Wimersma Greidanus *et al.* (1975a), with permission. By courtesy of Elsevier, Amsterdam.

1975a). Therefore, changes in motility and pain perception cannot be invoked as an explanation for the differences in avoidance behavior. Further, AVP or DGLVP, while restoring deficient passive avoidance performance, did not normalize pituitary–adrenal activation in HO-DI rats. This suggests that vasopressin can exert its behavioral effects independently from its control of ACTH released by stress (De Wied *et al.*, 1976).

The posttrial effectiveness of AVP and DGLVP suggests that these peptides normalized avoidance retention by a modulatory effect on memory storage. The time-dependence of the development of the retention deficit in HO-DI rats is also indicative of a disturbance in memory storage. However, this memory deficit is not an absolute one, for Bailey and Weiss (1978) found no difference between HO-DI and HE-DI rats with respect to acquisition of a one-trial step-through passive avoidance response. Under the conditions employed, however, both groups of animals avoided maximally for the limited duration of the first retention test, so that a ceiling effect cannot be excluded. Also, a sex difference might be important, since the Bailey and Weiss study differs from the other passive avoidance studies cited so far in that female animals were used. Our own work shows that male HO-DI rats, when trained in the step-through apparatus used by De Wied *et al.* (1975a, 1976), evidence normal retention of the passive avoidance response 24 hours after acquisition. They apparently forget more quickly, since performance is impaired when HO-DI animals are tested for the first time 72 hours after acquisition.

Brattleboro rats have been tested also for their ability to acquire a multitrial avoidance response. The available reports all concur that HO-DI rats are deficient in learning a shuttlebox response, but the estimates of the severity of the deficit vary. In two studies only about 30% of the HO-DI animals attained the acquisition criterion compared to 50–80% of the heterozygous or normal control animals (Celestian *et al.*, 1975; M. Miller *et al.*, 1976). In a third investigation HO-DI rats did learn a shuttlebox task, but at a slower rate than HE-DI animals. In a pole-jump avoidance test no difference in acquisition was found between HO-DI and HE-DI rats (Bohus *et al.*, 1975a). The results of these studies confirm that the acquisition deficit exhibited by HO-DI rats is not an absolute one.

Extinction data are contradictory. Celestian *et al.* (1975) found that those HO-DI rats that managed to reach acquisition criterion in a shuttlebox test exhibited retarded extinction. In contrast, Bohus and associates (1975a) reported that HO-DI rats showed somewhat accelerated extinction of both a shuttlebox and a pole-jump avoidance response. M. Miller *et al.* (1976) pointed out the difficulty of comparing extinction performance in groups of animals which differed in acquisition. In their data, the inferiority of HO-DI animals in extinction performance was eliminated when the differences in terminal acquisition performance were taken into account statistically by regression or covariance analysis.

D. OLD ANIMALS

Memory functions may deteriorate in aging animals and man (Botwinick, 1970; Gold and McGaugh, 1976; Thatcher, 1976). This is illustrated by the performance of young and old rats on a one-trial passive avoidance test (Gold and McGaugh, 1976). Young animals (60 days old) performed well after training-test intervals of 1, 7, or 21 days. After a 6-week training-test delay, test performance began to decline. Old rats (2 years old) already performed relatively poorly when tested 1 or 7 days after acquisition. Performance of 1-year-old rats was intermediate between that of young and old animals. A closer examination of the ability of 2-year-old rats to acquire and recall the passive avoidance response revealed that these rats retained the response for 2 hours, but not for 6 hours, after training. The poor retention performance of old rats could be due to deficient memory storage or deficient memory retrieval. Gold and McGaugh (1976) suggested that the age-related retention changes observed in old rats may be the result of impaired functioning of hormonal systems assumed to play a role in modulating memory storage.

Whatever the cause of the retention deficit shown by old rats may be, we have found this deficit to be reversible by treatment with an ACTH 4–9 analog before the retention test. This analog (Org 2766) has a profile of behavioral activity similar to the parent hormone and to ACTH 4–10 but its potency is enhanced (Greven and De Wied, 1973; Rigter *et al.*, 1976). We trained hungry young (9 weeks old) and old (110 weeks old) male rats to traverse a complex maze in order to obtain food pellets at the end of the maze (goal section). There was only one correct route from start to goal section. Entries in cul-de-sacs were recorded as errors. During the acquisition phase two trials per day were given, with an intertrial interval of 4–5 hours. Animals were trained until the criterion was attained, a maximum of one error during two subsequent trials. One week after achievement of criterion performance, the animals were retested in a 1-day session comprising four trials at 10-minute intervals. During acquisition, the rats were not treated; 1 hour before the start of the test session they received a subcutaneous injection of 0.1 μg of Org 2766 or placebo per rat.

Table IV shows that old rats did not differ significantly from young rats in their ability to learn the maze problem. However, old rats made more errors during the test than young animals. Org 2766 tended to improve test performance in both age groups, but this was statistically significant only for the old animals. This effect can be interpreted as a peptide-produced improvement of memory retrieval. It should be noted, though, that the old animals had no absolute memory deficit. Their performance on the *first* retention trial was as good as that of young rats. However, old animals made most of their errors during the remaining test trials. One should realize that these old rats, although housed in groups of 6–10 animals, had been kept for a long time in a deprived environment. Possibly, the resulting "boredom" could have resulted in an increased exploratory drive or general arousal that interfered with correct test performance. If so, Org 2766 may have protected old animals against distraction by stimuli irrelevant to the task. Conclusions cannot be drawn until possible effects on activity have been eliminated (see Table I).

TABLE IV

IMPROVEMENT OF TEST PERFORMANCE OF OLD RATS BY THE ACTH 4–9 ANALOG ORG 2766[a]

Animals	Acquisition performance[b]		Test performance[b]	
	Trials to criterion[d]	Errors to criterion[d]	First trial errors	Total errors[e]
Young rats, placebo[c]	13.1 ± 1.9	36.4 ± 7.3	0.9 ± 0.3	3.9 ± 1.2
Young rats, Org 2766	12.6 ± 1.5	32.7 ± 6.5	0.6 ± 0.2	2.1 ± 0.6
Old rats, placebo	15.3 ± 1.7	46.8 ± 7.5	1.0 ± 0.4	6.8 ± 0.9
Old rats, Org 2766	15.0 ± 1.2	42.2 ± 7.8	0.7 ± 0.2	3.8 ± 0.6

[a] Rats were placed on 23¼ hour food deprivation during acquisition, acquisition-test interval, and test. Reward/trial: five 37-mg Noyes food pellets. Six rats were tested in each old group; 7 rats, in each young group. Rats were matched in pairs within age groups on the basis of performance during acquisition.

[b] Mean ± SE.

[c] Treatment (1 ml of saline per rat or 0.1 μg of Org 2766 per rat) was given subcutaneously only once, 1 hour before test session. Within each pair one rat received placebo and the other Org 2766.

[d] Pooled young rats versus pooled old rats: no significant difference.

[e] Difference between placebo-treated young and old groups: $p < 0.05$ (Mann–Whitney U test). Difference between the control and peptide-treated young groups: nonsignificant. Difference between the control and peptide-treated old groups: $p = 0.05$ (Wilcoxon Matched-Pair Signed-Ranks Test). (Rigter, unpublished results.)

E. Experimental Amnesia

One of the most sensitive techniques for investigating the role of pituitary peptides in the amelioration of memory deficits is the induction of amnesia in normal animals. This approach allows clear identification of the aspects of memory processing affected by peptide treatment. We will devote Section VI to a detailed discussion of studies that employ experimentally induced amnesia.

F. Summary

In Section IV we have discussed some possible methods for assessing the role of pituitary principles in the maintenance of learned behavior in rats. Selective adenohypophysectomy or neurohypophysectomy has provided insight into the complexity of the behavioral substrate against which peptide effects are measured. Investigators have also examined animals with inherited vasopressin deficiency. The general difficulty in the interpretation of results from these models is inherent in the spectacular adaptive capacity of the laboratory rat; disturbance of the normal hormonal balance is undoubtedly compensated for in a variety of ways. We have reviewed evidence of the complexity of hormonal changes seen in hypophysectomized or HO-DI rats. Taken as a whole, however, these studies provide a number of working hypotheses with regard to hypophysial peptide effects

1. Adenohypophysectomy, or hypophysectomy, results in a deficiency in the acquisition of active avoidance responses in rats. Neurohypophysectomy results in deficient extinction of an active avoidance response. These deficiencies cannot be attributed solely to general physical malaise or to effects on motility and other performance factors; rather, specific deficits in some aspects of memory processing are implicated.

2. Inherited vasopressin deficiency results in impaired avoidance acquisition and, perhaps, extinction in Brattleboro rats.

3. Administration of ACTH-like peptides to animals with partial or complete pituitary lesions normalizes the lesion-induced deficit. This effect is limited to the period of treatment. If these peptides are given during acquisition, the amelioration does not clearly persist during later acquisition or extinction. If an ACTH-like peptide is given during extinction, however, the course of extinction is extended. These results can best be explained by assuming that ACTH-like peptides

exert a transient facilitation of processes necessary for optimal memory retrieval. Although the nature of the deficits seen in old animals is not known, ACTH-like peptides are able to reverse these deficits in a manner consistent with this hypothesis.

4. Administration of vasopressin-like peptides to pituitary-lesioned animals also normalizes behavioral deficits of both types. This effect, in contradistinction to the ACTH-like effects, persists long after treatment is discontinued. Vasopressin given during acquisition returns both acquisition and extinction responding to normal. Vasopressin given during extinction also ameliorates extinction responding. The persistent action of vasopressin strongly implicates this hormone in memory storage processes. The fact that posterior pituitary-lobectomized or diabetes insipidus animals are able to master some multitrial tasks indicates that lack of vasopressin produces a relative, not an absolute, memory deficit. The vasopressin effects discussed thus far may therefore be described as a modulation of memory storage.

5. The ability of fragments of these peptides that lack peripheral endocrine activity to mimic the effects of the parent hormones is strong evidence for direct actions on sites in the central nervous system.

V. Effects in Normal Animals

A. Treatments Administered after Training

1. *ACTH-like Peptides*

There are a few studies in which a possible memory modulatory effect of ACTH was examined by administering the hormone posttrial. Gold and Van Buskirk (1976) pretrained thirsty rats to lick from a water spout and then submitted their animals to an acquisition trial on which a footshock was administered while the animals were drinking. Immediately after this passive avoidance training, ACTH was administered subcutaneously. A retention test was conducted the next day. Animals injected with 0.03 or 0.3 IU of ACTH showed improved performance of the avoidance response at the test. A dose of 3.0 IU of ACTH impaired test performance. Furthermore, the doses of 0.3 IU of ACTH that effectively enhanced test performance when given immediately after training were ineffective when given 2 hours after training. In addition, Gold and Van Buskirk (1976) found that the nature of the modulatory effect of ACTH depended on the intensity of the aversive stimulus experienced during training. The dose of 3.0 IU of ACTH that was found to be disruptive in the first experiment both facilitated and impaired memory in a secondary study; at low foot-shock levels facilitation was observed, whereas at higher footshock levels disruption was seen.

These findings have important implications. First, the data indicate that the effect of a particular dose of ACTH is related to the intensity of the training experience. This suggests that the nature of the effect of exogenous ACTH may depend on the amount of endogenous ACTH that is mobilized by the training experience. Second, there is an inverted-U dose-response relationship between the dose of ACTH and later test performance. This suggests that the memory-modulatory process upon which ACTH may act has an optimal level of functioning; too much ACTH may disrupt rather than facilitiate the hypothetical process. Third, the effectiveness of ACTH in facilitating test performance diminished as the time between training and treatment was increased. In Section II we noted that it is commonly held that memory storage proceeds from a labile to a stable phase, modulatory treatments being effective only during the labile phase. The time-dependent nature of posttrial treatment with ACTH is, therefore, strong evidence for a modulatory effect of this hormone on memory storage.

Gold and McGaugh (1977) found posttrial injections of growth hormone, thyroid hormone, and thyroid-stimulating hormone to be ineffective in altering memory storage. Corticosterone was also without effect. The latter finding argues that ACTH did not exert its modulatory influence through its corticotropic properties. More direct evidence that ACTH, when given posttrial, may modulate memory storage independent of the adrenal cortex stems from experiments performed by Flood *et al.* (1976). These investigators showed that posttrial administration of the ACTH fragment ACTH 4–10 improved performance in mice on both passive and active avoidance tasks. Again, the facilitatory action was dose-related: a high dose of ACTH 4–10 (3 mg/kg) was less effective than a dose of 0.3 mg/kg (Fig. 8). In a passive avoidance task, it was demonstrated that the peptide had to be administered within 60 minutes of training for it to be clearly effective.

In contrast to the studies reported above, De Wied and associates have generally failed to find a posttrial effect of treatment with ACTH 4–10. For instance, when rats were trained in the pole-jump

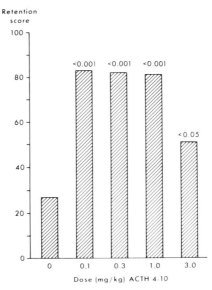

F IG. 8. Effects of ACTH 4–10 on retention for passive avoidance training in mice. The peptide was injected subcutaneously 30 minutes after training. Retention was tested 1 week later. Retention score is the percentage of mice attaining retention criterion. Significance levels given are with respect to control group. Adapted from Flood *et al.* (1976), with permission. By courtesy of ANKHO International Inc., Phoenix, Arizona.

test and subcutaneously injected with the peptide immediately after the first extinction session (in which responding remained high), extinction during subsequent sessions, 24 and 48 hours later, developed normally. The disagreement between investigators could be because of differences in procedures; nevertheless the design used in the De Wied laboratory was in itself sensitive to peptide effects, as exemplified by the finding that LVP delayed later extinction under the same circumstances (De Wied, 1971). Van Wimersma Greidanus (1977) reported that subcutaneous administration of either 15 or 50 μg of ACTH 4–10 immediately after a passive avoidance acquisition trial did not affect subsequent retention. Posttrial treatment with antiserum against either ACTH 1–24 or α-MSH or a combination of both antisera also failed to alter retention (Van Wimersma Greidanus *et al.*, 1978). Similarly, Martinez *et al.* (1979) failed to find a posttrial effect of Org 2766 over a dose range of 0.005-5.0 mg/kg given immediately after training in a one-trial passive avoidance test. Rather, these authors found Org 2766 to be active only when injected in a high dose (5.0 mg/kg) 1 hour before acquisition; this treatment facilitated retention of the response. Martinez *et al.* suggested that Org 2766 acts by influencing sensory, motivational, or attentional variables rather than directly by affecting memory storage.

To this point, we have surveyed behavioral studies in which animals were prompted to learn a new response by the delivery of an electric shock. In order to draw more general conclusions, we need information about the effect of hormones on the performance of subjects on a variety of tests. A recent series of experiments with ACTH employed an aversive stimulus other than electric shock (Leshner and Roche, 1977). Basically, these investigators trained mice on a multiple-trial step-through passive avoidance test in which entry of a mouse into a compartment was punished by the attack of a trained fighter of the same strain. ACTH administered immediately after the passive avoidance criterion was achieved increased performance of the avoidance response at retention tests 24 and 48 hours later. An effect of the hormone was no longer observed at the third retention test, which was conducted 240 hours after training. It was concluded that ACTH had a short-lived effect on retention of the avoidance response.

Although many ACTH effects could be explained by a short-acting influence on processes associated with retrieval, it may be necessary to postulate that the hormone occasionally may exert an additional effect on storage. Only one study that employed fragments of ACTH has yielded significant posttrial effects (Flood *et al.*, 1976). The other effective posttrial studies used ACTH itself (Gold and Van Buskirk, 1976; Gold and McGaugh, 1977; Leshner and Roche, 1977). Therefore, posttrial efficacy may be a property of full-molecule ACTH and to a (much) less extent of ACTH fragments or analogs. If true, a contribution from a peripheral mechanism cannot be excluded. Alternatively, facilitation of memory storage might have structure-activity requirements that differ from those for facilitation of retrieval.

2. Vasopressin-like Peptides

De Wied (1971) studied the posttrial efficacy of LVP in influencing extinction of a pole-jump response. After successful acquisition of the avoidance response, rats were given an extinction session of 10 trials. Only rats that made 8 or more avoidance responses during this initial session were selected for further extinction testing. ACTH 4–10 (100 μg per rat) or LVP (1 μg per rat) was injected subcutaneously immediately after the selection session and extinction performance was observed in a series of sessions conducted 2, 4, 24, 48, and 72 hours after injection. ACTH 4–10 had its usual short-term effect; it retarded extinction 2 and 4 hours after administration, but the effect had become dissipated by 24 hours. In contrast, LVP delayed extinction persistently; even at 72 hours LVP-treated animals failed to show appreciable extinction. The specificity of LVP in this respect was indicated by the lack of effect of a number of structurally and physiologically related peptides (oxytocin, angiotensin II, insulin, and growth hormone, all in the single subcutaneous dose of 1 μg per rat). Even stronger evidence for posttrial efficacy of LVP was obtained in a subsequent experiment. Rats were again treated with LVP or ACTH 4–10 on termination of the selection session, but extinction tests were not performed until 24 hours after selection, rendering it likely that any effect of treatment would be on storage rather than retrieval. This particular experiment also sought to assess the time-dependence of the LVP effect. For this purpose, separate groups of animals received LVP either immediately, 1 hour, or 6 hours after the selection session. Whereas a posttrial action of ACTH 4–10 was not observed, LVP treatment was effective in delaying extinction. The LVP effect was time-dependent; postponement of treatment for 1 hour slightly diminished the efficacy of LVP, and no effect was seen when LVP was given 6 hours after the selection session.

Vasopressin has also been examined in the one-trial passive avoidance paradigm. The results of these studies meet the two criteria for the assessment of treatment effects on memory storage, i.e., posttrial efficacy and time-dependence of the posttrial effect. Thus, systemic or intracerebroventricular administration of LVP or AVP immediately after acquisition facilitated performance during a later retention test (Ader and De Wied, 1972; Bohus *et al.*, 1978b; Krejči and Kupková, 1978; but see also Gold and McGaugh, 1976). AVP was still effective when injected 3 hours after training, but not when given 6 hours after training (Bohus *et al.*, 1978b).

The capability of vasopressin administered posttrial to influence later test performance is not restricted to avoidance learning. In a study by Bohus (1977), male rats were trained to traverse a wooden maze to gain access to a sexually receptive female. After leaving the start box and traversing the connected alley, the animals arrived at a T-shaped choice point. Essentially, the rats had to learn to take either the left or the right turn in order to arrive at the goal box containing the female. Some males were rewarded for making the correct choice by being allowed to copulate with the female; other males were prevented from contacting the female by a wire-mesh partition. The male rats received injections of placebo or DGLVP after the last trial of each acquisition session. DGLVP treatment facilitated retention in the rewarded groups as evidenced by a larger number of correct choices. Males that were prevented from copulation showed no signs of acquisition, and the peptide was ineffective in this group.

A further illustration of the generality of the posttrial efficacy of vasopressin is provided by data from the report of Leshner and Roche (1977), who examined LVP in their avoidance-of-attack model. LVP administered immediately after the mice had attained the learning criterion improved test performance; this improvement was most pronounced in a late (240 hours) retention test. These investigators agreed with the view that the behavioral effect of LVP is of longer-term consequence than that of ACTH.

If exogenously administered vasopressin facilitates memory storage, one might expect that inactivation of endogenous vasopressin should impair memory. There is experimental support for this supposition. Rats treated intracerebroventricularly with antibodies against AVP directly on termination of training displayed virtually no passive avoidance in tests conducted 24 hours and 48 hours later (Van Wimersma Greidanus et al., 1975a). Intravenous injection of 100 times as much AVP antiserum removed the hormone from the circulation, as indicated by absence of AVP in the urine and by increased urine production, but failed to affect passive avoidance behavior (Van Wimersma Greidanus et al., 1975b). This indicates that interference with central, but not peripheral, vasopressin impairs memory storage. The time-dependence of this effect was reflected in an amnesia gradient; when intracerebroventricular injection of AVP antiserum was delayed for 1–6 hours after training, the effectiveness of the treatment progressively diminished. Furthermore, onset of amnesia was gradual. Central administration of AVP antiserum immediately after the acquisition trial did not prevent animals from displaying passive avoidance for the first few hours after training, but impairment of retention was apparent 3 hours after training and at the time of later retention tests (Van Wimersma Greidanus and De Wied, 1976a).

Recent observations have revealed that oxytocin may have behavioral effects opposite from those of vasopressin. Schulz et al. (1974) reported that systemically administered vasopressin and oxytocin delayed and accelerated, respectively, extinction of an avoidance response. Relatively small quantities of oxytocin applied intracerebroventricularly immediately after training affected performance of a passive avoidance test after 24 hours in a manner opposite to that of AVP (Bohus et al., 1978a). Reduced avoidance latencies were measured in rats given oxytocin in doses as low as 0.1 and 1.0 ng. The fact that a higher dose of oxytocin (10.0 ng) did not alter test performance in comparison with control rats suggests that the peptide may have a dose-related bimodal effect. In contrast, doses of 1.0 and 10.0 ng of AVP facilitated test performance; the high dose produced a long-term effect that extended to the 48-hour test. Furthermore, posttrial intracerebroventricular injection of AVP antiserum and oxytocin antiserum also exerted opposite actions. Whereas, in agreement with previous findings (Van Wimersma Greidanus et al., 1975a), antibodies against AVP reduced passive avoidance behavior, oxytocin antiserum increased avoidance behavior. The intracerebroventricular route of administration appeared to be important for demonstrating the inhibitory action of oxytocin. A single posttrial systemic (subcutaneous) injection of oxytocin failed to affect later test performance unequivocally; some of the peptide-treated animals showed attenuated, and others showed enhanced, passive avoidance (Bohus et al., 1978a). However, another group of investigators (Kovács et al., 1978) reported impaired retention of a multitrial passive avoidance response after systemic (intraperitoneal) administration of oxytocin. In this study, the hormone was given before acquisition (and also before the retention test); its effects, therefore, are less clearly interpretable as an action on memory storage.

That memory storage is the behavioral substrate of the posttrial effect of oxytocin is further suggested by a time-dependence study in rats (Bohus et al., 1978b). Oxytocin was given intracerebroventricularly in a dose of 1.0 ng at various times after acquisition of a one-trial passive avoidance response. The hormone impaired retention when given immediately or 3 hours after training, but not when given 6 hours after training.

Attempts have also been made to demonstrate memory-modulatory effects of vasopressin and oxytocin in multitrial active avoidance tests (Bohus et al., 1978a). Rats were trained in the pole-jump test and received intracerebroventricular injections of AVP or oxytocin immediately after each acquisition session (consisting of 10 daily trials). Treatment with oxytocin did not affect acquisition on days 1 and 2 of the experiment but lowered the terminal level of acquisition assessed at day 3. Treatment with AVP did not influence acquisition scores, but, despite the cessation of treatment after the last training session, AVP-treated rats were more resistant to subsequent extinction than control animals.

An elegant attempt to elucidate the nature of the modulatory effect of vasopressin on memory storage was undertaken by King and De Wied (1974). These investigators trained rats in the pole-jump test. The animals received LVP immediately after making their first avoidance response. Training was then interrupted for 6 hours in order to ensure that the behavioral substrate for the hormone effect was restricted to a single avoidance response. Nevertheless, LVP delayed later extinction. Weaker resistance to extinction was produced when the substrate behavior was confined to the classically conditioned component of the pole-jump response. In other words, vasopressin was less, but still significantly, effective in retarding extinction when administered at a time when the rats had not yet responded to the warning signal by jumping onto the pole but had already developed a classically conditioned fear for this signal. The hormone had no effect when given at a time when conditioning, in whatever form, had not yet taken place. King and De Wied proposed that some minimum of associative strength must be present before vasopressin could be effective in modulating memory storage.

In a later series of experiments, De Wied (1976b) employed the pole-jump test to study the structure-activity relationships of intracerebroventricularly administered vasopressin congeners on extinction. The peptides were injected immediately after the last acquisition session. Extinction sessions were conducted 1, 2, and 5 days after treatment. Posttrial administration of picogram and nanogram quantities of AVP produced a persistent delay in extinction. The ring structure of AVP, pressinamide, appeared to be more potent in producing the posttrial effect than the tail amino acid sequence, Pro-Arg-Gly (the structures of vasopressin, oxytocin, and fragments of these hormones are given in Table V).

The posttrial effectiveness of vasopressin and the time-dependence of this posttrial effect are strong arguments in favor of the view that this hormone modulates memory storage. Apparently, this hormone-

TABLE V

STRUCTURE OF VASOPRESSINS, OXYTOCIN, AND SOME CONGENERS[a]

LVP	H-Cys-Tyr-Phe-Gln-Asn-Cys-Pro-Lys-Gly-NH$_2$
AVP	H-Cys-Tyr-Phe-Gln-Asn-Cys-Pro-Arg-Gly-NH$_2$
DGLVP	H-Cys-Tyr-Phe-Gln-Asn-Cys-Pro-Lys-OH
DGAVP	H-Cys-Tyr-Phe-Gln-Asn-Cys-Pro-Arg-OH
Pressinamide	H-Cys-Tyr-Phe-Gln-Asn-Cys-NH$_2$
Oxytocin	H-Cys-Tyr-Ile-Gln-Asn-Cys-Pro-Leu-Gly-NH$_2$
Tocinamide	H-Cys-Tyr-Ile-Gln-Asn-Cys-NH$_2$

[a] LVP, lysine vasopressin; AVP, arginine vasopressin; DGLVP, deglycinamide LVP; DGAVP, deglycinamide AVP.

produced modulation is not demonstrable under all experimental conditions. The extent and nature of the modulation probably depends upon dose level and test characteristics. Thus, modulation of memory storage by vasopressin seems easier to assess in one-trial than in multitrial learning tasks. The results further suggest that there may be a variety of modulatory influences on memory traces, some influences being beneficial, some influences being detrimental to an optimal consolidation of memory items. For instance, in contrast to vasopressin, oxytocin tends to disrupt memory storage. Again, this inhibitory influence is not an absolute one; the effect of oxytocin varies with dose level and type of experimental measure.

Opposite biological effects of oxytocin and vasopressin are not limited to these behavioral findings. For example, small doses of oxytocin induced diuresis (Pickford, 1961) and antagonized the antidiuretic responses to vasopressin in the rat (Brunner *et al.*, 1956; Sawyer and Valtin, 1965). Similarly, AVP facilitated, while oxytocin suppressed, spontaneous nerve activity of *Periplaneta americana* (Schulz, 1970). Oxytocin shortened the reaction time to an acoustic stimulus in the rat, and LVP prolonged the reaction time (Schwarzberg and Unger, 1970). Finally, oxytocin increased and vasopressin decreased the rate of brain self-stimulation in rats (Schwarzberg *et al.*, 1976).

B. TREATMENTS ADMINISTERED BEFORE TESTING FOR RETENTION

1. *Introduction*

The most logical approach to the assessment of a possible effect of a peptide on memory retrieval is to administer the substance before the retention test. Provided that the test is conducted after a time sufficient for the completion of memory storage, any effect seen should most likely be limited to retrieval processes.

In the present section experiments pertinent to this approach will be discussed. In many studies effects of peptides on extinction of acquired responses have been examined. Resistance to extinction may be regarded as a measure of retention of the acquired response. Accordingly, if treatment with a peptide before extinction sessions results in an alteration of extinction performance, such an effect could be interpreted as a modulation of processes associated with or underlying memory retrieval. However, as we discussed in Section II, "extinction" is a descriptive term; the underlying process or processes are far from clear (see Mackintosh, 1974). Specifically, it is often held that extinction measurements not only reflect the strength of retention of the original response, but also reflect the acquisition by the animal of new information. These and perhaps other factors are easily confounded when extinction is assessed over many trials; these objections are invalid if testing is confined to a single trial. For these reasons, De Wied and associates have adopted, in addition to extinction paradigms, the one-trial passive avoidance test shown in Fig. 3. The advantage of this test is not only that a single trial usually suffices for a rat to acquire the passive avoidance response, but also that retrieval of the response can reliably be determined at a single retention test trial.

2. ACTH-like Peptides

Treatment of intact rats with ACTH analogs during the extinction phase leads to a delay in extinction. We and others have observed that this is true not only for shock-motivated responses (De Wied, 1969; Greven and De Wied, 1973), but also for nonshock aversively motivated (Hennessy et al., 1976; Rigter and Popping, 1976) or food-motivated (Garrud et al., 1974; Kastin et al., 1974) and sexually motivated responses (Bohus et al., 1975b). The general picture for appetitive learning is essentially the same as for aversive learning. Thus, it has been reported that administration of ACTH or ACTH 4–10 during acquisition of an appetitively motivated response, traversing a runway to obtain a food reward, does not change later extinction; injections are effective only when given during the period of extinction (Gray and Garrud, 1977).

Bohus and colleagues (1968) examined in normal rats what happened if ACTH treatment were postponed until extinction of an avoidance response had already substantially progressed. ACTH was able to delay extinction if given during early extinction, a time when control animals were still performing the original response at 70% level. ACTH given later during extinction was ineffective. Apparently, when the tendency to execute the original response is displaced, either by the experience that nonresponding remains unpunished or by interfering behavioral activities, the efficacy of ACTH in retarding extinction disappears.

Another remarkable study that should be mentioned in this context was conducted by De Wied and Bohus (1966). After normal rats had acquired a shuttlebox avoidance response, the animals were subjected to daily extinction tests for 14 days. Treatment during acquisition with Pitressin, a crude posterior lobe extract that contains vasopressin, delayed later extinction in accordance with previous studies. Administration of α-MSH during the acquisition period failed to alter later extinction. In a second experiment, treatment with peptides was restricted to the first extinction period of 14 days. After a rest of 14 days, a second set of extinction sessions was conducted for 3 subsequent days. Pitressin prevented extinction of the shuttlebox response during the extensive first extinction period. Treatment with Pitressin was able to retard extinction even during the second extinction period, 21–24 days after discontinuation of treatment. In contrast, α-MSH delayed extinction only during the actual period of treatment. Thus, α-MSH inhibited extinction during the first extinction period, but its influence did not endure for the interval between the first and second extinction period. During the second extinction period, animals previously treated with α-MSH performed as poorly as control animals.

Using the pole-jump test (Fig. 1), the structure–activity relationships for the inhibitory effect of ACTH-like peptides on extinction have been studied. A consistent finding has been that peptides that share the amino acid sequence Met-Glu-His-Phe-Arg-Trp-Gly (= ACTH 4–10) all retard extinction of the pole-jump response. These peptides include α-MSH and β-MSH. The view that the minimal requirements crucial for behavioral activity reside in the amino acid sequence 4–10 received support from the finding that ACTH 4–10 is as active as the parent hormone or ACTH 1–24 in delaying extinction, whereas ACTH 11–24 is far less active (Greven and De Wied, 1973). Subsequent studies revealed that ACTH 4–7 contains the essential requirements for the inhibitory effect on extinction; the sequences 7–9 and 11–13 seem to possess some behavioral properties in a dormant form (De Wied et al., 1975b; Greven and De Wied, 1977). Structural modifications of ACTH fragments may lead to potentiation (cf., Org 2766) or alteration of behavioral activity. An example of the latter is 7-D-Phe-ACTH 4–10, in which the phenylalanine residue in position 7 is replaced by its D-isomer. This peptide facilitated rather than inhibited extinction of avoidance responses (De Wied, 1969; Greven and De Wied, 1973; Wiegant et al., 1978). When treatment with this D-peptide was terminated, extinction performance returned to control levels (De Wied, 1969).

Kamin (1957) trained rats in a shuttlebox avoidance task and then tested their retention immediately, after 1 to several hours, or 24 hours later. Their retention was relatively poor at intermediate intervals. This phenomenon has become known as the Kamin effect. Klein (1972) showed that the Kamin effect could be blocked by implantation of ACTH into the lateral anterior hypothalamus; that is, ACTH restored normal avoidance behavior at the intermediate retest interval. Klein interpreted the Kamin effect deficit to be due to a failure of retrieval processes associated with a hypo- rather than a hyperfunction of the pituitary–adrenal system. If this were the case, one would expect hypophysectomy to potentiate the Kamin effect. Oddly enough, the fact that ablation of the pituitary gland (Klein and Kopish, 1975; Marquis and Suboski, 1969) does not alter the Kamin effect was interpreted as evidence that a normal pituitary–adrenal system does not seem to be a necessary prerequisite for the retrieval deficit assumed to be the cause of the Kamin effect (Klein and Kopish, 1975).

We now turn to studies that employed the single-trial passive avoidance test. In general, a training-test interval of 24 hours has been used in these studies, since the length of this interval renders it improbable that effects of administration of peptides before the retention test are caused by modulation of memory storage. In experiments designed to assess a facilitatory effect of peptides on retrieval of the passive avoidance response, a relatively mild shock intensity of short duration has been employed that produces in control animals a low level of avoidance. The duration of the shock, and consequently the avoidance level in control animals, was increased in studies designed to measure inhibitory effects on retrieval of the passive avoidance response.

Subcutaneous injection of ACTH-like peptides 1 hour before the retention test raised the entrance latencies (Greven and De Wied, 1973; De Wied, 1974). ACTH 11–24 and ACTH 25–39 were less active than ACTH 1–10 or ACTH 4–10. Control animals hardly avoided at all. This means that the peptide-treated rats probably were more attentive to some conditional stimulus or set of stimuli or were quicker to recognize the motivational value of these stimuli. In the terms of the present chapter, ACTH-related peptides promoted memory retrieval. The possibility that the peptide-treated animals were less active is not likely since ACTH 1–10 did not affect ambulation in the open field test and ACTH 4–10 did not affect entrance latencies in nonshocked rats (Rigter et al., 1974).

The effect of administration of ACTH 1–10 before the first passive avoidance test is of a short-term nature, since potentiation of avoidance was observed 1 hour after a single injection of the peptide but not at a second test 24 hours after the first one (De Wied, 1974). It is difficult to see why peptide-enhanced avoidance performance at the first test would not carry over to the second test. If ACTH 1–10-treated animals, despite an increased avoidance tendency, eventually entered the avoidance box during the first test, the delaying effect of ACTH 1–10 on extinction nevertheless should have prevented the extinction of the avoidance response; these animals should still have displayed avoidance behavior in the second test. On the other hand, if the majority of ACTH 1-10-treated animals did not enter the avoidance box within the time limits of the first test, one could assume (a) that extinction was not a confounding factor; (b) that ACTH 1-10 has a transient effect on memory retrieval; and (c) that the memory that was activated by the peptide during the first test did not sufficiently increase in strength as a result of this activation to be retrieved at the second test. All these assumptions make the interpretation very difficult. What is needed is a separate analysis of data from those peptide-treated rats that did enter at the first test and those that did not.

One more study should be mentioned in the present context. Van Wimersma Greidanus et al. (1978) showed that administration of antiserum against ACTH 1-24 interfered with retrieval of a passive avoidance response in the first and second test sessions in rats, while antiserum against α-MSH reduced the latency only in the second test. The antisera were given before the first test.

3. *Vasopressin-like Peptides*

Subcutaneous administration of Pitressin before acquisition sessions in a shuttlebox test did not enhance the rate of avoidance learning, but produced a delay in later extinction (De Wied and Bohus, 1966). Conversely, intracerebroventricular injection of AVP antiserum before acquisition sessions in the pole-jump test either did not affect (Van Wimersma Greidanus et al., 1975a) or improved (Bohus et al., 1978a) the rate of acquisition; in both experiments subsequent extinction was accelerated. Oxytocin antiserum enhanced acquisition of the pole-jump response, but, in contrast to AVP antiserum, delayed later extinction (Bohus et al., 1978a). These findings indicate that in normal rats changes in vasopressin do not systematically influence multitrial avoidance learning.

We have suggested that the inhibitory action of vasopressin on extinction can, in principle, be explained by assuming that this peptide facilitates memory storage. Such an assumption might account for the similar effects of treatment with vasopressin-like peptides during acquisition and extinction, respectively. Thus, De Wied and Bohus (1966) found that Pitressin delayed extinction of a shuttlebox task when administered during acquisition but also when injected prior to extinction sessions. A single injection of DGLVP also retarded extinction (De Wied et al., 1974).

We doubt, however, that a memory storage hypothesis is sufficient to account fully for the extinction effect of vasopressin and related peptides. An experiment performed by King and De Wied (1974) may serve to illustrate this point. Rats were trained in the pole-jump test. Subsequently, these animals were subjected to forced extinction before the usual extinction sessions were run by placing them in the box with the pole absent. During forced extinction a new experience is acquired because nonresponding is no longer punished by shock. As a rule, forced extinction accelerates regular extinction. The crucial question was what would happen if vasopressin were administered before the start of forced extinction. If the hormone supported the memory of behavior with which it was primarily associated (the experience gained during forced extinction), the effect of forced extinction should be enhanced; instead of retarding the development of normal extinction, vasopressin should even further precipitate extinction. This prediction was proved to be incorrect. In fact, vasopressin partially blocked the effect of forced extinction. The authors concluded that memory storage is not invariably promoted by vasopressin. A possible interpretation of this result is that as a consequence of treatment with the hormone the original memory of aversive experiences was revived to such an extent that acquisition of new material was being blocked. In other words, the forcefulness of a possible retrieval-promoting effect of vasopressin could have prevented optimal processing of new information.

Vasopressin-like peptides also promote the retrieval of a passive avoidance response when given 1 hour before the retention test. This effect has been reported for LVP (Ader and De Wied, 1972), AVP (Bohus et al., 1978b), and DGLVP (De Wied et al., 1974). The action of the vasopressin-like peptides was long-lasting; avoidance responses were still augmented at the second retention test. Furthermore, intracerebroventricular injection of antivasopressin serum 1 hour before the test in the passive avoidance paradigm resulted in a passive avoidance deficit (Van Wimersma Greidanus and De Wied, 1976a). We have outlined above that vasopressin and oxytocin may have opposite effects on memory storage; these hormones also have opposite effects in the present paradigm. Thus, oxytocin administered 1 hour before the retention test impaired passive avoidance behavior (Bohus et al., 1978b).

There is an indication here of a dual effect of both vasopressin and oxytocin. In addition to their effects on memory storage, the preretention test efficacy of vasopressin and oxytocin suggests that they may influence memory retrieval. The long-term nature of the effect of vasopressin suggests that, in addition to a facilitation of retrieval, vasopressin-like peptides may promote the integration of the aversive experience of the retention test with the original learning experience, thus strengthening memory storage.

C. SUMMARY OF EFFECTS IN NORMAL ANIMALS

1. In general, the peptide effects initially explored in hypophysec-tomized animals have been extended to normal rats.

2. Posttrial administration of ACTH has been reported to enhance, or disrupt, subsequently tested retention; both time- and dose-dependent effects have been demonstrated. Together, these findings implicate ACTH as an effective agent in the modulation of memory storage. However, if ACTH were to have a consistent effect on memory storage, one would expect that the effect would persist beyond the actual period of treatment. It remains to be seen how a possible effect of ACTH on memory storage can be reconciled with the often observed short nature of ACTH effects. At present, the view that ACTH modulates processes associated with memory retrieval is more consistently supported but does not preclude a possible effect on memory storage. Evidence for the memory retrieval hypothesis can be derived from preretention test efficacy of ACTH-like peptides.

3. Vasopressin-like peptides exert long-lasting effects on condi-tioned responses; given during acquisition or retention testing, they strengthen responding (e.g., they delay extinction). Posttrial ad-ministration clearly demonstrates their efficacy in promoting storage processes. In the preceding section, however, we have reviewed studies in normal animals in which vasopressin given before retention testing directly affected performance at the retention test. In single-trial passive avoidance studies, for example, retention is tested during a single trial; thus, the enhancement of performance with vasopressin given before the retention trial cannot be explained as a storage effect. Rather, it would seem that vasopressin exerts a role in both storage and retrieval or a process common to both. It remains to be estab-lished under what circumstances vasopressin predominantly affects storage and under what circumstances it affects retrieval.

VI. EFFECTS ON EXPERIMENTAL AMNESIA

A. INTRODUCTION

We have discussed the efficacy of posttraining administration of a compound as a paradigm for differentiating effects on storage from those on performance factors unrelated to memory. Comparison of posttrial with preretention administration allowed us to distinguish storage from retrieval effects. We now turn to a body of related research in which an animal learned a conditioned response and was then subjected to an amnesic treatment. The efficacy of peptide treatment in affecting the amnesia was assessed. In this paradigm, the peptide may be given at about the time of the amnesic treatment; efficacy in the prevention of amnesia may be interpreted as a strengthening of storage processes or as a specific interference with the disruptive influence of the amnesic agent. Alternatively, the peptide may be given prior to retention testing. In this case, a facilitatory action would be most likely because of enhancement of some process associated with retrieval.

B. Prevention of Amnesia

1. ACTH-like Peptides

We have usually employed carbon dioxide (CO_2) to induce amnesia for a one-trial passive avoidance response. Rats were trained in the apparatus shown in Fig. 3. Immediately after the acquisition trial, they were subjected to amnesic treatment by anesthesia with CO_2. Passive avoidance was measured in a single test 24 hours after training. Subcutaneous administration of the peptide ACTH 4–10 1 hour before the acquisition trial failed to prevent amnesia (Rigter et al., 1974). A similar finding was reported by Lande et al. (1972). These investigators, who employed an active avoidance task in which amnesia was induced by the protein synthesis inhibitor puromycin failed to find a preventive action of ACTH. In contrast to these results, however, Flood et al. (1976) presented evidence that under particular experimental conditions ACTH 4–10 may be able to prevent amnesia. Mice were trained in a passive avoidance task, and amnesia was produced by treatment with the protein synthesis inhibitor anisomycin. The degree of amnesia was varied by varying the number of anisomycin injections. A high dose of 3 mg/kg of ACTH 4–10 injected subcutaneously 30 minutes after training lessened partial amnesia. ACTH 4–10 did not alter cerebral protein synthesis measured by the incorporation of valine into protein nor did the peptide influence the inhibition of protein synthesis caused by anisomycin. Flood et al. mentioned the possibility that ACTH 4–10 may play a role in memory storage, perhaps by facilitating essential protein synthesis at sites specific for the memory being established.

2. Vasopressin-like Peptides

In contrast to ACTH, DGLVP administered in a high dose (0.1 mg per mouse) markedly protected animals against the amnesic effect of puromycin (Lande et al., 1972). Mice were trained in a single session to select the correct arm in a Y-maze. A footshock was given for failure to move from the stem of the Y within 5 seconds and for errors of left–right discrimination. Training was terminated when a mouse scored 9 correct responses in 10 consecutive trials. Amnesia was induced by intracerebral injection of puromycin 1 day later. A test of retention of memory was conducted 1 week after administration of puromycin. Puromycin-induced amnesia was almost completely prevented when the mice were treated with DGLVP between 20 hours before and 12 hours after the acquisition of the avoidance response. In a subsequent series of experiments (Walter et al., 1975), an attempt was made to determine structure–activity relationships. Peptides were injected subcutaneously in a single dose of 0.1 mg per mouse immediately after termination of training. The AVP was similar to LVP in efficacy against amnesia; DGLVP was 20% less active. Vasotocin and oxytocin were ineffective. The investigators suggested that the structural properties that appear to be important for the antiamnesic effect of vasopressin congeners include the combination of a cyclic moiety containing the Tyr and Phe residues along with a basic residue in position 8. However, the tail amino acid sequence of oxytocin, Pro-Leu-Gly NH_2 (PLG) was also active. Structural modifications of PLG yielded highly potent peptides, such as Z-Pro-Leu-Gly-NH_2, cyclo (Leu-Gly), and the L and D isomers of Leu-Gly-NH_2. The last two peptides have a low potency in the pole-jump extinction test (Walter et al., 1978), which suggests that different structure–activity relationships may exist for peptide effects in the two paradigms. Another explanation for these discrepancies may be the differences in dose levels employed in the various studies.

In the study by Walter et al. (1975) a single dose of the peptides under examination was used. A recent report on dose-response relationships (Flexner et al., 1977) revealed that AVP was most active in preventing the puromycin effect, followed in order of potency by LVP, DGLVP, PLG, and oxytocin. Oxytocin was active only at high dose levels. We have extended the series of experiments of Flexner and associates by examining the action of vasopressin-like peptides on CO_2-induced amnesia for a passive avoidance response (Rigter et al., 1974; Rigter, unpublished results). AVP and LVP, injected in amounts of 0.3–30 μg per rat 1 hour before training, were able to prevent CO_2-induced amnesia to a marked degree. DGLVP and DGAVP were also active in this respect but somewhat less potent than the parent hormones. In the doses used, oxytocin was without effect (Figs. 9–11). Time-dependence studies have been conducted with DGLVP (Rigter et al., 1975). DGLVP prevented CO_2-induced amnesia if injected subcutaneously less than 4 hours before the acquisition trial or immediately after the acquisition trial and amnesic treatment.

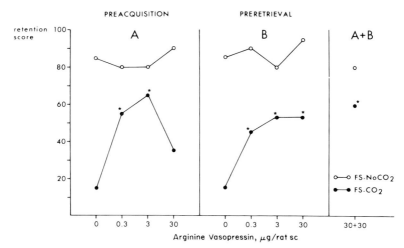

FIG. 9. Effect of arginine vasopressin on CO_2-induced amnesia for a passive avoidance response. FS-CO_2: groups of rats that received amnesic treatment with CO_2 immediately after avoidance training. FS-NoCO_2: groups of rats that were not subjected to amnesic treatment. Retention was tested 24 hours after acquisition. Placebo or peptide was injected subcutaneously 1 hour before acquisition (panel A), 1 hour before retention (panel B), or at both times (A + B). Retention scores are based on categorization of avoidance latencies. Weights were assigned to the performance of the rats: 0 = no avoidance; 1 = incomplete avoidance; 2 = complete avoidance. For each group of 10 animals the individual weights were summed, the maximum for a group being 10 × 2 = 20. The retention score is expressed as the percentage of the maximum score. Asterisks indicate statistically significant difference with respect to similarly treated control group. Statistical analysis was performed by means of the two-tailed randomization test for independent samples.

A variety of agents are able to elicit amnesia in rodents. Another amnesic treatment consists of administering a convulsive dose of pentylenetetrazole. Using this technique, Bookin and Pfeifer (1977) found that 1 µg of LVP per rat, injected subcutaneously 1 hour before training in a passive avoidance task, prevented amnesia in rats. It therefore appears that there is general agreement that vasopressin-like peptides protect animals against the amnesic effect of a variety of agents. The antiamnesic effect of these peptides may result from a facilitation of memory storage or, alternatively, from a reduction of the adverse effects of the amnesic treatment. This latter possibility is rendered improbable by the finding that the antiamnesic effect of vasopressin congeners is not dependent on the type of amnesic agent used.

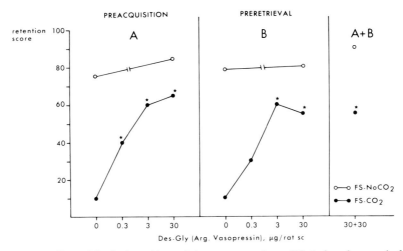

Fig. 10. Effect of deglycinamide arginine vasopressin on CO_2-induced amnesia for a passive avoidance response. See legend to Fig. 9.

C. Reversal of Amnesia

1. *ACTH-like Peptides*

In the preceding section we stated that ACTH 4–10 is ineffective in preventing CO_2-induced amnesia in rats if injected prior to the acquisition trial and the subsequent administration of the amnesic agent. However, we have found that ACTH 4–10 (but not 11–24) attentuates CO_2-induced amnesia when injected 1 hour before the retention test (Rigter *et al.*, 1974, 1977a). This improvement in test performance is probably not due to a general change in locomotor behavior of the rats since the peptide did not change the entrance latencies of rats at the test trial from those of nonshocked control groups, whether CO_2 had been given or not. Neither did ACTH 4–10 alter the avoidance responses exhibited by the rats that had received footshock but no amnesic treatment. This latter finding may seem to be inconsistent with the data discussed earlier, but in this series of experiments the shock intensity was high enough for control animals to show near-optimal avoidance behavior. It is clear that under those circumstances a facilitation of avoidance behavior could not be detected. Still, it could be argued that in the animals subjected to amnesic treatment the avoidance tendency had been reduced sufficiently to allow for an assessment of a possible effect of the ACTH fragment on passive avoidance per se. This explanation is too limited, as we have shown that CO_2-induced amnesia for a thirst-motivated response could also be reversed by pretest treatment with ACTH 4–10 (Rigter and Van

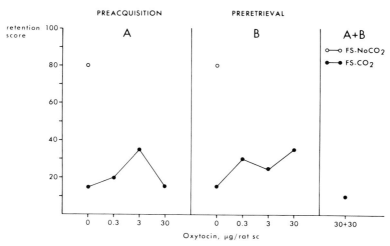

Fɪɢ. 11. Lack of effect of oxytocin on CO_2-induced amnesia for a passive avoidance response. See legend to Fig. 9.

Riezen, 1975). In this study, water-deprived rats were placed one at a time in a circular box. A Perspex pillar was located against the wall of the box, and the spout of an empty water bottle protruded through a niche in the bottom of the pillar. On the acquisition day the bottle was filled with water and the subjects were allowed to drink for a short period. The retention test was conducted 1 day later; during this test the water bottle was empty. Animals that did not receive amnesic treatment explored the niche much more frequently than CO_2-treated animals. The apparent amnesia of the CO_2-treated rats was alleviated by pretest administration of ACTH 4–10.

Various other explanations are possible to account for the antiamnesic effect of ACTH 4–10. It could be surmised that the peptide did antagonize some of the aftereffects of the amnesic agent. This possibility can easily be discounted. First, we have never noticed aftereffects of CO_2 on the test performance of nonshocked control animals. Second, ACTH 4–10 attenuates amnesia induced by a variety of amnesic agents, including electroconvulsive shock (Rigter and Van Riezen, 1975), the protein synthesis inhibitor cycloheximide (Quinton, 1972), and intracerebroventricularly administered vasopressin antiserum (Van Wimersma Greidanus and De Wied, 1976b). Third, in one study we considerably extended the training-test interval. Animals were not tested until 14 days after training and amnesic treatment, at a time when dissipation of any aftereffects of CO_2 would be expected. Amnesia was seen in the placebo-treated control animals, whereas pretest treatment with ACTH 4–10 still resulted in a reversal of amnesia (Rigter et al., 1975).

In our opinion, two possibilities remain as an explanation for the antiamnesic action of ACTH 4–10; either ACTH 4–10 promotes by some process the retrieval of weak memory items spared by the amnesic agent, or the peptide promotes memory retrieval by reversing a retrieval deficit induced by the amnesic treatment. A clear decision between these possibilities must await a definite answer to the question whether amnesia produces faulty storage or faulty retrieval.

2. *Vasopressin-like Peptides*

We have reported that vasopressin congeners prevent amnesia. We have also examined the possibility that these peptides may also reverse amnesia. Subcutaneous injection of DGLVP 1 hour before the retention test diminished CO_2-amnesia for the passive avoidance response (Rigter *et al.*, 1974). Other vasopressin-like peptides have a similar effect (Fig. 9 and 10). This antiamnesic effect of pretest administration of DGLVP does not dissipate when there is an interval of 2 weeks between training and test (Rigter *et al.*, 1975).

D. SUMMARY OF EFFECTS ON AMNESIA

1. Results of studies on experimentally induced amnesia strongly reinforce hypotheses derived from studies in normal animals.

2. ACTH-like and vasopressin-like peptides reverse a previously established amnesia, probably through an enhancement of processes associated with retrieval. In most studies ACTH-like peptides fail to prevent amnesia. Thus, a retrieval effect of ACTH-like peptides is probable, but an effect on storage is less certain.

3. Vasopressin-like peptides are able both to reverse and to prevent amnesia, and therefore seem to influence both retrieval and storage or a process common to both.

VII. THE ENDORPHINS: A NEW FIELD OF RESEARCH

A. INTRODUCTION

In preceding sections we emphasized studies on ACTH-like and vasopressin-like peptides, since for these classes of peptides sufficient data are available to enable a critical analysis of memory effects. Interpretations were facilitated by the fact that both ACTH- and vasopressin-like peptides have been examined in a wide variety of behavioral tests. As yet, only a limited number of neuropeptides have been studied in a sufficiently large battery of animal tests to allow conclusions about the nature and relative importance of their behavioral effects. The use of only a few tests for the evaluation of peptides clearly poses some problems. A subject in a test situation is usually quite restricted in its behavioral repertoire, so behavioral changes assessed in a particular test may be caused by a variety of factors. Thus, the capacity of peptides such as TRH and LHRH to delay transiently extinction of the pole-jump response in rats (De Wied *et al.*, 1975b) cannot simply be taken to indicate that these substances and ACTH exert identical behavioral effects.

The same caveat applies when one considers results obtained with endorphins. Nevertheless, we feel that a section on endorphins should not be omitted from the present review, for we are convinced that memory research will devote much attention to this class of peptides in the next few years. One reason for this attention is the existence of physiological interactions between endorphins and ACTH and vasopressin. Such interactions raise the expectation that endorphins may have some role in memory.

B. INTERACTIONS BETWEEN ENDORPHINS AND ACTH AND VASOPRESSIN

1. *Endorphins and ACTH*

Endorphins were named for their affinity to opiate receptors. A number of endorphins have been isolated from brain and pituitary tissues of a variety of animal species (Hughes *et al.*, 1975; Guillemin *et al.*, 1976; Simantov and Snyder, 1976). These peptides are structurally related to the polypeptide lipotropic hormone (β-lipotropin or β-LPH). β-LPH is present in the pituitary glands of many species, including man (Li and Chung, 1976). This hormone has 91 residues; the C-terminus comprises the sequences 61–91 (= β-endorphin). With the exception of Leu-enkephalin, other endorphins of known composition are identical with part of the amino acid sequence of β-endorphin (Fig. 12) [for a detailed review the reader is referred to the contribution of Miller and Cuatrecasas (1978) in Volume 36 of this series]. It is of interest to note that β-LPH also contains the amino acid sequence of β-MSH and ACTH 4–10 (= β-LPH 47–53).

Several relatively independent endorphin systems have been de-

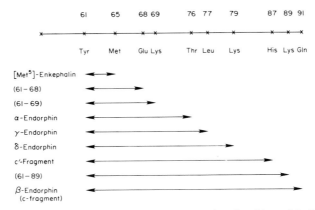

F IG. 12. Correspondence of amino acid sequence of endorphins with C-terminal of polypeptide lipotropic hormone (β-LPH). From Miller and Cuatrecasas (1978), with permission.

tected, some systems being present in brain and others in the pituitary gland. Some systems are closely linked with ACTH, which is not surprising in view of the fact that ACTH and β-LPH derive from a common 31K precursor (Mains *et al.*, 1977; Roberts and Herbert, 1977). This precursor has been named pro-opiocortin (Rubinstein *et al.*, 1978). In rat brain cell bodies of a single hypothalamic group with axons to midbrain and limbic system were found that probably contain β-LPH, β-endorphin ACTH, and the biosynthetic machinery for these peptides (Watson *et al.*, 1977, 1978b; Barchas *et al.*, 1978; Bloom *et al.*, 1978; Akil *et al.*, 1978b). Thus, there is evidence for related brain β-LPH/β-endorphin and ACTH biosynthetic mechanisms and for parallelism in their distribution.

It remains to be seen, however, whether there are multiple brain ACTH systems that perhaps contain different portions of the ACTH molecule. This possibility was raised by reports of differential levels (Krieger *et al.*, 1977b) or localization (Tramu *et al.*, 1977) of ACTH and β-endorphin in brain. However, Akil and co-workers (1978b) were unable to detect any ACTH-like immunoreactivity outside the β-LHP–β-endorphin–ACTH system.

Enkephalin has been detected in many cell groups in brain, in contrast to the single group described for β-LPH–β-endorphin–ACTH. In general, enkephalin cells have relatively short axons, and at least some of them may serve as interneurons (Lamotte *et al.*, 1976; Cuello, 1978; Johansson *et al.*, 1978). So far, immunocytochemical mapping of

Leu- and Met-enkephalin failed to delineate clearly different cerebral distributions for these two peptides (Watson *et al.*, 1977; Akil *et al.*, 1978a; Johansson *et al.*, 1978; Miller and Cuatrecasas, 1978). Differences in brain distribution of enkephalin and β-endorphin cell bodies and fibers indicate the existence of at least two separate opioid peptide neuronal systems (Rossier *et al.*, 1977; Watson *et al.*, 1978a). This view is further supported by the finding that brain lesions differentially affect the enkephalin and endorphin cerebral systems (Watson *et al.*, 1978a).

In addition to these cerebral systems, endorphins were detected in the pituitary. Confusion exists as to the relative distribution of β-LPH and β-endorphin. Guillemin *et al.* (1977) suggested that the anterior lobe of the rat contains much more β-endorphin than β-LPH, but in other studies β-LPH was found to be the major adenohypophysial peptide, and β-endorphin predominated in the intermediate lobe (Rubinstein *et al.*, 1977; Liotta *et al.*, 1978). This difference may be due to differential conversion of β-LPH into β-endorphin in the two pituitary tissues. Lowry and colleagues (Lowry and Scott, 1975; Lowry *et al.*, 1977) proposed that corticotropic cells in both the anterior and the intermediate hypophysial lobes synthesize β-LPH. This hormone presumably is secreted in intact form from the anterior lobe, whereas in the pars intermedia β-LPH serves as a precursor for smaller fragments such as β-endorphin and β-MSH. With respect to the intermediate lobe of the pituitary gland of the rat, experimental support for this proposition was provided by Chretien *et al.* (1978), whose results suggest that β-LPH in the pars intermedia is very rapidly cleaved to form β-endorphin. Bloom (1978) also suggested that the anterior lobe and the intermediate lobe β-LPH–β-endorphin stores are functionally different systems because of his finding that the latter could be depleted by reserpine and the former could not.

Pro-opiocortin is also present in the pituitary gland in concentrations approximately equimolar to those found for β-LPH (Rubinstein *et al.*, 1978). In the intermediate lobe of the rat, β-LPH and ACTH are probably cleaved from this precursor. Such common origin suggests functional interrelationships. This suggestion is even more compelling in view of the finding that β-LPH–β-endorphin are seen only in the corticotropic cells of the anterior and intermediate lobes of all species studied and that they are probably stored in the same secretory granules as ACTH (Bloom *et al.*, 1977; Pelletier *et al.*, 1977; Weber *et al.*, 1978). Joint storage of β-LPH–β-endorphin and ACTH (and possibly other related peptides, cf. Bloom *et al.*, 1977; Bloch *et al.*,

1978) indicates that both classes of peptides are released together. Accordingly, several studies examined the effect of treatments known to produce the release of ACTH-like peptides on their ability to release β-LPH–β-endorphin. Thus, both acute stress and prior adrenalectomy produced concomitant pituitary release of ACTH and β-endorphin in rats while dexamethasone inhibited secretion of both peptides (Guillemin et al., 1977; Akil et al., 1978b). In vitro, purified hypothalamic corticotropin-releasing factor and other putative regulatory agents had similar effects on secretion of β-endorphin- and ACTH-like immunoreactivities (Vale et al., 1978). ACTH and β-LPH are secreted concomitantly in the human after insulin-induced hypoglycemia or vasopressin administration (Krieger et al., 1979). A target organ for the secreted β-LPH–β-endorphin is not yet known.

There is evidence for physiological interaction between ACTH-like peptides and endorphins. Some actions of ACTH-like peptides suggest morphinomimetic properties; others indicate that these peptides are antagonists. Intracerebroventricular administration of ACTH fragments induces a behavioral syndrome that includes excessive grooming, and this is blocked by opiate antagonists (Gispen and Wiegant, 1976). Fragments of β-LPH also elicit excessive grooming (Gispen et al., 1976b). ACTH fragments mimic the effect of morphine in the mouse vas deferens assay and show affinity for morphine antibodies (Plomp and Van Ree, 1978). The nature of the affinity of ACTH 1–24 for brain opiate receptors is suggestive of mixed agonist–antagonist properties (Terenius, 1976). Further, ACTH and related peptides counteract morphine-induced analgesia (Gispen et al., 1976a) and reverse the reduction of spinal reflex activity produced by morphine (Zimmermann and Krivoy, 1973). The structure–activity requirements for activity of ACTH-fragments in these tests may differ somewhat from requirements for activity in learning and vigilance tests (cf. Plomp and Van Ree, 1978).

A recent study by Jacquet (1978) provided further support for functional interrelationships between ACTH and endorphin. Injections of ACTH into the periaqueductal gray area of the brain of rats mimicked an opiate abstinence syndrome characterized by hyperactivity and explosive motor behavior. α-MSH and ACTH 4–10 caused attenuated forms of this syndrome. Injections of β-endorphin at the same brain site caused different responses: sedation, catatonia, and analgesia. Jacquet (1978) proposed that there are distinct ACTH and endorphin receptors, with some degree of interaction. Morphine is thought to activate both receptors; the peptides, therefore, mimic only parts of the morphine syndrome.

2. *Vasopressin and Endorphins*

Recent findings indicate that physiological interactions also exist between vasopressin and endogenous opioid peptides. Intravenous administration of β-endorphin caused the release of vasopressin (Weitzman *et al.*, 1977). Distinct fiber-like processes within the neurohypophysis reacted to enkephalin antiserum (Bloom *et al.*, 1978). Bloom (1978) reported the existence of an enkephalinergic supraoptic–neurohypophysial tract. The nerve terminals of this tract do not contain enkephalin in HO-DI Brattleboro rats. All these data suggest a role for endorphins in the modulation of vasopressin release. On the other hand, vasopressin (an agent known to cause discharge of ACTH from the adenohypophysis) induced release of β-endorphin from the anterior lobe of pituitaries of rats (Przewlocki *et al.*, 1978).

Further support for functional interactions between vasopressin and endorphins is provided by the finding of impaired development of tolerance to the analgetic effects of morphine in HO-DI rats (De Wied and Gispen, 1976). Also, the regional distribution of stereospecific opiate-binding sites was found to be altered in HO-DI rats, when compared to HE-DI and normal Brattleboro animals (Rigter *et al.*, 1979).

C. POSSIBLE EFFECTS OF OPIOIDS ON MEMORY

1. *Opiates and Opiate Antagonists*

Morphine has been studied in one-trial passive avoidance experiments in rats, using posttrial administration. The results are controversial. Belluzzi and Stein (1977) found that intracerebroventricular administration of morphine facilitated retention of the avoidance response. Another group of investigators, however, reported that morphine, administered immediately after training, impaired, while the opiate antagonist naloxone enhanced, retention (Messing *et al.*, 1979). These latter workers injected the drugs intraperitoneally, so that one may surmise that route of administration might explain the discrepancy between the studies of Belluzzi and Stein (1977) and those of Messing *et al.* (1979). It is doubtful if such an explanation would suffice, since Gallagher and Kapp (1978) found results similar to those of Messing and co-workers after intracerebral administration. Posttrial treatment with levorphanol and naloxone impaired and facilitated, respectively, retention of the passive avoidance response. Levorphanol and naloxone were effective when injected into the amygdala, but not when administered into the putamen, which is just dorsal to the amygdala (Gallagher and Kapp, 1978). An interesting aspect of the data of Messing *et al.* (1979) was that low and moderate doses of naloxone and morphine were effective whereas high doses were not. This suggests that, as in the case of many peptides, behavioral activity may disappear or even reverse at doses above an optimal dose.

2. *Endorphins*

The results of posttrial studies with opiate agonists and antagonists raised the expectation that endorphins might influence memory storage. At the time of preparation of this review only one publication on posttrial efficacy of endorphins was available. Subcutaneous injection of α-endorphin immediately after training of a one-trial passive avoidance response facilitated performance in a later retention test. In contrast, γ-endorphin had no effect while posttrial treatment with des-Tyr-γ-endorphin impaired performance in the retention test. All peptides were tested at the single dose of 1.5 μg per rat (De Wied *et al.*, 1978b). Rigter (1978) found that subcutaneous administration to rats of 3–30 μg of Met-enkephalin 1 hour before the acquisition trial of a one-trial passive avoidance response partially prevented CO_2-induced amnesia. Even doses in the nanogram range were slightly effective. Leu-enkephalin did not affect amnesia when given before acquisition. Kastin *et al.* (1976) demonstrated that Met-enkephalin administered intraperitoneally before acquisition sessions facilitated acquisition of an appetitively motivated maze task. Rats given the peptide negotiated the maze faster and made fewer errors than controls. Two analogs, one with and the other without opiate activity, also enhanced acquisition. Although the authors offered some evidence that these peptides, in the doses used, did not affect perception and motility, an effect on other performance factors cannot be excluded. Thus, without further posttrial data and without time-dependence studies, it would be premature to postulate a role of endorphins in memory storage.

There is suggestive, though scanty, support for the notion that endorphins may influence memory retrieval in rats. Rigter (1978) observed that subcutaneous administration of Met-enkephalin of Leu-enkephalin prior to retention testing partially reversed CO_2-induced amnesia for a one-trial passive avoidance response. The results suggest differential activity of Met-enkephalin and Leu-enkephalin. Since the effect of Met-enkephalin (both prevention and reversal of amnesia) resembles that of vasopressin-like peptides and the effect of Leu-enkephalin resembles that of ACTH-like peptides (reversal of amnesia only), it is important to assess possibly differential interactions between these endorphin pentapeptides and ACTH and vasopressin.

De Wied and co-workers examined the potential of endorphins to affect retention test performance when given subcutaneously 1 hour before the first retention test in the one-trial passive avoidance paradigm. α-Endorphin facilitated test performance at the first retention test; as with ACTH 4–10, the effect had disappeared at the time of the second test, which was performed 24 hours after the first one. α-Endorphin also augmented motility in the open field ambulation test, but such an effect cannot explain facilitated performance at the passive avoidance retention test, since one would rather expect increased motility to interfere with test performance (De Wied et al., 1978a). In a subsequent study, the effect of α-endorphin was replicated, although in this experiment the effect of the peptide carried over to the second retention test (De Wied et al., 1978b). This study also examined some other peptides. Pretest administration of γ-endorphin, as in the case of α-endorphin, enhanced avoidance behavior at the first retention test, but the effect had become dissipated by the time of the second test. Also, γ-endorphin was active in only half of the animals tested. Des-Tyr-γ-endorphin attenuated avoidance behavior, with the effect still present at the second retention test. This particular study also included control groups that were tested in the open field. In this case, no effect on ambulation was seen with α-endorphin, γ-endorphin, or des-Tyr-γ-endorphin. Thus, motility changes probably did not confound the effects of these peptides on performance in the avoidance tests.

Endorphins were also tested in the pole-jump extinction paradigm (De Wied, 1977; De Wied et al., 1978a,b). α-Endorphin, β-endorphin, β-LPH 61–69, and Met-enkephalin consistently delayed extinction; γ-endorphin, and even more so des-Tyr-γ-endorphin, facilitated extinction.

In the above studies, the peptides were effective after both subcutaneous and intracerebroventricular routes of administration. The endorphins affected extinction and passive avoidance in doses generally lower than those necessary for the elicitation of analgesia (De Wied, 1977). An interesting lead for future studies is the possibility that the behavioral effects of endorphins, as assessed in tests of learning and memory, are not associated with the opioid activity of these peptides. This is suggested by the behavioral efficacy of peptides that have no affinity for opiate binding sites, such as des-Tyr-γ-endorphin

(De Wied *et al.*, 1978b) and D-4-Phe-Met-enkephalin amide (Kastin *et al.*, 1976) and also by the failure of naloxone to counteract the antiamnesic effects of the enkephalins (Rigter *et al.*, 1977a).

In conclusion, we have summarized evidence that endorphins may modulate memory processes. However, more studies are needed to exclude alternative hypotheses.

VIII. Peptides and Memory Processes: Human Data

A. Introduction

Virtually nothing is known about the possible physiological role of peptides in human mental performance. Clinical reports on psychological and electroencephalographic changes in hyper- and hypocorticoid patients (Cleghorn, 1957; Delay *et al.*, 1954; Goulon and Aubert, 1959) suggest that pituitary–adrenal hormones may influence brain activity in man, but these observations have not led to sufficient attempts to characterize the possible behavioral activity of these and other hormones in man.

One experimental approach would be to study possible psychological deficits exhibited by patients subjected to hypophysectomy or with altered pituitary function. An obvious problem is that disturbances of pituitary function may give rise to marked metabolic disorders that easily mask alterations in mental performance. Conversely, improvements in mental performance after hormonal correction of the metabolic disorders cannot simply be ascribed to a direct beneficial effect of a hormone on some mental process, since such improvements may also result from restored feelings of well-being. Therefore, it is difficult to evaluate a report by Luria (1976) that patients with pituitary tumors often exhibited memory disturbances. These memory deficits were more severe in cases where there was proliferation of the tumor from the pituitary gland to adjacent brain areas. Patients with tumors restricted to the pituitary gland itself had no difficulty in memorizing various types of information, as long as they were not distracted. Recall of simple items was impaired, however, when the learning experience was followed by interfering activity, such as conversation or the requirement to perform an arithmetical task. This finding suggests that in patients with pituitary tumors memory processing may be abnormally susceptible to interference by distraction. If true, such an interpretation has important theoretical implications, and an independent repetition of Luria's study is therefore clearly needed.

Another approach would be to administer peptides, preferably peptides without marked peripheral endocrine activity, to healthy subjects. A disadvantage of this approach is that these subjects are often already highly motivated to perform optimally on psychological tests. Under such conditions, it is difficult to assess the potential of a peptide to enhance performance. This objection may account for the failure of initial human studies to demonstrate clear-cut peptide effects on most tests of memory (see below).

Consequently, research efforts in man are presently concentrated on two strategies. The first is to give normal subjects tests that are so demanding that control subjects fail to maintain an optimal performance level over time. This type of investigation attempts to counteract the resulting performance decrement with peptide treatment. The second strategy is to assess peptide effects in subjects with specific deficits in mental performance. Such studies used retardates, elderly people with memory complaints, or hyperactive learning-disabled children as subjects. Ideally, for both strategies one would like to see correlations between endogenous hormonal function, initial performance deficit, and efficacy of treatment with exogenous peptides. However, such elaborate studies have not yet been conducted.

B. STUDIES IN NORMAL SUBJECTS

1. *Introduction*

The hypothesis that ACTH 4–10 may modulate memory processes prompted a number of studies in man. In the majority of the experiments, subjects were required to complete a battery of memory tests shortly after a (usually) acute treatment with ACTH 4–10. As a rule, only seconds or minutes intervened between the "acquisition" and "test" phases. In general, these studies do not, therefore, allow a distinction between short-term peptide effects on memory storage and memory retrieval; moreover, most of these studies provide no information about the possible efficacy of the peptide in altering longer-term aspects of memory processing.

2. *ACTH-like Peptides*

a. Effects on Memory. Effects of ACTH 4–10 on short-term recall of verbal material have been assessed in a number of ways. For instance, various kinds of association learning tests have been applied. Ex-

amples of association learning tests are paired-associate learning and
the first and last names test. In paired-associate learning, word pairs
are presented until a list is learned. Retention is tested by presentation of only the first member of each pair, and the subject must respond with the appropriate word associate. The first and last names
test employs a list of paired first and last names. Shortly after inspec-
tion of this list, a list of only the last names is presented and the subject is asked to recall the corresponding first names.

Miller *et al.* (1976) examined ACTH 4–10 in healthy male volunteers
in a complete crossover, double-blind design. A single subcutaneous
injection of 30 mg of the peptide failed to influence paired-associate
learning in this study. The first and last names test also yielded
negative results with ACTH 4–10 in a study with healthy volunteers
(Sannita *et al.*, 1976). Other tests of short-term recall of verbal items
have similarly failed to yield consistent effects of ACTH 4–10. Dornbush and Nikolovski (1976) used short-term memory tests in which
consonant trigrams (series of three consonants such as "DKG") were
presented either auditorily or visually to healthy volunteers. Subjects
were required to recall each trigram after intervals of 0, 6, 12, and 18
seconds. During the retention intervals, subjects were given a 3 digit
number from which they had to count backward. The procedure
prevented subjects from rehearsing the trigram, so that relatively un-
confounded measures of duration of short-term memory could be obtained. Strength and duration of short-term memory were similar
after peptide and control treatment. Two studies in normal subjects
reported facilitatory effects of ACTH 4–10 on memory span for series
of digits (Miller *et al.*, 1976; Sannita *et al.*, 1976). This finding was not
confirmed in a third investigation (Sandman *et al.*, 1975).

Ashton *et al.* (1977) gave normal male subjects 10 mg of α-MSH,
β-MSH 1–22, or placebo intravenously in a double-blind crossover
design. Several tests of memory were given, and the contingent
negative variation, an EEG index sensitive to stimulant and depres-
sant drugs, was measured. α-MSH facilitated and β-MSH 1–22
disrupted performance on verbal scales of the Wechsler Memory
Scale. Tests of mental arithmetic, mood, and the contingent negative
variation were not affected. Veith *et al.* (1978) found a similar facilitation of verbal memory in normal females after 30 mg of ACTH 4–10
had been given subcutaneously. In a concept learning task, acquisition of a discrimination was not affected, but reversal learning was impaired by peptide treatment.

Another line of research has employed tests of visual memory. In
four studies the effect of ACTH 4–10 on performance of healthy sub-

jects on the Benton Visual Retention Test was determined. This test involves the presentation of sets of geometric forms of varying complexity. Fifteen seconds after removal of each picture, subjects are instructed to reproduce it. Whereas one study reported a beneficial effect of the peptide on visual retention (Miller *et al.*, 1976), the other studies failed to establish a significant effect of ACTH 4–10 (Sannita *et al.*, 1976; Sandman *et al.*, 1977; Veith *et al.*, 1978). α-MSH similarly failed to affect the Benton test (Ashton *et al.*, 1977). ACTH 4–10 was also inactive in another test of short-term retention of visual items (Dornbush and Nikolovski, 1976).

In summary, a number of studies have attempted to assess effects of ACTH 4–10 on learning and retention in man. The conditions used in these investigations were rather restricted. In most of the experiments the peptide was acutely injected in a single dose. Correlations between endogenous levels of ACTH-like peptides, control performance, and performance of subjects after treatment with ACTH 4–10 or MSH have not yet been studied. In general, the tests employed focused on short-term retention. Within this limited framework, ACTH 4–10 did not have consistent effects on normal memory.

b. Effects on Vigilance. ACTH-like peptides have been stated to enhance performance by increasing selective attention (Sandman and Kastin, 1977) or by increasing arousal in response to motivationally relevant stimuli (De Wied, 1976a). In our opinion, the available data cannot clearly distinguish between these related concepts. Selective attention suggests responding to relevant stimuli and ignoring those that have no behavioral significance. It seems clear that selective attention cannot be maintained without both adequate arousal and motivation. Whether ACTH-like peptides affect retrieval processes by influencing attention, motivation, or arousal is not easily distinguishable within existing animal research paradigms (see Table I). In human research, the maintenance of selective attention is usually termed vigilance; we will consider performance attributable to sustained attention (and the presumed adequacy of motivational and arousal levels) under this descriptive common denominator.

Initial suggestion of a possible influence of peptides on vigilance came from a study in healthy volunteers in which ACTH 4–10 was found to delay the development of electroencephalographic signs of habituation in a "go–no go" reaction time task (Miller *et al.*, 1974). Subjects were requested to respond to a "go" signal by pressing a lever and to refrain from pressing when the "no go" signal was presented. Peptide-treated subjects habituated normally to the "no go" signal, but, in contrast to placebo-treated subjects, exhibited no habituation to the "go" signal. This was considered to be evidence for an enhancement of selective attention by ACTH 4–10. In a subsequent double-blind crossover investigation, performance of healthy subjects on a continuous vigilance task was evaluated. This task required subjects to view an oscilloscope screen on which letters appeared briefly and press a button whenever the letter X appeared. The difficulty of the task was varied by decreasing the relative frequency of occurrence of the letter X. ACTH 4–10 led to improved performance on the first occasion when the difficulty level of the task was changed. Subjects at this time detected more Xs and responded incorrectly to other letters less frequently. Since the peptide-induced facilitation could not have been caused simply by increased response rate, it was interpreted as an improvement of attention (L. Miller *et al.,* 1976).

Another study with the same peptide reinforces this type of hypothesis. Gaillard and Sanders (1975) gave two groups of normal subjects subcutaneous injections of either placebo or 30 mg of ACTH 4–10. The subjects were then tested for reaction time in a continuous session. In this task, the subject was instructed to respond to one of six lights by pressing the appropriate key as quickly as possible. Shortly after each response, a new light appeared; therefore, in order to perform well, the subject had to monitor the light panel continuously. Performance was measured by accuracy of response (whether the correct key was pressed) and reaction time (latency to press the key). As training progressed on this task, the average reaction time remained stable, but two tendencies developed. First, there was a gradual shortening of reaction time because of learning. On the other hand, there was an increased incidence of long reaction times, which was attributed to mental fatigue or loss of motivation (but which also could have been decreased arousal or a loss of attention). These two counterbalancing trends resulted in stable average performance in the control group. However, the number of errors increased as training progressed. ACTH 4–10 prevented the increase in the incidence of long reaction time trials seen in the placebo group. In addition, it prevented the elevation in error rate normally seen. Gaillard and Varey (1977) obtained similar results with orally administered Org 2766. In both studies, the effects of the peptide had become dissipated at the time of a short retest 35 minutes later. This was taken as strong evidence of a specific effect on motivation as opposed to an effect on learning.

Further support for the view that ACTH-like peptides influence vigilance in man comes from a study by O'Hanlon (personal communication). Normal subjects were given an oral placebo, 40 mg of Org

2766, or 10 mg *d*-amphetamine and then were tested in a visual signal-detection task. Each subject was tested three times and served as his own control. Signal detection deteriorated in the subjects given the placebo as the test progressed. This decline was blocked by Org 2766. Amphetamine also prevented the decline in signal detection and improved performance in the middle of the test as well. Subsequent analysis showed that the drug effects were more clear-cut in those subjects who had performed most poorly when given the placebo. Subjective state was also assessed by questionnaire; peptide and *d*-amphetamine treatments could be distinguished from each other as well as from placebo. Finally, only amphetamine depressed EEG theta energy. The effect of Org 2766, however, was not confirmed in a subsequent experiment with elderly subjects.

3. *Vasopressin*

In one preliminary study (Legros *et al.*, 1978) vasopressin was administered by nasal spray to men aged 50–65 years. Subjects were given either lysine vasopressin or placebo three times daily for 3 days. The approximate total daily dose of vasopressin was 16 IU. Performance on a variety of psychometric tests was assessed before and after the period of treatment. Vasopressin-treated subjects showed significant improvement in tests of attention, concentration, and motor speed [K.T. attention test and the digit-symbol substitution subscale of the Wechsler Adult Intelligence Scale (W.A.I.S.)]. Further, improvement was seen on the digit span scale of the W.A.I.S. and in several visual and verbal memory tests of Rey. The design of the study did not allow detection of a possible effect of vasopressin on memory storage.

C. STUDIES IN COGNITIVELY IMPAIRED SUBJECTS

1. *Introduction*

A problem in assessing peptide effects in humans has been that normal subjects in general exhibit a memory capacity sufficiently strong that a "ceiling" effect makes it very difficult to induce a measurable improvement. Indeed, most of the tasks employed in the research surveyed in the preceding section are more sensitive for the assessment of impaired than enhanced function. As a consequence of this limitation, subsequent studies have turned to subjects with specific or general cognitive deficits in the hope that the lower baseline performance of such subjects might allow the expression of peptide effects.

2. ACTH 4–10

a. Effects on Memory. Ferris *et al.* (1976) gave 15 or 30 mg of ACTH 4–10 subcutaneously to cognitively impaired elderly subjects. Mildly impaired patients were less deficient in paired-associate learning than severely impaired patients. ACTH 4–10 was ineffective in both groups of subjects in modulating learning. However, the peptide had a dose-related effect on the first and last names test. Patients with severe cognitive impairment improved with 15 mg of ACTH 4–10, but not with 30 mg; mildly impaired patients improved with 30 mg of ACTH 4–10, but not with 15 mg. The peptide has also been investigated in children suffering from minimal brain dysfunction (Rapoport *et al.,* 1976). Features of this syndrome include hyperactivity and impaired learning. A single subcutaneous dose of 30 mg of ACTH 4–10 was also without effect on paired-associate learning in this group of subjects. However, this study suffered from the fact that it was difficult to motivate the children to perform stably on the tests.

Two studies assessed delayed recall of a problem after ACTH treatment. In the study by Ferris *et al.* (1976) previously described, day-later recall for visual material was assessed in geriatric patients with mild cognitive impairment. Test performance was impaired on the day following subcutaneous injection of 30 mg of ACTH 4–10. On the other hand, the recognition of visual items was improved in severely impaired subjects given 30 mg of ACTH 4–10. In another study, retention was tested 48 hours after training (Small *et al.* 1977). This study attempted to assess whether subcutaneous ACTH 4–10 could counteract or reduce memory impairments induced in psychiatric patients by electroconvulsive shock (ECS). Observations after a single ECS suggested some positive effects, but studies between seizures after 5 or 6 ECS treatments showed no significant peptide effects. Although these findings were largely negative, the authors did not rule out positive effects of ACTH 4–10 on memory. Possibly the design and timing of the experiments, which were different from the parameters usually employed in animal experiments, were unsuitable for demonstrating influences of ACTH 4–10.

Finally, Branconnier *et al.* (1978) tested volunteers over the age of 60 who exhibited neuropsychological impairment of visual reaction time and memory. ACTH 4–10 (30 mg subcutaneously) was tested against placebo in a double-blind crossover design with 14 days between test sessions. No significant peptide effects were found for the Perceptual Trace, Bender-Gestalt, or Wechsler Memory Scale. A tendency toward an improvement in reaction time was seen briefly after peptide treatment, and the peptide significantly reduced the percentage of α-EEG time. The peptide also reduced confusion, anger, and depression while enhancing vigor on the Profile of Mood States.

b. *Effects on Vigilance.* One study undertook to study vigilance in the mentally retarded (Sandman *et al.*, 1976). Adult retardates were trained on a visual discrimination task and subsequently on reversal, intradimensional, and extradimensional shifts. The visual stimuli differed in two dimensions, e.g., color and shape. If during original acquisition the subjects had learned to choose between stimuli on the basis of color (blue versus green) and to disregard shape, color remained the relevant dimension during reversal training (green instead of blue). On the intradimensional shift, a new set of stimuli with new colors and shapes was presented, color still being the relevant cue (e.g., red). The extradimensional shift required a subject to ignore the previously correct cue (color) and start to respond on the basis of shape. Performance of subjects on both intra- and extradimensional shift was improved after treatment with ACTH 4–10. These results were attributed to an improvement in attention. The effect of ACTH 4–10 on reaction time reported by Branconnier *et al.* (1978) may also indicate an effect on attention.

3. *Vasopressin*

In the first investigation of the efficacy of vasopressin in cognitively impaired subjects (Moeglen *et al.*, 1977; Oliveros *et al.*, 1978), vasopressin was administered to three amnesic patients by means of intranasal spray. One male patient suffered from a syndrome reminiscent of Korsakoff's disease. This syndrome is often seen in subjects with a prior history of excessive and prolonged alcohol intake, and its primary feature is amnesia. The patient concerned suffered from severe retrograde amnesia (inability to recall experiences that occurred in a particular time period before the onset of illness) and from anterograde amnesia (inability to memorize experiences after the onset of illness). Treatment with vasopressin was prescribed at a dose of 11 IU/day, divided among 4 nasal sprays. There was an improvement in both retrograde and anterograde amnesia within days. The patient became hypomanic under treatment; this subsided approximately 4 days after cessation of treatment. Memory functions did not relapse after treatment was stopped. The second patient was a female with retrograde and anterograde amnesia resulting from the trauma associated with a car accident 6 years earlier. The severity of her retrograde amnesia was illustrated by loss of memory for English although she had spoken it fluently as a second language for many years. Her anterograde amnesia was apparent, for instance, in the difficulty she had in remembering where she had placed pieces of furniture at home. Vasopressin was given for 9 days in a daily dose of about 13.5 IU. At the end of treatment clinical assessment showed considerable improvement. For example, her knowledge of the English language had returned. There was no marked relapse after cessation of treatment. As the result of a car accident the third patient presented severe retrograde and anterograde amnesia for the 3 months before the accident and the 3.5 months afterward. Vasopressin was administered in a daily dose of about 13.5 IU. Seven days after the start of treatment memory had completely recovered and remained stable after cessation of treatment.

A second report has since appeared (Blake *et al.*, 1978) about a study in which 16 IU of vasopressin were given daily via nose spray to two alcoholic patients. Both patients (one male, one female) expressed global confusional states making it impossible to assess specific memory deficits. High doses of thiamine alleviated the global confusion, leaving Korsakoff-type amnesic syndromes. Treatment with vasopressin for 15 or 21 days, respectively, induced no further improvement. In a third report, Le Boeuf *et al.* (1978) gave 22.5 IU of LVP per day to a single Korsakoff patient in a crossover design. They reported a dramatic improvement in several memory tests; they also noted clinical improvement to such an extent that outpatient status was considered. Success with one other patient studied in less controlled fashion was also reported. Finally, the authors noted that vasopressin was much less effective in senile dementia; this suggests that some unknown number of patients had failed to respond to the drug.

These findings must be considered to be merely of anecdotal value. The possible therapeutic action of vasopressin on amnesia suggests that also in man vasopressin is able to facilitate memory storage or retrieval. However, further investigations under stringently controlled conditions in a larger number of patients are clearly called for.

D. SUMMARY OF PEPTIDE EFFECTS IN HUMANS

The evaluation of the human psychopharmacology of ACTH 4–10 has yielded unclear results. Given the consistency with which ACTH affects several aspects of memory in animals, the most striking feature of the literature on human subjects reviewed in the previous section is the inconsistency with which effects appear. We do not understand the basis for this discrepancy of results in the two populations, but more than one factor probably contributes. Insofar as normal human subjects have adequately functioning memory systems, a ceiling effect may have prevented the expected expression of peptide enhancement in these studies. The more consistently positive results seen in studies that employed fatiguing tests or that used subjects suffering from some form of cognitive impairment tend to support this hypothesis. It should be noted, however, that even in impaired subjects the results were equivocal. Thus, it seems unlikely that experimental and methodological limitations alone could explain the difference. A second possibility is that ACTH-like peptides favor a process that is relatively more important in the expression of animal memory than human memory. In Section II we outlined some differences between human and animal memory processes. The complexity of memory functioning in man and the presumed high degree of adaptability that human subjects bring to an experimental situation make it likely that there will be compensation for experimental conditions that might relatively impair cognitive functioning. Without such a background of impairment, one might expect it to be difficult to display effects of peptide treatment. If this is true, then tasks that measure more specifically noncognitive performance capability should be more amenable to manipulation with peptides. In support of this notion is the fact that tests of vigilance have shown the most reliable peptide effects in man.

IX. POSSIBLE SITES AND MECHANISMS OF ACTIONS

A. NEUROANATOMY

1. *ACTH-like Peptides*

One technique that has been exploited to examine possible sites of action of ACTH fragments is the local application of crystalline peptide into various brain areas. Van Wimersma Greidanus and De Wied (1971) fixed stainless steel plates on the skull of rats; these plates contained 12 holes through which hollow needles could be lowered to specified brain areas. After recovery from surgery, the animals were trained in the pole-jump task. ACTH 1-10 was administered before extinction. Unilateral microinjections of the peptide into the posterior thalamic area, including the parafascicular nucleus, mimicked the inhibitory effect of systemic administration on extinction of the avoidance response. Implantation of ACTH 1–10 into the ventral thalamic nucleus, the anterior medial nucleus reuniens, the fasciculus retroflexus, the globus pallidus, the caudate or the preoptic nucleus was without effect.

The results of implantation indicate that the posterior thalamic area may be involved in the regulation of the behavioral activity of ACTH-like peptides. However, this does not mean that other brain sites are not involved. Apart from the fact that in the implantation study only a limited number of sites were studied and unilateral application of relatively small amounts of peptide was employed, it is probable that the function of ACTH-sensitive areas is critically dependent on the activity of a number of interconnected brain sites. In an attempt to obtain additional information, it was therefore decided to examine the effects of brain lesions. Bilateral lesions in the parafascicular area did not substantially affect acquisition of an active response but produced a facilitation of extinction. The lesions rendered rats insensitive to the action of ACTH 4–10 and α-MSH on extinction. Similarly, ACTH 4–10 was ineffective in delaying extinction in rats bearing lesions in the anterodorsal hippocampus and the rostral septum (Bohus and De Wied, 1967; Van Wimersma Greidanus, 1977). The importance of the septum for the mediation of behavioral activity of ACTH and related peptides is further exemplified by the preferential uptake of the ACTH 4–9 analog, Org 2766, by septal nuclei (Verhoef et al., 1977). Finally, ACTH has been identified in the amygdala by radioimmunoassay (Pacold et al., 1978) and systemic administration of ACTH to amygdalectomized rats restored the surgically induced deficit in shuttlebox responding to normal (Bush et al., 1973). On the basis of these data we conclude that the integrity of several midbrain-limbic brain structures is a prerequisite for at least some of the behavioral actions of ACTH-like peptides (Fig. 13).

2. Vasopressin

A growing body of data indicates that there may be vasopressin-containing pathways in the brain other than the hypothalamo-neurohypophysial connection. Vasopressin is synthesized in hypothalamic neurons, notably the nucleus supraopticus, the nucleus paraventricularis, and the nucleus suprachiasmaticus (Vandesande et al., 1975; Buys, 1978). From there the hormone is transported to the

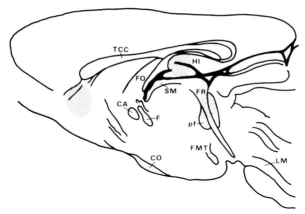

FIG. 13. Brain areas (stippled) implicated in the behavioral actions of ACTH-like and vasopressin-like peptides (rostroseptal area, anterodorsal hippocampus and the parafascicular nuclei). CA, commissura anterior; CO, chiasma opticum; F, columna fornicis; FMT, fasciculus mamillothalamicus; FO, fornix; FR, fasciculus retroflexus; HI, hippocampus; LM, lemniscus medialis; pf, nucleus parafascicularis; SM, stria medullaris thalami; TTC, truncus corpus callosi. Adapted from Van Wimersma Greidanus (1977), with permission. By courtesy of S. Karger, Basel, Switzerland.

posterior pituitary, but this is not the only route of transport. Vasopressin is probably released also into the hypophysial portal vessels. Furthermore, axons that originate in vasopressin-containing hypothalamic areas run to the walls of the brain ventricular system, and there is evidence for direct secretion of vasopressin into the cerebrospinal fluid. Indeed, it has been proposed that the cerebrospinal fluid is the preferential route of transport for vasopressin to accomplish its behavioral actions (see review by Van Wimersma Greidanus and De Wied, 1977). It is also possible that the behavioral actions of vasopressin are mediated through postulated networks of neurosecretory fibers originating in the hypothalamus and coursing to the limbic system (amygdala, hippocampus, and septum), medulla oblongata, and spinal cord (Sterba, 1974; Brownfield and Kozlowski, 1977; Buys, 1978).

Attempts to detect vasopressin-sensitive brain sites have followed the same approaches as employed for ACTH. Implantation of crystalline LVP into the posterior thalamic area produced delayed extinction of the pole-jump response. Microinjections into other brain structures, including ventromedial and anteromedial parts of the thalamus, posterior hypothalamus, substantia nigra, retricular formation, substantia grisea, putamen, and dorsal hippocampus were ineffective

in this regard (Van Wimersma Greidanus *et al.*, 1975c). The brain lesion approach revealed that, as in the case with ACTH, the septum
and the dorsal hippocampus may have a role in behavioral actions of
vasopressin (Fig. 13). Extensive electrolytic destruction of the preoptic rostral area or the dorsal hippocampal complex prevented
vasopressin-induced retardation of extinction. Surprisingly, lesions in
the posterior thalamus, notably the parafascicular nuclei, had a lesser
effect on vasopressin-induced delay of extinction. Although these
latter lesions reduced the behavioral action of the hormone, they did
not completely prevent it. Thus, while the parafascicular region was
sensitive to the action of vasopressin, it did not seem to be crucial.
Such lesioned rats only required more vasopressin to exhibit delayed
extinction (Van Wimersma Greidanus *et al.*, 1975c).

3. *Possible Functions of Peptide-Sensitive Brain Areas*

a. Posterior Thalamus. Delacour (1971) reviewed studies in rats on
the behavioral consequences of electrolytic destruction of the centrum
medianum–parafascicular complex. Lesions in this area decreased performance in a shuttlebox test both in rats operated before the beginning of training and in rats trained before operation and tested by
postoperative retraining. This performance deficit could not be ascribed to changes in motility or pain sensitivity. The lesion did not interfere with memory in general since it had no or only a slight effect
on passive avoidance behavior or on acquisition and retention of appetitively motivated responses. It is of interest that destruction of
this part of the thalamus in cats and monkeys failed to affect performance. This suggests that there may be species differences in the
relative importance of this brain structure in the mediation of
particular responses. Delacour (1971) proposed that the centrum
medianum–parafascicular complex is involved either in arousal or in
motor control, with the result that adaptive behavior is protected
against interference by competing responses. If so, the role of the
ACTH-sensitive substrate in this area might be dampening of arous-
ing properties of distracting stimuli.

b. Septum. The septal area in rats subserves at least four dis-
sociable behavior patterns; of these, the control of responding to
reinforcing stimuli seems most relevant to the present discussion. Mc-
Cleary (1966) developed the influential theory that septal damage produces a lack of response inhibition. However, it is apparent from many
subsequent studies (reviewed by Fried, 1972) that disinhibition is not

an inevitable consequence of injury to the septum. Fried proposed that septal dysfunction results in a release of those behaviors that are highest in habit strength for a particular situation, thereby preventing new responses from stabilizing. Animals with septal damage overrespond to motivating stimuli in a variety of situations; for example, increasing their rate of responding if reinforcement is received or expected. Further, they are impaired in their ability to suppress responses that have been reinforced in the past; thus, they exhibit delayed extinction and deficient passive avoidance behavior. It should be stressed that septally lesioned animals certainly do not exhibit a general deficit (Fried, 1972), although it is not impossible that a further fractionation of the behavioral syndrome shown by such animals may reveal that this area, or part of it, is involved in aspects of memory.

c. Hippocampus. Classic reviews on the behavioral functions of the hippocampus in animals have concluded that this area, like the septum, may be involved in the control of response suppression, although it certainly has no unitary function. In agreement with this view, most workers have found delayed extinction and impaired passive avoidance behavior after hippocampectomy (Douglas, 1967; Kimble, 1968).

Experimental interest in the behavioral functions of the hippocampus in animals has been stimulated by reports that human subjects with hippocampal lesions, in addition to damage to adjoining temporal lobe structures, have impaired memory (Scoville and Milner, 1957; Drachman and Hughes, 1971). The finding that hippocampectomized animals have no generalized memory impairment (Douglas, 1967; Kimble, 1968) has been considered to be an embarrassing discrepancy with the results of clinical studies that show amnesia after medial temporal (including hippocampal) lesions in man. Recent attempts to reconcile the animal and human data have yielded some promising hypotheses. The amnesia shown by subjects with temporal lobe damage had traditionally been interpreted as a failure of memory storage, but there is now evidence that at least part of the difficulty exhibited by these subjects in tests of memory is due to a disruption of memory retrieval. This faulty memory retrieval could result from an increased susceptibility to interfering memory material. Warrington and Weiskrantz (1973) advanced the theory that amnesic patients fail to inhibit or dissipate irrelevant information. In support of this view, these authors found that amnesic subjects demonstrated normal retention when memory was tested by means of a partial information method, either cueing with the first three letters of the five-letter test words or cueing with a perceptually fragmented form of the test words. Warrington and Weiskrantz argued that cueing reduced interference by decreasing the number of response alternatives, and thus alleviated the retrieval deficit. This view has been weakened somewhat by others (Marslen-Wilson and Teuber, 1975), who confirmed the efficacy of the cueing procedure but also found evidence for faulty storage in amnesic subjects.

Nevertheless, with this reinterpretation of at least part of the syndrome exhibited by patients with temporal lobe damage, the prospect of a reconciliation of animal and human data has been opened. Correll and Scoville (1970) have presented evidence that hippocampectomized monkeys show a retrieval deficit attributable to interference from antecedent memory. Further, an attempt has been made to discriminate two types of retrieval, an "associative" and a "contextual" retrieval system (Hirsh, 1974). According to this theory, hippocampal dysfunction would not lead to deficits in performance in situations where associative retrieval would be sufficient to maintain adequate responding; however, when an experimental situation demanded the use of contextual retrieval, the hippocampectomized animal would fail. One prediction derived from this theory is that animals with the hippocampus ablated will be less distracted than normal animals by irrelevant stimuli when these stimuli are clearly distinct from task-relevant stimuli, but will be more distracted when the irrelevant stimuli are similar to task-relevant stimuli. Hirsh (1974) cited evidence in favor of this prediction. The relevance of the theoretical constructs used by Hirsh remains to be determined. His analysis offers promise, however, that the bewildering gap between animal and human data eventually may be bridged. Further, it is possible that the relative inefficacy of peptide treatment in man as opposed to animals may result from the differential nature of the information processing between the species.

In sum, peptide-sensitive brain areas are involved in the mediation of a variety of behavioral functions. Among these functions are attention and memory processing. There is, therefore, a semblance of logic in the attempt to relate the normal function of these active sites to the action of the peptides. Such an analysis is hampered, however, by the hypothetical character of the theoretical constructs employed (e.g., "(selective) attention," "memory retrieval"). The picture is further complicated by the possible existence of species differences in the roles of these brain structures.

B. NEUROPHYSIOLOGY

ACTH-like and vasopressin-like peptides have been reported to influence a host of electrophysiological indices (reviewed by Bohus and De Wied, 1978; Urban, 1977), of which only a limited number may be inferred to be of importance within the context of a discussion on memory. In general, ACTH has been found to increase the firing rate of neurons in the hypothalamus and the hippocampus of rats or rabbits (Steiner, 1970; Pfaff *et al.*, 1971; Van Delft and Kitay, 1972; Baldwin *et al.*, 1974). In cats treatment with ACTH decreased firing in the septum and the preoptic area (Korányi *et al.*, 1971a,b). Presumably, dose, species, and brain region are crucial variables. Also, it is not clear at present whether the neurophysiological responses to ACTH can be mimicked by fragments and analogs, such as ACTH 4–10. Such knowledge is essential to decide whether and which neurophysiological effects of ACTH are relevant for an understanding of its behavioral activity.

Our knowledge of possible actions of ACTH-like peptides on the electrical activity of the human brain is equally sketchy. Nevertheless, the dramatic effects of ACTH on petit mal epilepsy in some children (Klein, 1970) suggest a role for this hormone, and possibly for related peptides, in the regulation of brain electrical activity. In some studies in man (Section VIII,B), EEG measures have been included as an adjunct to behavioral testing. ACTH 4–10 retarded habituation of EEG arousal (α-activity) in response to meaningful repetitive stimulation (Miller *et al.*, 1974). Similarly, Endröczi *et al.* (1970) reported prolonged EEG arousal in response to a repetitive sound stimulus in subjects treated with ACTH 1–10. In another paradigm, somatosensory evoked responses were augmented after infusion of α-MSH (Kastin *et al.*, 1971).

In view of the involvement of septum and hippocampus in the mediation of behavioral actions of peptides, we will present here in some detail investigations of theta rhythm. The septum contains pacemaker cells that drive hippocampal slow rhythmic electrical activity, the theta rhythm. The theta rhythm has attracted a good deal of experimental interest and has been the subject of vastly differing theories. Functions hypothesized to be associated with theta rhythm include arousal, attention, initiation of voluntary movement, and also memory processes (cf. reviews by Landfield, 1976; Schacter, 1977).

A number of observations led Landfield (1976) to conclude that the theta rhythm plays an important, active role in both memory storage and memory retrieval. Posttrial low frequency septal stimulation driving the theta rhythm facilitated acquisition in rats of both active and passive avoidance responses in contrast to high-frequency stimulation, which blocked theta rhythm. Low-frequency stimulation during the retention test promoted memory retrieval in the active, but not in the passive, avoidance task. The amnesic effect of ECS was correlated with a disruption of theta rhythm. Further, the amount of posttraining theta rhythm in the half hour following acquisition of a one-trial passive avoidance response was correlated with retention test performance 2 days later. An indispensable role of the theta rhythm in memory processes in animals seems improbable in the absence of dramatic changes in memory processes produced by hippocampal damage. The less farfetched proposition that the hippocampal theta rhythm may be associated with memory-modulatory events seems to be more in keeping with the surveyed data.

To test such a hypothesis it is obvious to seek interrelationships between the theta rhythm and the proposed memory-modulators, ACTH- and vasopressin-like peptides. These interrelationships have been explored by Urban and De Wied. Normal rats injected subcutaneously with ACTH 4–10 showed accelerated theta rhythm, as evidenced by increased percentages of the high-frequency components of hippocampal activity. In this study, theta activity was induced by electrical stimulation of the reticular formation in freely moving rats. The effect of the peptide was similar to the effect seen when the intensity of the electrical stimulation was increased. This was taken as evidence that in the presence of ACTH 4–10 the excitability of the theta generating system was enhanced (Urban and De Wied, 1976).

The possible role of vasopressin and related peptides was examined in diabetes insipidus Brattleboro rats. Theta rhythm was studied during paradoxical sleep, a sleep phase characterized by the frequent occurrence of theta activity. The absence of vasopressin in homozygous diabetes insipidus rats did not prevent the occurrence of paradoxical sleep. However, it was found that the theta rhythm of these animals contained lower frequencies than the hippocampal theta activity of their heterozygous or normal littermates. The anomalous frequency distribution of the theta rhythm of HO-DI animals could be transiently corrected by intracerebroventricular injection of DGAVP or ACTH 4–10. This electrophysiological investigation failed to provide evidence for a difference in action between the latter two peptides. The effect of ACTH 4–10 and DGAVP followed an almost identical timecourse. The effect reached its maximum between 60 and 120 minutes after injection; thereafter it declined over a period of several hours and returned to control levels within 24 hours. Administration of AVP antiserum into the brain ventricular system of normal rats induced hippocampal rhythmicity of the same frequency composition as that of HO-DI animals (Urban and De Wied, 1978). In a third experiment, oxytocin and its antiserum were intracerebroventricularly injected into normal Wistar rats. Oxytocin affected the theta rhythm generated during paradoxical sleep episodes in an opposite manner from its antiserum. Oxytocin administration led to a shift in the power spectrum in the direction of lower frequencies. Conversely, oxytocin antiserum increased the incidence of higher frequencies in the theta rhythm (Bohus et al., 1978).

Together, these results suggest that peptides may alter the frequency distribution of the hippocampal theta rhythm. These alterations seem to be correlated with the effect of these peptides on avoidance responses; ACTH 4–10, DGAVP, and oxytocin antiserum facilitate performance of avoidance responses and increase the incidence of higher theta frequencies, while oxytocin and anti-AVP serum impede behavioral performance and promote the occurrence of lower theta frequencies. The effects of peptides on the theta rhythm have been interpreted to be the result of either increased or decreased excitability along reticuloseptohippocampal pathways. These excitability changes might represent memory-modulatory events. In agreement with our analysis, Urban (1977) was careful to note that alterations in hippocampal rhythmic activity indeed may modulate memory processes but that the frequency pattern of the theta rhythm and paradoxical sleep itself are not indispensable for memory function.

C. NEUROCHEMISTRY

A massive body of research has been devoted to neurochemical effects of ACTH-like peptides and to a lesser extent to neurochemical actions of vasopressin. It is not clear at present whether and to what extent neurochemical alterations brought about by these peptides are associated with their action on memory processes. An increase in cerebral norepinephrine and dopamine turnover has been reported in ACTH 4–10-treated rats and mice (Versteeg, 1973; Leonard, 1974; Dunn et al., 1976; but see Iuvone et al., 1978). Surprisingly, α-MSH and β-MSH seem to be inactive in this regard (Spirtes et al., 1975; Dunn et al., 1976; Iuvone et al., 1978). We have undertaken a series of experiments in an attempt to relate one of the behavioral effects of

ACTH 4-10 to changes in hippocampal amine metabolism. Training in a passive avoidance task was followed by an increase in hippocampal serotonin levels that persisted for at least 24 hours. This increase was not seen in rats rendered amnesic with CO_2. ACTH 4-10, but not ACTH 11-24, reinstated the elevation in hippocampal serotonin levels (Ramaekers et al., 1978).

Progress in this field of research is hampered by the failure to identify receptors for ACTH in the brain in contrast to the adrenal cortex. Perhaps the finding that the septum preferentially binds ACTH analogs (Verhoef et al., 1977) may be helpful in identifying cerebral ACTH receptors.

It is generally assumed that peptide hormones interact with receptors on the outer surface of effector cells and do not penetrate these cells. After such receptor-binding, an intracellular adenylate cyclase is presumed to be activated; the cyclic AMP (cAMP) so produced acts as an intracellular second messenger, which promotes various metabolic activities, principally by changing the phosphorylation state of crucial proteins (Dunn and Gispen, 1977). This concept is derived from the postulated sequence of events in cells of the adrenal cortex but is challenged by recent suggestions that cGMP may be engaged in the mediation of adrenal cortex responses rather than cAMP (Honn and Chavin, 1975). Nevertheless, ACTH 1-10 has been found to enhance cAMP levels in slices from rat posterior hypothalamus (Wiegant and Gispen, 1975), and α-MSH has been reported to increase cAMP concentrations in the occipital cortex of normal and hypophysectomized rats (Christensen et al., 1976). Schneider et al. (1977) reported that Org 2766 (40 μg/kg) increased cAMP levels in many brain regions in male mice. These authors related their findings to the ability of Org 2766 to alter cerebral blood flow in male, but not in female, mice (Goldman and Murphy, 1977).

These data do not preclude the possibility that ACTH-related peptides may exert effects independent of cAMP. For instance, ACTH 1-24 has been shown to modify the phosphorylation of synaptic plasma membrane proteins in vitro, but differences were noted in the protein bands affected by cAMP and the peptide (Zwiers et al., 1976). It is noteworthy that alterations in the phosphorylation of synaptic plasma membranes have been observed during avoidance training (Perumal et al., 1975).

Changes in cyclic nucleotides may be reflected in changes in brain macromolecule metabolism. Hypophysectomized rats have impaired brain RNA and protein metabolism (Gispen and Schotman, 1973), which suggests that peptides are involved in the regulation of these processes. The available data suggest that behaviorally active ACTH-like peptides influence brain macromolecule metabolism at the translational (ribosome) rather than the transcriptional level (genome). A recent review (Dunn and Gispen, 1977) indicates that the rate of cerebral protein synthesis in hypophysectomized as well as intact animals can be altered by ACTH or ACTH 4–10. This review concludes that, whereas the ACTH 4–10 sequence is sufficient to produce translational effects, the full ACTH 1–24 sequence is necessary for transcriptional effects. There is little information about exactly which proteins are affected, but according to one study the effect of ACTH fragments seems to be general in nature, i.e., not restricted to particular protein species (Reith *et al.*, 1975). Dunn and Gispen (1977) attempted to enumerate the various neurochemical actions of ACTH-like peptides (Fig. 14). They postulated that there must be at least two types of cell surface receptors in view of the diversity in neurochemical actions of these peptides. Receptor interaction was proposed to stimulate the synthesis of cyclic nucleotides and perhaps prostaglandins. The ionic environment may also be affected. The cyclic nucleotides then act through protein kinases to activate or inhibit specific cellular processes, such as RNA synthesis, protein synthesis, neurotransmitter synthesis, and processes controlling the permeability of the membrane.

Neurochemical actions of vasopressin are less well documented than those of ACTH-related peptides. The little work reported has for the greater part failed to show significant effects of vasopressin on a limited number of neurochemical measurements. We are convinced that attempts to correlate neurochemical and behavioral actions of vasopressin and other peptides will fail if the analysis is restricted to crude brain samples. Fortunately, increasing sophistication of dissection techniques and neurochemical assays now allows for the assessment of neurochemical alterations in discrete brain areas. Using such techniques, Tanaka *et al.* (1977) were able to show that after intracerebroventricular injection of a 30-ng dose of AVP into rats catecholamine metabolism was changed in a restricted number of brain nuclei. Disappearance of norepinephrine after pretreatment with the synthesis inhibitor α-methylparatyrosine was accelerated in AVP-treated animals in the dorsal septal nucleus, the anterior hypothalamic nucleus, the medial forebrain bundle, the parafascicular nucleus, the dorsal raphe nucleus, the locus coeruleus, the nucleus tractus solitarii, the A1 region, and, to a lesser extent, parts of the hippocampal complex. Disappearance of norepinephrine was retarded in the supraoptic nucleus and the nucleus ruber. Further, the hormone facilitated disap-

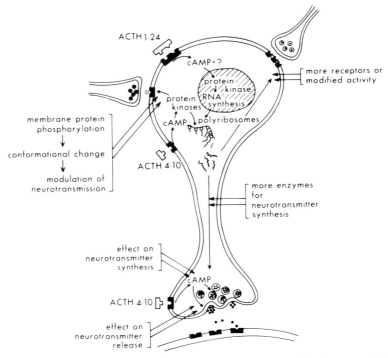

F<small>IG</small>. 14. Mechanisms of ACTH action on neurons, as proposed by Dunn and Gispen (1977). ACTH interacts with specific receptors on the outside of the cell membrane, thus activating adenylate (or perhaps guanylate) cyclase. The cyclic nucleotides then activate protein kinases, which may activate messenger RNA synthesis in the nucleus, activate protein synthesis by polyribosomes in the perikaryon, modify the properties of postsynaptic receptors, stimulate neurotransmitter synthesis, modulate neuro-transmitter release, or any combination of these. Not all cells respond to ACTH; even responsive cells may show only one or a few of these responses. Adapted from Dunn and Gispen (1977), with permission. By courtesy of ANKHO International Inc., Phoenix, Arizona.

pearance of dopamine in the caudate, the median eminence, the dorsal raphe nucleus, and the A8 region. In all the other areas studied, the peptide did not influence catecholamine metabolism. These results were taken as support for the view that vasopressin participates in the regulation of a variety of physiological processes by modulating neurotransmission in specific brain nuclei. It is noteworthy that those brain areas implicated in the modulatory actions of vasopressin on memory (parafascicular nucleus, septum, and hippocampus) all showed altered norepinephrine disappearance after hormonal treat-ment. In most of these regions another peptide, PLG, failed to affect catecholamine metabolism (Versteeg *et al.*, 1978). The PLG mimicked the effect of AVP in the caudate, the supraoptic nucleus, and the nucleus ruber. PLG increased the disappearance of norepinephrine in the A8 region and the nucleus commissuralis and decreased that of norepinephrine and dopamine in the A9 region.

The sophisticated microdissection approach outlined above has not yet been applied to the study of possible effects of vasopressin on protein metabolism. It is therefore not surprising that the first few preliminary studies failed to yield consistent results. Lysine vasopressin was found to be ineffective in altering the incorporation of radioactively labeled lysine into brain protein in mice (Dunn *et al.*, 1976). Similarly, DGLVP did not influence consistently the incorporation of labeled valine into protein in a number of large brain areas in intact, hypophysectomized, and diabetes insipidus rats (Reith *et al.*, 1977).

X. CONCLUDING COMMENTS

The variety of results reviewed in the preceding sections makes it difficult to formulate any unassailable generalizations about peptide effects on memory. This, in turn, renders a discussion of possible modes of action of the peptides somewhat speculative. Nonetheless, we feel that the data we reviewed support a number of conclusions and give rise to several testable hypotheses.

ACTH-like peptides facilitate retrieval of memory in animals. This effect derives from sites of action within the central nervous system. The facilitated retrieval is transient and does not generally persist beyond the period of treatment.

ACTH-like peptides enhance vigilance in humans. This effect also derives from sites of action within the central nervous system. The lack of consistent effects on human memory suggests that ACTH-like peptides do not significantly affect cognitive abilities. Consequently, the enhancement of memory retrieval in animals by ACTH and related peptides may be attributable to a modulation of the prerequisite sustaining processes—motivation and attention—processes that in animals are not easily distinguishable from "cognitive" aspects of retrieval. How such effects may relate to the action of these substances on human vigilance remains to be seen.

ACTH-like peptides may facilitate memory storage as well, but evidence for this proposition is conflicting in both humans and animals.

We mentioned the possibility that different structure–activity requirements may underlie a possible effect of ACTH on memory storage or that another mechanism of action, perhaps involving a peripheral component, is implicated, or both.

In the absence of central stores of vasopressin, animals are greatly impaired in the acquisition of a one-trial passive avoidance response but less so in learning a multitrial active avoidance response. We may safely conclude that vasopressin and related peptides have no indispensable role in memory functioning. It is clear, on the other hand, that vasopressin can *modulate* memory storage. Such modulatory influences are long-lasting. Vasopressin-like peptides can also enhance memory retrieval in animals. There is suggestive, but not yet conclusive, evidence for a role for vasopressin in the modulation of human memory processes.

Animal data allow for a further specification of the modulatory effect of vasopressin on memory storage. Diabetes insipidus rats and rats treated with vasopressin antiserum show normal retention of a passive avoidance response for the first few hours after the acquisition trial, indicating that short-term retention is unaffected. Conceivably, vasopressin does not facilitate short-term memory per se, but rather favors the consolidation process.

The relative resistance of acquisition of multitrial tasks by animals to changes in vasopressin is reminiscent of a phenomenon in human memory processing. Humans tend, overtly or covertly, to rehearse new information. In fact, this strategy is assumed to aid in the consolidation of labile short-term memory (Deutsch and Deutsch, 1975; Klatzky, 1975). One may expect that repetitive experience provided by multitrial tasks may aid in overcoming a relative consolidation deficit associated with vasopressin deficiency.

We reviewed evidence for specific modulatory influences, both enhancing and disrupting, of a variety of peptides. The disruptive effects of oxytocin and the facilitatory effects of vasopressin on memory suggest that if endogenous peptides are active in normal memory functioning they interact in a complex fashion. That is, a balance of facilitatory and inhibitory influences may be presumed to exist. Such a supposition is further supported by the fact that the effects of exogenous peptide administration are often bimodal, depending on the dosage used.

We further discussed evidence that vasopressin-like peptides, and perhaps also ACTH-like peptides, have dual effects in animals, i.e., they modulate both storage and retrieval processes. Although it might be argued that vasopressin congeners must, therefore, have a dual mechanism of action, this is not necessarily the case. We propose that some effect of vasopressin may serve as an additional conditional stimulus. That is, it may be itself incorporated into the learning experience, resulting in strengthened storage. Similarly, vasopressin given before retention testing may serve as a reminder of the training experience, thereby facilitating the retrieval of other components of the learning experience. We also reviewed evidence for a possible role for endorphins in the modulation of memory processes. Undoubtedly, the next few years will see attempts to replicate and extend the initial promising findings. This line of research may further delineate components of the complex neurohormonal balance that enables an organism to cope adaptively with changes in its environment.

Research activity in these areas is growing. As it does so, we gain a clearer picture of the role of normal functioning in the establishment of memory. As well, the subtlety with which we are able to manipulate memory processes by employing small peptides as experimental tools has led to theoretical advances in the area of the neurobiology of memory. It seems likely that this interface between endocrinology and the neurobiology of memory will continue to expand, enriching both parent fields in the process.

ACKNOWLEDGMENTS

We wish to express our gratitude for the patience and care with which Monique van der Borg and Jeannette Jordens assisted us in the preparation of the manuscript.

REFERENCES

Ader, R., and De Wied, D. (1972). *Psychon. Sci.* **29**, 46.

Akil, H., Watson, S. J., Berger, P. A., and Barchas, J. D. (1978a). *In* "The Endorphins" (E. Costa and M. Trabucchi, eds.) (*Adv. Biochem. Pharmacol.* 18), p. 125. Raven, New York.

Akil, H., Watson, S. J., Levy, R. M., and Barchas, J. D. (1978b). *In* "Characteristics and Function of Opioids" (J. M. Van Ree and L. Terenius, eds.) (*Dev. Neurosc.* 4) p. 123. Elsevier/North-Holland, Amsterdam.

Allen, J. P., Kendall, J. W., McGilvra, R., and Vancura, C. (1974). *J. Clin. Endocrinol.* **38**, 586.

Anderson, D. C., Winn, W., and Tam, T. (1968). *J. Comp. Physiol. Psychol.* **66**, 497.

Applezweig, M. H., and Baudry, F. D. (1955). *Psychol. Rep.* **1**, 417.

Applezweig, M. H., and Moeller, G. (1959). *Acta Psychol.* **15**, 602.

Arimura, A., Sawano, S., Redding, T. W., and Schally, A. V. (1968). *Neuroendocrinology* **3**, 187.

Ashton, H., Millman, J. E., Telford, R., Thompson, J. W., Davies, T. F., and Hall, R. (1976). *Br. J. Clin. Pharmacol.* **3**, 423.

Bailey, W. H., and Weiss, J. M. (1978). *Horm. Behav.* **10**, 22.

Baldwin, D. M., Haun, C. K., and Sawyer, C. H. (1974). *Brain Res.* **80**, 291.

Barchas, J. D., Akil, H., Elliott, G. R., Holman, R. B., and Watson, S. J. (1978). *Science* **200**, 964.

Barondes, S. H., and Cohen, H. D. (1968). *Proc. Natl. Acad. Sci. U.S.A.* **61**, 923.

Bélanger, D. (1958). *Can. J. Psychol.* **12**, 171.

Belluzzi, J. D., and Stein, L. (1977). *Soc. Neurosci. Abstr.* **3**, 230.

Bergland, R. M., and Page, R. B. (1978). *Endocrinology* **102**, 1325.

Blake, D. R., Dodd, M. J., and Evans, J. G. (1978). *Lancet* **1**, 608.

Bloch, B., Bugnon, C., Fellmann, D., and Lenys, D. (1978). *Neurosci. Lett.* **10**, 147.

Bloom, F. (1978). Paper presented at 8th Annual Meeting of the Society for Neuroscience, St. Louis, Missouri.

Bloom, F., Battenberg, E., Rossier, J., Ling, N., Leppaluoto, J., Vargo, T. M., and Guillemin, R. (1977). *Life Sci.* **20**, 43.

Bloom, F. E., Rossier, J., Battenberg, E. L. F., Bayon, A., French, E., Henriksen, S. J., Siggins, G. R., Segal, S., Browne, R., Ling, N., and Guillemin, R. (1978). *In* "The Endorphins" (E. Costa and M. Trabucchi, eds.) (*Adv. Biochem. Pharmacol.* **18**), p. 89. Raven, New York.

Bohus, B. (1977). *Horm. Behav.* **8**, 52.

Bohus, B., and De Wied, D. (1967). *Physiol. Behav.* **2**, 221.

Bohus, B., and De Wied, D. (1980). *In* "General, Comparative and Clinical Endocrinology of the Adrenal Cortex" (I. Chester Jones and I. W. Henderson, eds.), Vol. 3. Academic Press, New York. In press.

Bohus, B., Nyakas, Cs., and Endröczi, E. (1968). *Int. J. Neuropharmacol.* **7**, 307.

Bohus, B., Gispen, W. H., and De Wied, D. (1973). *Neuroendocrinology* **11**, 137.

Bohus, B., Van Wimersma Greidanus, T. B., and De Wied, D. (1975a). *Physiol. Behav.* **14**, 609.

Bohus, B., Hendrickx, H. H. L., Van Kolfschoten, A. A., and Krediet, T. G. (1975b). *In* "Sexual Behavior: Pharmacology and Biochemistry" (M. Sandler and G. L. Gessa, eds.), p. 269. Raven, New York.

Bohus, B., Urban, I., Van Wimersma Greidanus, T. B., and De Wied, D. (1978a). *Neuropharmacology* **17**, 239.

Bohus, B., Kovács, G., and De Wied, D. (1978b). *Brain Res.* **157**, 414.

Bookin, H. B., and Pfeifer, W. D. (1977). *Pharmacol. Biochem. Behav.* **7**, 51.

Botwinick, J. (1970). *Annu. Rev. Psychol.* **21**, 239.

Branconnier, R. J., Cole, J. O., and Gardos, G. (1978). *Psychopharmacol. Bull.* **14**, 27.

Brownfield, M. S., and Kozlowski, G. P. (1977). *Cell Tissue Res.* **178**, 111.

Brunner, H., Kuschinsky, G., and Peters, G. (1956). *Naunyn-Schmiedebergs Arch. Exp. Pathol. Pharmakol.* **228**, 457.

Brush, F. R., and Froelich, J. C. (1975). *In* "Psychopharmacogenetics" (B. E. Eleftheriou, ed.), p. 777. Plenum, New York.

Brush, F. R., and Levine, S. (1966). *Physiol. Behav.* **1**, 309.

Bush, D. F., Lovely, R. H., and Pagano, R. R. (1973). *J. Comp. Physiol. Psychol.* **83**, 168.

Buys, R. M. (1978). *Cell Tissue Res.* **192**, 423.

Celestian, J. F., Carey, R. J., and Miller, M. (1975). *Physiol. Behav.* **15**, 707.

Cherkin, A. (1969). *Proc. Natl. Acad. Sci. U.S.A.* **63**, 1094.

Chretien, M., Crine, P., Lis, M., Gianoulakis, C., Gossard, F., Benjannet, S., and Seidak, N. G. (1978). *In* "Characteristics and Function of Opioids" (J. M. Van Ree and L. Terenius, eds.), (*Dev. Neurosci.* **4**), p. 245. Elsevier/North-Holland, Amsterdam.

Christensen, C. W., Hartston, C. T., Kastin, A. J., Kostrzewa, R. M., and Spirtes, M. A. (1976). *Pharmacol. Biochem. Behav.* **5**, Suppl. 1, 117.

Cleghorn, R. A. (1957). *In* "Hormones, Brain Function and Behavior" (H. Hoagland, ed.), p. 3. Academic Press, New York.

Correll, R. E., and Scoville, W. B. (1970). *J. Comp. Physiol. Psychol.* **70**, 464.

Cuello, A. C. (1978). *In* "The Endorphins" (E. Costa and M. Trabucchi, eds.) (*Adv. Biochem. Pharmacol.* **18**), p. 111. Raven, New York.

Delacour, J. (1971). *Neuropsychologia* **9**, 157.

Delay, J., Bertagna, L., and Lanvas, A. (1954). *Presse Med.* **62**, 1037.

Deutsch, D., and Deutsch, J. A. (eds.) (1975). "Short Term Memory." Academic Press, New York.

De Wied, D. (1964). *Am. J. Physiol.* **207**, 255.

De Wied, D. (1965). *Int. J. Neuropharmacol.* **4**, 157.

De Wied, D. (1968). *Excerpta Med. Found. Int. Congr. Ser.* n184, 310.

De Wied, D. (1969). *In* "Frontiers in Neuroendocrinology, 1969" (W. F. Ganong and L. Martini, eds.), p. 97. Oxford Univ. Press, London and New York.

De Wied, D. (1971). *Nature (London)* **232**, 58.

De Wied, D. (1974). *In* "The Neurosciences. Third Study Program" (F. O. Schmitt and F. G. Worden, eds.), p. 653. MIT Press, Cambridge, Massachusetts.

De Wied, D. (1976a). *Hosp. Pract.*, January 1976, 123.

De Wied, D. (1976b). *Life Sci.* **19**, 685.

De Wied, D. (1977). *Ann. N. Y. Acad. Sci.* **297**, 263.

De Wied, D., and Bohus, B. (1966). *Nature (London)* **212**, 1484.

De Wied, D., and Gispen, W. H. (1976). *Psychopharmacologia* **46**, 27.

De Wied, D., Greven, H. M., Lande, S., and Witter, A. (1972). *Br. J. Pharmacol.* **45**, 118.

De Wied, D., Bohus, B., and Van Wimersma Greidanus, T. B. (1974). *In* "Integrative Hypothalamic Activity" (D. F. Swaab and J. P. Schadé, eds.) (*Prog. Brain Res.* **41**), p. 417. Elsevier, Amsterdam.

De Wied, D., Bohus, B., and Van Wimersma Greidanus, T. B. (1975a). *Brain Res.* **85**, 152.

De Wied, D., Witter, A., and Greven, H. M. (1975b). *Biochem. Pharmacol.* **24**, 1463.

De Wied, D., Bohus, B., and Van Wimersma Greidanus, T. B. (1976). *In* "Cellular and Molecular Bases of Neuroendocrine Processes" (E. Endröczi, ed.), p. 547. Akadémiai Kiadó, Budapest.

De Wied, D., Bohus, B., Van Ree, J. M., and Urban, I. (1978a). *J. Pharmacol. Exp. Ther.* **204**, 570.

De Wied, D., Kovács, G. L., Bohus, B., Van Ree, J. M., and Greven, H. M. (1978b). *Eur. J. Pharmacol.* **49**, 427.

Dogterom, J., Van Wimersma Greidanus, T. B., and Swaab, D. F. (1977). *Neuroendocrinology* **24**, 108.

Dogterom, J., Snijdewint, F. G. M., and Buys, R. M. (1978). *Neurosci. Lett.* **9**, 341.

Dornbush, R. L., and Nikolovski, O. (1976). *Pharmacol. Biochem. Behav.* **5**, Suppl. 1, 69.

Douglas, R. J. (1967). *Psychol. Bull.* **67**, 416.

Drachman, D. A., and Hughes, J. R. (1971). *Neurology*, **21**, 1.

Duncan, C. P. (1949). *J. Comp. Physiol. Psychol.* **42**, 32.

Dunn, A. J., and Gispen, W. H. (1977). *Biobehav. Rev.* **1**, 15.

Dunn, A. J., Iuvone, P. M., and Rees, H. D. (1976). *Pharmacol. Biochem. Behav.* **5**, Suppl. 1, 139.

Endröczi, E., Lissák, K., Fekete, T., and De Wied, D. (1970). *In* "Pituitary, Adrenal and the Brain (D. De Wied and J. A. W. M. Weijnen, eds.), *Prog. Brain Res.* **32**, p. 254. Elsevier, Amsterdam.

Ferris, S. H., Sathananthan, G., Gershon, S., Clark, C., and Moshinsky, J. (1976). *Pharmacol. Biochem. Behav.* **5**, Suppl. 1, 73.

Flexner, J. B., Flexner, L. B., Hoffman, P. L., and Walter, R. (1977). *Brain Res.* **134**, 139.

Flexner, L. B., and Flexner, J. B. (1968). *Science* **159**, 330.

Flood, J. F., Jarvik, M. E., Bennett, E. L., and Orme, A. E. (1976). *Pharmacol. Biochem. Behav.* **5**, Suppl. 1, 41.

Fried, P. A. (1972). *Psychol. Bull.* **78**, 292.

Gaillard, A. W. K., and Sanders, A. F. (1975). *Psychopharmacologia* **42**, 201.

Gaillard, A. W. K., and Varey, C. A. (1977). IZF report 1977–18. TNO-Soesterberg, The Netherlands.

Gallagher, M., and Kapp, B. S. (1978). *Soc. Neurosci. Abstr.* **4**, 258.

Garrud, P., Gray, J. A., and De Wied, D. (1974). *Physiol. Behav.* **12**, 109.

George, J. M., and Jacobowitz, D. M. (1975). *Brain Res.* **93**, 363.

Gispen, W. H., and Schotman, P. (1973). *In* "Drug Effects on Neuroendocrine Regulation" (E. Zimmermann *et al.*, eds.) (*Prog. Brain Res.* **39**), p. 443. Elsevier, Amsterdam.

Gispen, W. H., and Wiegant, V. M. (1976). *Neurosci. Lett.* **2**, 159.

Gispen, W. H., Van Wimersma Greidanus, T. B., and De Wied, D. (1970). *Physiol. Behav.* **5**, 143.

Gispen, W. H., Van der Poel, A., and Van Wimersma Greidanus, T. B. (1973). *Physiol. Behav.* **10**, 345.

Gispen, W. H., Buitelaar, J., Wiegant, V. M., Terenius, L., and De Wied, D. (1976a). *Eur. J. Pharmacol.* **39**, 393.

Gispen, W. H., Wiegant, V. M., Bradbury, A. F., Hulme, E. C., Smyth, D. G., Snell, C. R., and De Wied, D. (1976b). *Nature (London)* **264**, 794.

Glickman, S. E. (1961). *Psychol. Bull.* **58**, 218.

Gold. P. E., and McGaugh, J. L. (1975). *In* "Short Term Memory" (D. Deutsch and J. A. Deutsch, eds.), p. 356. Academic Press, New York.

Gold, P. E., and McGaugh, J. L. (1976). *In* "Neurobiology of Aging" (J. M. Ordy and K. R. Brizzee, eds.), p. 145. Plenum, New York.

Gold, P. E., and McGaugh, J. L. (1977). *In* "Neuropeptide Influences on the Brain" (L. H. Miller *et al.*, eds.), p. 127. Raven, New York.

Gold, P. E., and Van Buskirk, R. B. (1976). *Behav. Biol.* **16**, 387.

Goldman, H., and Murphy, S. (1977). *Pharmacologist* **19**, 154 (abstract).

Goulon, M., and Aubert, P. (1959). *Rev. Neurol.* **100**, 596.

Gray, J. A., and Garrud, P. (1977). *In* "Neuropeptide Influences on the Brain" (L. H. Miller *et al.*, eds.). p. 201. Raven, New York.

Greven, H. M., and De Wied, D. (1973). *In* "Drug Effects on Neuroendocrine Regulation" (E. Zimmermann *et al.*, eds.) (*Prog. Brain Res.* **39**), p. 429. Elsevier, Amsterdam.

Greven, H. M., and De Wied, D. (1977). *In* "Melanocyte-Stimulating Hormone: Control, Chemistry and Effects" (F. J. H. Tilders *et al.*, eds.) (*Front. Horm. Res.* **4**), p. 140. Karger, Basel.

Guillemin, R., Ling, N., and Burgus, R. (1976). *C. R. Acad. Sci. Ser. D* **282**, 783.

Guillemin, R., Vargo, T., Rossier, J., Minick, S., Ling, N., Rivier, C., and Bloom, F. (1977). *Science* **197**, 1367.

Hebb, D. O. (1949). "The Organization of Behavior." Wiley, New York.

Hennessy, J. W., Smotherman, W. P., and Levine, S. (1976). *Behav. Biol.* **16**, 413.

Hirsh, R. (1974). *Behav. Biol.* **12**, 421.

Honn, K. V., and Chavin, W. (1975). *Gen. Comp. Endocrinol.* **26**, 374.

Hughes, J., Smith, T. W., Kosterlitz, H. W., Fothergill, L. A., Morgan, B. A., and Morris, H. R. (1975). *Nature (London)* **258**, 577.

Iuvone, P. M., Morasco, T., Delanoy, R. L., and Dunn, A. J. (1978). *Brain Res.* **139**, 131.

Jacquet, Y. F. (1978). *Science* **201**, 1032.

Johansson, O., Hökfelt, T., Elde, R. P., Schultzberg, M., and Terenius, L. (1978). *In* "The Endorphins" (E. Costa and M. Trabucchi, eds.) (*Adv. Biochem. Pharmacol.* **18**), p. 51. Raven, New York.

Kamin, L. J. (1957). *J. Comp. Physiol. Psychol.* **50**, 457.

Kastin, A. J., Miller, L. H., Gonzáles-Bárcena, D., Hawley, W. D., Dyster-Aas, K., Schally, A. V., Velasco de Para, L., and Velasco, M. (1971). *Physiol. Behav.* **7**, 893.

Kastin, A. J., Dempsey, G. L., Le Blanc, B., Dyster-Aas, K., and Schally, A. V. (1974). *Horm. Behav.* **5**, 135.

Kastin, A. J., Scollan, E. L., King, M. G., Schally, A. V., and Coy, D. H. (1976). *Pharmacol. Biochem. Behav.* **5**, 691.

Kimble, D. P. (1968). *Psychol. Bull.* **70**, 285.

King, A. R., and De Wied, D. (1974). *J. Comp. Physiol. Psychol.* **86**, 1008.

Klatzky. R. L. (1975). "Human Memory. Structures and Processes." Freeman, San Francisco, California.

Klein, R. (1970). *In* "Pituitary, Adrenal and the Brain" (D. De Wied and J. A. W. M. Weijnen, eds.) (*Prog. Brain Res.* **32**), p. 263. Elsevier, Amsterdam.

Klein, S. B. (1972). *J. Comp. Physiol. Psychol.* **79**, 341.

Klein, S. B., and Kopish, R. M. (1975). *Behav. Biol.* **13**, 377.

Korányi, L., Beyer, C., and Guzmán-Flores, C. (1971a). *Physiol. Behav.* **7**, 321.

Korányi, L., Beyer, C., and Guzmán-Flores, C. (1971b). *Physiol. Behav.* **7**, 331.

Kovács, G. L., Vécsei, L., and Telegdy, G. (1978). *Physiol. Behav.* **20**, 801.

Krejči, I., and Kupková, B. (1978). *Activ. Nerv. Super.* **20**, 11.

Krieger, D. T., Liotta, A., and Brownstein, M. J. (1977a). *Proc. Natl. Acad. Sci. U.S.A.* **74**, 648.

Krieger, D. T., Liotta, A., Suda, T., Palkovits, M., and Brownstein, M. J. (1977b). *Biochem. Biophys. Res. Commun.* **73**, 930.

Krieger, D. T., Liotta, A. S., and Suda, T. (1979). *In* "Endorphins in Mental Health Research" (E. Usdin *et al.*, eds.), p. 561. Macmillan, New York.

Lamotte, C., Pert, C. B., and Snyder, S. H. (1976). *Brain Res.* **112**, 407.

Lande, S., Witter, A., and De Wied, D. (1971). *J. Biol. Chem.* **246**, 2058.

Lande, S., Flexner, J. B., and Flexner, L. B. (1972). *Proc. Natl. Acad. Sci. U.S.A.* **69**, 558.

Landfield, P. W. (1976). *In* "Molecular and Functional Neurobiology" (W. H. Gispen, ed.), p. 390. Elsevier, Amsterdam.

Lashley, K. (1917). *Psychobiology* **1**, 141.

Le Boeuf, A., Lodge, J., and Eames, P. (1978). *Lancet* **2**, 8104, 1370.

Legros, J. J., Gilot, P., Seron, X., Claessens, J., Adam, A., Moeglen, J. M., Audibert, A., and Berchier, P. (1978). *Lancet* **2**, 41.

Leonard, B. E. (1974). *Arch. Int. Pharmacodyn. Ther.* **207**, 242.

Leshner, A. I., and Roche, K. E. (1977). *Physiol. Behav.* **18**, 879.

Levine, S. (1968). *In* "Nebraska Symposium on Motivation (W. Arnold, ed.), p. 85. Univ. of Nebraska Press, Lincoln.

Levine, S., and Levin, R. (1970). *Horm. Behav.* **1**, 105.

Li, C. H., and Chung, D. (1976). *Nature (London)* **260**, 622.

Liotta, A. S., Suda, T., and Krieger, D. T. (1978). *Proc. Natl. Acad. Sci. U.S.A.* **75**, 2950.

Lissák, K., and Endröczi, E. (1965). "The Neuroendocrine Control of Adaptation." Pergamon, Oxford.

Lowry, P. J., and Scott, A. P. (1975). *Gen. Comp. Endocrinol.* **26**, 16.

Lowry, P. J., Silman, R. E., and Hope, J. (1977). In "ACTH and Related Peptides: Structure, Regulation and Action" (D. T. Krieger and W. F. Ganong, eds.) (*Ann. N. Y. Acad. Sci.* 297), p. 49. New York Academy of Sciences, New York.

Luria, A. R. (1976). "The Neuropsychology of Memory." Holt (Winston), New York.

McCleary, R. A. (1966). In "Progress in Physiological Psychology" (E. Stellar and J. M. Sprague, eds.), Vol. 1, p. 209. Academic Press, New York.

McGaugh, J. L. (1961). *Psychol. Rep,* **8**, 99.

McGaugh, J. L., and Dawson, R. G. (1971). *Behav. Sci.* **16**, 45.

McGaugh, J. L., and Herz, M. J. (1972). "Memory Consolidation." Albion, San Francisco, California.

McGaugh, J. L., and Petrinovich, L. F. (1965). *Int. Rev. Neurobiol.* **8**, 139.

Mackintosh, N. J. (1974). "The Psychology of Animal Learning." Academic Press, New York.

Mains, R. E., Eipper, B. A., and Ling, N. (1977). *Proc. Natl. Acad. Sci. U.S.A.* **74**, 3014.

Marquis, H. A., and Suboski, M. D. (1969). *Proc. 77th Annu. Conv. APA* **4**, 207.

Marslen-Wilson, W. D., and Teuber, H.-L. (1975). *Neuropsychologia* **13**, 353.

Martinez, Jr., J. L., Vasquez, B. J., Jensen, R. A., Soumireu-Mourat, B., and McGaugh, J. L. (1979). *Pharmacol. Biochem. Behav.* **10**, 145.

Messing, R. B., Jensen, R. A., Martinez, Jr., J. L., Spiehler, V. R., Vasquez, B. J., Soumireu-Mourat, B., Liang, K. C., and McGaugh, J. L. (1979) *Behav. Neural. Biol.* **27**, 266.

Mezey, E., Palkovits, M., De Kloet, E. R., Verhoef, J., and De Wied, D. (1978). *Life Sci.* **22**, 831.

Miller, L. H., Kastin, A. J., Sandman, C. A., Fink, M., and Van Veen, W. J. (1974). *Pharmacol. Biochem. Behav.* **2**, 663.

Miller, L. H., Harris, L. C., Van Riezen, H., and Kastin, A. J. (1976). *Pharmacol. Biochem. Behav.* **5**, Suppl. 1, 17.

Miller, M., Barranda, E. G., Dean, M. C., and Brush, F. R. (1976). *Pharmacol. Biochem. Behav.* **5**, Suppl. 1, 35.

Miller, R. J., and Cuatrecasas, P. (1978). *Vitam. Horm. (New York)* **36**, 297.

Mirsky, I. A., Miller, R., and Stein, M. (1953). *Psychosom. Med.* **15**, 574.

Moeglen, J. M., Audibert, A., Timsit-Berthier, M., and Oliveros, J. C. (1977). In "Seminario di Neuroendocrinologia. Aspetti biologici e clinici" (A. Polleri, ed.), p. 18. Biodata, Genoa.

Moll, J., and De Wied, D. (1962). *Gen. Comp. Endocrinol.* **2**, 215.

Morris, J. F., Sokol, H. W., and Valtin, H. (1977). In "Neurohypophysis" (A. M. Moses and L. Share, eds.), p. 58. Karger, Basel.

Oliveros, J. C., Jandeli, M. K., Trimsit-Berthier, M., Remy, R., Benghezal, A., Audibert, A., and Moeglen, J. M. (1978). *Lancet* **2**, 42.

Pacold, S. T., Kirsteins, L., Hoyvat, S., Lawrence, A., and Hagen, T. (1978). *Science* **199**, 804.

Pelletier, G., Leclerc, R., Labrie, F., Cote, J., Chretien, M., and Lis, M. (1977). *Endocrinology.* **100**, 770.

Perumal, R., Gispen, W. H., Wilson, J. E., and Glassman, E. (1975). In "Hormones, Homeostasis and the Brain" (W. H. Gispen *et al.*, eds.) (*Prog. Brain Res.* **42**), p. 201. Elsevier, Amsterdam.

Pfaff, D. W., Silva, M. T. A., and Weiss, J. M. (1971). *Science* **172**, 394.

Pickford, M. (1961). In "Oxytocin" (R. Caldeyro-Barcia and H. Heller, eds.), p. 68. Pergamon, Oxford.

Plomp, G. J. J., and Van Ree, J. M. (1978). Br. J. Pharmacol. 64, 223.

Przewlocki, R., Höllt, V., and Herz, A. (1978). In "Characteristics and Function of Opioids" (J. M. Van Ree and L. Terenius, eds.) (Dev. Neurosci. 4), p. 285. Elsevier/North-Holland, Amsterdam.

Quinton, E. (1972): Paper presented at meeting of Rocky Mountain Psychological Association.

Ramaekers, F., Rigter, H., and Leonard, B. E. (1978). Pharmacol. Biochem. Behav. 8, 547.

Rapoport, J. L., Quinn, P. O., Copeland, A. P., and Burg, C. (1976). Neuropsychobiology 2, 291.

Reith, M. E. A., Schotman, P., and Gispen, W. H. (1975). Neurobiology 5, 355.

Reith, M. E. A., Schotman, P., and Gispen, W. H. (1977). In "Mechanisms, Regulation and Special Function of Protein Synthesis in the Brain" (Roberts et al., eds.), p. 383. Elsevier, Amsterdam.

Rigter, H. (1978). Science 200, 83.

Rigter, H., and Popping, A. (1976). Psychopharmacologia 46, 255.

Rigter, H., and Van Riezen, H. (1975). Physiol. Behav. 14, 563.

Rigter, H., and Van Riezen, H. (1978). In "Psychopharmacology: A Generation of Progress" (M. A. Lipton et al., eds.), p. 677. Raven, New York.

Rigter, H., and Van Riezen, H. (1979). In "Current Developments in Psychopharmacology" (W. B. Essman and L. Valzelli, eds.), Vol. 5. Spectrum, New York. In press.

Rigter, H., Van Riezen, H., and De Wied, D. (1974). Physiol. Behav. 13, 381.

Rigter, H., Elbertse, R., and Van Riezen, H. (1975). In "Hormones, Homeostasis and the Brain" (W. H. Gispen et al., eds.) (Prog. Brain Res. 42), p. 163. Elsevier, Amsterdam.

Rigter, H., Janssens-Elbertse, R., and Van Riezen, H. (1976). Pharmacol. Biochem. Behav. 5, Suppl. 1, 53.

Rigter, H., Greven, H., and Van Riezen, H. (1977a). Neuropharmacology 16, 545.

Rigter, H., Shuster, S., and Thody, A. J. (1977b). J. Pharm. Pharmacol. 29, 110.

Rigter, H., Messing, R. B., Vasquez, B. J., Jensen, R. A., Martinez, Jr., J. L., Crabbe, J. C., and McGaugh, J. L. (1979). Life Sci. 25, 1137.

Roberts, J. L., and Herbert, E. (1977). Proc. Natl. Acad. Sci. U.S.A. 74, 5300.

Roberts, R., Flexner, J. B., and Flexner, L. B. (1970). Proc. Natl. Acad. Sci. U.S.A. 66, 310.

Rosenbloom, A. A., and Fisher, D. A. (1975). Neuroendocrinology 17, 354.

Rossier, J., Vargo, T. M., Minick, S., Ling, N., Bloom, F. E., and Guillemin, R. (1977). Proc. Natl. Acad. Sci. U.S.A. 74, 5162.

Rubinstein, M., Stein, S., Gerben, L. D., and Udenfriend, S. (1977). Proc. Natl. Acad. Sci. U.S.A. 74, 3052.

Rubinstein, M., Stein, S., and Udenfriend, S. (1978). Proc. Natl. Acad. Sci. U.S.A. 75, 669.

Sandman, C. A., and Kastin, A. J. (1977). In "Neurobiology of Sleep and Memory" (R. R. Drucker-Colin and J. L. McGaugh, eds.), p. 347. Academic Press, New York.

Sandman, C. A., George, J. M., Nolan, J. D., Van Riezen, H., and Kastin, A. J. (1975). Physiol. Behav. 15, 427.

Sandman, C. A., George, J. M., Walker, B. B., Nolan, J. D., and Kastin, A. J. (1976). Pharmacol. Biochem. Behav. 5, Suppl. 1, 23.

Sandman, C. A., George, J., McCanne, T. R., Nolan, J. D., Kaswan, J., and Kastin, A. J. (1977). *J. Clin. Endocrinol. Metabol.* **44**, 884.

Sannitta, W. G., Irwin, P., and Fink, M. (1976). *Neuropsychobiology* **2**, 283.

Sawyer, W. H., and Valtin, H. (1965). *Endocrinology* **76**, 991.

Schacter, D. L. (1977). *Biol. Psychol.* **5**, 47.

Schneider, D. R., Felt, B. T., and Goldman, H. (1977). *Pharmacologist* **19**, 154 (abstract).

Schulz, H. (1970). *Arch. Int. Pharmacodyn. Ther.* **186**, 108.

Schulz, H., Kovács, G. L., and Telegdy, G. (1974). *Acta Physiol. Acad. Sci. Hung.* **45**, 211.

Schwarzberg, H., and Unger, H. (1970). *Acta Biol. Med. Ger.* **24**, 507.

Schwarzberg, H., Hartmann, G., Kovács, G. L., and Telegdy, G. (1976). *Acta Physiol. Acad. Sci. Hung.* **47**, 127.

Scoville, W. B., and Milner, B. (1957). *J. Neurol. Neurosurg. Psychiat.* **20**, 11.

Simantov, R., and Snyder, S. H. (1976). *Life Sci.* **18**, 781.

Small, J. G., Small, I. F., Milstein, V., and Dian, D. A. (1977). *Acta Psychiat. Scand.* **55**, 241.

Spirtes, M. A., Kostrzewa, R. M., and Kastin, A. J. (1975). *Pharmacol. Biochem. Behav.* **3**, 1011.

Steiner, F. A. (1970). *In* "Pituitary, Adrenal and the Brain" (D. De Wied and J. A. W. M. Weijnen, eds.) (*Prog. Brain Res.* **32**), p. 102. Elsevier, Amsterdam.

Sterba, G. (1974). *Zool. Jahrb. Abt. Allg. Zool. Physiol. Tiere* **78**, 409.

Tanaka, M., De Kloet, E. R., De Wied, D., and Versteeg, D. H. G. (1977). *Life Sci.* **20**, 1799.

Terenius, L. (1976). *Eur. J. Pharmacol.* **38**, 211.

Thatcher, R. W. (1976). *In* "Neurobiology of Aging" (R. D. Terry and S. Gershon, eds.), p. 43. Raven, New York.

Tramu, G., Leonardelli, J., and Dubois, M. P. (1977). *Neurosci. Lett.* **6**, 305.

Urban, I. (1977). Ph.D. Thesis, University of Utrecht.

Urban, I., and De Wied, D. (1976). *Exp. Brain Res.* **24**, 325.

Urban, I., and De Wied, D. (1978). *Pharmacol. Biochem. Behav.* **8**, 51.

Vale, W., Rivier, C., Yang, L., Minick, S., and Guillemin, R. (1978). *Endocrinology* **103**, 1910.

Valtin, H., Schroeder, H. A., Bernischke, K., and Sokol, H. W. (1962). *Nature (London)* **196**, 1109.

Valtin, H., Sokol, H. W., and Sunde, D. (1975). *Recent Prog. Horm. Res.* **31**, 447.

Van Delft, A. M. L. (1970). *In* "Pituitary, Adrenal and the Brain" (D. De Wied and J. A. W. M. Weijnen, eds.) (*Prog. Brain Res.* **43**), p. 192. Elsevier, Amsterdam.

Van Delft, A. M. L., and Kitay J. I. (1972). *Neuroendocrinology* **9**, 188.

Vandesande, F., Dierickx, K., and DeMay, J. (1975). *Cell Tissue Res.* **156**, 377.

Van Wimersma Greidanus, T. B. (1977). *In* "Melanocyte-Stimulating Hormone: Control, Chemistry and Effects" (F. J. H. Tilders *et al.*, eds.) (*Front. Horm. Res.* **4**), p. 129. Karger, Basel.

Van Wimersma Greidanus, T. B., and De Wied, D. (1971). *Neuroendocrinology* **7**, 291.

Van Wimersma Greidanus, T. B., and De Wied, D. (1976a). *Behav. Biol.* **18**, 325.

Van Wimersma Greidanus, T. B., and De Wied, D. (1976b). *Proc. Int. Congr. Endocrinol. 5th*, No. 225.

Van Wimersma Greidanus, T. B., and De Wied, D. (1977). *In* "Biochemical Correlates of Brain Structure and Function" (A. N. Davidson, ed.), p. 284. Academic Press, New York.

Van Wimersma Greidanus, T. B., Bohus, B., and De Wied, D. (1975a). *In* "Hormones, Homeostasis and the Brain" (W. H. Gispen *et al.*, eds.) (*Prog. Brain Res.* **42**), p. 135. Elsevier, Amsterdam.

Van Wimersma Greidanus, T. B., Dogterom, J., and De Wied, D. (1975b). *Life Sci.* **16**, 637.

Van Wimersma Greidanus, T. B., Bohus, B., and De Wied, D. (1975c). *In* "Anatomical Neuroendocrinology" (W. E. Stumpf and L. D. Grant, eds.), p. 284. Karger, Basel.

Van Wimersma Greidanus, T. B., Van Dijk, A. M. A., De Rotte, A. A., Goedemans,

Veith, J. L., Sandman, C. A., George, J. M., and Stevens, V. C. (1978). *Physiol. Behav.* **20**, 43.

Verhoef, J., and Witter, A. (1976). *Pharmacol. Biochem. Behav.* **4**, 583.

Verhoef, J., Witter, A., and De Wied, D. (1977). *Brain Res.* **131**, 117.

Versteeg, D. H. G. (1973). *Brain Res.* **49**, 483.

Versteeg, D. H. G., Tanaka, M., De Kloet, E. R., Van Ree, J. M., and De Wied, D. (1978). *Brain Res* **143**, 561.

Walter, R., Hoffman, P. L., Flexner, J. B., and Flexner, L. B. (1975). *Proc. Natl. Acad. Sci. U.S.A.* **72**, 4180.

Walter, R., Van Ree, J. M., and De Wied, D. (1978). *Proc. Natl. Acad. Sci. U.S.A.* **75**, 2493.

Warrington, E. K., and Weiskrantz, L. (1973). *In* "The Physiological Basis of Memory" (J. A. Deutsch, ed.), p. 365. Academic Press, New York.

Watson, S. J., Barchas, J. D., and Li, C. H. (1977). *Proc. Natl. Acad. Sci. U.S.A.* **74**, 5155.

Watson, S. J., Akil, H., Richard, C. W., III, and Barchas, J. D. (1978a). *Nature (London)* **275**, 226.

Watson, S. J., Richard, C. W., III, and Barchas, J. D. (1978b). *Science,* **200**, 1180.

Weber, E., Voigt, K. H., and Martin, R. (1978). *Brain Res.* **157**, 385.

Weijnen, J. A. W. M., and Slangen, J. L. (1970). *In* "Pituitary, Adrenal and the Brain" (D. De Wied and J. A. W. M. Weijnen, eds.) (*Prog. Brain Res.* **32**), p. 221. Elsevier, Amsterdam.

Weiss, J. M., McEwen, B. S., Silva, M. T. A., and Kalkut, M. F. (1970). *Am. J. Physiol.* **218**, 864.

Weitzman, R. E., Fisher, D. A., Minick, S., Ling, N., and Guillemin, R. (1977). *Endocrinology* **101**, 1643.

Wertheim, G. A., Conner, R. L., and Levine, S. (1969). *Physiol. Behav.* **4**, 41.

Wiegant, V. M., and Gispen, W. H. (1975). *Exp. Brain Res.* **23**, Suppl., 219.

Wiegant, V. M., Colbern, D., Van Wimersma Greidanus, T. B., and Gispen, W. H. (1978). *Brain Res. Bull.* **3**, 167.

Wolthuis, O. L., and De Wied, D. (1976). *Pharmacol. Biochem. Behav.* **4**, 273.

Zimmermann, E., and Krivoy, W. (1973). *In* "Drug Effects on Neuroendocrine Regulation" (E. Zimmermann *et al.*, eds.) (*Prog. Brain Res.* **39**), p. 383. Elsevier, Amsterdam.

Zwiers, H., Veldhuis, H. D., Schotman, P., and Gispen, W. H. (1976). *Neurochem. Res.* **1**, 669.

VITAMINS AND HORMONES, VOL. 37

Inhibin: From Concept to Reality*

P. FRANCHIMONT, J. VERSTRAELEN-PROYARD,
M. T. HAZEE-HAGELSTEIN, Ch. RENARD, A. DEMOULIN,
J. P. BOURGUIGNON, AND J. HUSTIN

*Radioimmunoassay Laboratory, Institute of Medicine, University
of Liège, Liège, Belgium*

I. Relationship between Gametogenesis and FSH Secretion:
Definition of Inhibin 244
II. Sources of Inhibin and Techniques for Purification 246
   A. Extraction of Inhibin from Human Seminal Plasma 247
   B. Extraction of Inhibin from Ram Rete Testis Fluid 247
III. Detection and Measurement of Inhibin 249
   A. *In Vivo* Tests 251
   B. *In Vitro* Assays 254
   C. Radioligand Assays 256
   D. Present Position of Inhibin Assays and Outlook for the Future . 257
IV. Physicochemical and Immunological Characteristics of Inhibin 260
V. Biological Properties of Inhibin 267
   A. Sites of Action of Inhibin 267
   B. Mechanism of Action of Inhibin at the Pituitary Level 272
   C. Kinetics of the Action of Inhibin on Gonadotropin Secretion *in Vivo* .. 274
   D. Interactions between Inhibin, Androgens, and Estrogens 279
   E. Effects of Inhibin on Gonadal Function 280
VI. Origin and Transport of Inhibin 287
   A. Testicular Origin 287
   B. Follicular Origin 290
   C. Similarity of Ovarian and Testicular Inhibin 291
   D. Transport of Inhibin to the Hypothalamopituitary Axis 293
VII. Possible Roles of Inhibin 293
   A. Negative Feedback of FSH Secretion 294
   B. Negative Feedback on LH Secretion 296
   C. Is Inhibin a Cybernine? 296
VIII. Summary and Conclusions 298
References 299

In numerous physiological and pathological conditions, the levels of two gonadotropins, follicle-stimulating hormone (FSH) and luteinizing hormone (LH), change independently (see review by Franchimont and Burger, 1975).

The secretion of LH is controlled by positive and negative feedback

*Work subsidized by grant 74.039 de l-Organisation Mondiale de la Santé, Geneva, Switzerland and by grant 3.4501.80 du FRSM.

243

mechanisms induced by androgens and estrogens (see review by Set-chell *et al.*, 1977).

In contrast, the secretion of FSH in both men and women, correlates inversely with gametogenesis.

I. Relationship between Gametogenesis and FSH Secretion: Definition of Inhibin

The concept of a gonadal hormone regulating FSH secretion and related directly or indirectly to gametogenesis originated many years ago. The hormone was called androhormone by Martins and Rocha (1931), inhibin by McCullagh (1932), and X hormone by Klinefelter *et al.* (1942). The concept has been strengthened by recent studies in both humans and animals that show an inverse relationship between gamatogenesis and the secretion of FSH.

Before puberty, the basal secretion of FSH and its response to exogenous LH-releasing hormone (LH-RH) are greater than those of LH. In contrast, as puberty develops, the levels of FSH, after a transitory rise, level off and may even fall. Thus, during pubertal development in the rat, the levels of LH increase in parallel with the development of spermatogenesis and testosterone secretion. In contrast, the level of FSH is high at the prepubertal stage when compared to adult levels. Serum FSH begins to fall coincidentally with the appearance of the first mature sperm and reaches adult levels at the time of complete spermatogenesis (Swerdloff *et al.*, 1971). Similarly, in boys and in girls the levels of FSH increase progressively from the first to the third stage of puberty and then level off from the third to the fifth stage. Moreover, if an LH-RH test is performed in males prior to the onset of puberty (stage 1), during puberty (stages 2 and 3), and after completion of sexual maturation (stage 5) it can be shown that the cumulative FSH response to 25 μg of LH-RH, reflecting the available pituitary reserve of FSH, diminishes significantly from stage 1 to stage 5 (adult) (Franchimont *et al.*, 1975a).

In women, the level of FSH increases at the beginning of the menstrual cycle, when the follicles are small. As the development of the follicle progresses, the level of FSH falls. Moreover, in women approaching the menopause, the level of FSH is greatly increased, sometimes up to five times the values observed at midcycle, whereas estradiol secretion remains normal and LH concentrations are unchanged (Korenman and Sherman, 1976). When the menopause becomes established, the levels of FSH increase further to values that are clearly higher than those seen at the midcycle peak in menstruating women. LH, on the other hand, usually rises less dramatically and may not exceed midcycle peak levels. The changes observed at this stage of a woman's life are accompanied by a marked reduction of ovarian follicles and failure of their normal maturation.

In men suffering from germinal cell failure without damage of Leydig cells, due to various causes, the levels of FSH are often increased, whereas LH levels are frequently normal (Franchimont, 1972; Franchimont et al., 1975b). In these patients, there is a linear relationship between the level of FSH and both qualitative (Franchimont et al., 1972) and quantitative (De Kretser et al., 1972) aspects of spermatogenesis observed in testicular biopsies. Thus, when spermatogenesis is arrested before the spermatid stage, the level of FSH is always elevated. When spermatids are present in the seminiferous tubules, the levels of FSH are usually normal (Franchimont et al., 1972). This relationship does not occur with LH.

To interpret the consistently high FSH levels when spermatids are absent, one may postulate that spermatid maturation induces or permits the formation of a factor that controls FSH secretion. This interpretation would be consistent with the view that there is a specific stage in the process of spermatogenesis involved in testicular feedback on FSH secretion—at spermatid formation (Franchimont et al., 1972) or at the point of maturation of spermatozoa (Johnsen, 1970). Alternatively, spermatids may have no specific function in FSH regulation. The depletion of these cells may merely be a reflection of a severe depression of the basal germinal cell population. The germinal cells could, under these conditions, produce less inhibitory factor, and FSH levels would increase as a result. The studies of De Kretser et al., (1972) support this latter interpretation. These investigators have shown that there is an inverse correlation between FSH levels and the severity of reduction in germinal cells from spermatogonia to late spermatids. The most significant correlation was that found with the number of spermatogonia per tubular cross section.

Paulsen et al. (1972) suggested an additional explanation for the elevation in FSH observed in oligospermic men. The depletion of germinal cell elements may correlate with abnormalities of another process, such as Sertoli cell function, that actually controls FSH secretion. Since germinal cell depletion and Sertoli cell dysfunction are probably interrelated, the apparent correlation between FSH levels and germinal cell depletion may, in fact, reflect concomitant Sertoli cell abnormalities.

The regulating factor for FSH, related directly or indirectly to gametogenesis, in this review, will be called "inhibin" as proposed by McCullagh in 1932.

DEFINITION OF INHIBIN

Inhibin can be defined as a peptidic factor of gonadal origin that specifically or selectively lowers the rate of secretion of FSH.

Other names have been given to substances isolated from a variety of biological fluids and possessing similar properties: folliculostatin (Schwartz and Channing, 1977), follitropin-suppressing principle (Sairam *et al.*, 1978), Sertoli cell factor (Steinberger and Steinberger, 1976).

We will nevertheless give the same name "inhibin" to all the various preparations described in the literature that meet the definition of this hormone, although we cannot exclude differences in their physiocochemical properties or physiological significance.

II. SOURCES OF INHIBIN AND TECHNIQUES FOR PURIFICATION

Inhibin has been detected and partially purified from human seminal fluid (Franchimont, 1972; Franchimont *et al.*, 1975b), bovine seminal fluid (Franchimont *et al.*, 1975c; Sairam *et al.*, 1978; Chari *et al.*, 1978), ram rete testis fluid (RTF) (Setchell and Sirinathsinghji, 1972; Setchell and Jacks, 1974; Baker *et al.*, 1976; Davies *et al.*, 1978; Franchimont *et al.*, 1977, 1978; Cahoreau *et al.*, 1979), extracts of spermatozoa (Lugaro *et al.*, 1974; Setchell and Main, 1974), testicular extracts (Lee *et al.*, 1974; Keogh *et al.*, 1976; Baker *et al.*, 1976; Moodbidri *et al.*, 1976), ovarian extracts (Hopkinson *et al.*, 1975, 1977a; Chappel *et al.*, 1978), bovine follicular fluid (De Jong and Sharpe, 1976; Welschen *et al.*, 1977), porcine follicular fluid (Welschen *et al.*, 1977; Marder *et al.*, 1977; Lorenzen *et al.*, 1978), human follicular fluid (Chari *et al.*, 1979), as well as the culture medium of Sertoli cells (Steinberger and Steinberger, 1976) and granulosa cells (Erickson and Hsueh, 1978).

The extraction techniques used include homogenization in aqueous media (Lee *et al.*, 1974; Nandini *et al.*, 1976; Moodbidri *et al.*, 1976), precipitation with organic solvents (ethanol, acetone, ether) (Franchimont *et al.*, 1975b,c; Hopkinson *et al.*, 1977a; De Jong and Sharpe,

1976), and Deae-cellulose chromatography with elution by pH gradient (Franchimont *et al.*, 1977) or molarity gradient (Baker *et al.*, 1978), carboxymethyl chromatography (Baker *et al.*, 1978), precipitation with ammonium sulfate (Baker *et al.*, 1978; Chari *et al.*, 1979), and filtration using various molecular sieves.

In this review, experiments will be concerned with active material extracted from human seminal plasma and ram rete testis. Some details of the extraction will be given to provide the reader with information concerning the nature of the material used.

A. Extraction of Inhibin from Human Seminal Plasma (HSP) (Franchimont *et al.*, 1979a)

Human seminal plasma is centrifuged at 4°C for 10 minutes to remove spermatozoa. The supernatant is chromatographed in 3-ml fractions on a Sephadex G-100 column (2.6 × 92 cm), previously equilibrated with Sorensen phosphate buffer (0.05 M, pH 7.5). HSP elutes in three main peaks on Sephadex G-100. The first peak (HSP$_1$) elutes just after the void volume of the column. The second (HSP$_3$) and third (HSP$_4$) are markedly delayed. Fractions eluted between HSP$_1$ and HSP$_3$ are pooled to form fraction HSP$_2$. Fraction HSP$_{3-4}$ consists of the tail of peak HSP$_3$ and the beginning of HSP$_4$ (Fig. 1). The fractions corresponding to these different zones are pooled and lyophilized. In the example, the protein concentrations estimated by Folin's method were 922 mg for HSP$_1$, 262 mg for HSP$_2$, 448 mg for HSP$_3$, 56.4 mg for HSP$_{3-4}$, and 13 mg for HSP$_4$ from 100 ml of HSP. Only HSP$_3$ and HSP$_{3-4}$ fractions contained the inhibin-like substance capable of selectively inhibiting the secretion of FSH both *in vivo* (reduction of serum levels of FSH in rats 24 hours after castration) and *in vitro* (reduction of the FSH released in culture medium by LH-RH in rat pituitary cell culture).

B. Extraction of Inhibin from Ram Rete Testis Fluid (RTF) (Franchimont *et al.*, 1978, 1979a)

Ram rete testis fluid is centrifuged to eliminate spermatozoa and other cells and then lyophilized. A quantity of lyophilyzate corresponding to 300 ml of RTF is dissolved in 20 ml of eluting buffer and submitted to gel. filtration on Sephadex G-100 (90 × 5 cm). The

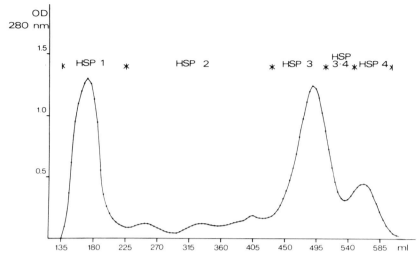

F IG . 1. Elution profile of human seminal plasma (HSP) filtered on Sephadex G-100. Abscissa: volume of elution; ordinate: optical density at 280 nm. External volume: 145 ml; salt peak (KI) is eluted from 566 ml. Reproduced from Franchimont *et al.* (1979a), with permission of the publisher.

Sephadex is equilibrated, and the elution is performed with ammonium bicarbonate buffer, 0.05 M, pH 7.5, at a constant flow of 60 ml/hour. In the *in vivo* and *in vitro* bioassays, RTF_{1a} and RTF_3 both possessed biological activity (Fig. 2).

Seventy milligrams of fraction 1a were submitted to preparative isotachophoresis Uniphor LKB 7900 on acrylamide–bisacrylamide

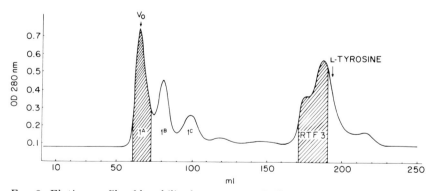

F IG . 2. Elution profile of lyophilized ram rete testis fluid (RTF) on Sephadex G-100 column (88 × 5 cm). Abscissa: milliliters of elution; ordinate: optical density at 280 nm. The hatched area represents biological activity.

(3.3%) gel containing riboflavin, 0.8 mg/dl; TEMED, 30 μl/dl; and ammonium persulfate, 10 mg/dl. The gel is polymerized in the leading buffer Tris-HCl, pH 7.5, with a final concentration of 0.01 M. The anodic and elution buffer is constituted by Tris 0.02 M added with HCl 1 M to reach pH 8. The terminating solution is constituted of Tris 0.02 M and valine 0.01 M, pH 9. The following discrete spacers, each 125 μmol, are used: ACES, MOPS, HEPES, Bicine, TAPS, Histidine. A constant current of 85 μA is applied, and voltage at the beginning of isotachophoresis is 0.350 kV. The elution rate is 10 ml/hour.

By optical density at 280 nm, seven peaks were obtained, one of which, RTF$_{38}$, was biologically active (Fig. 3).

RTF$_{38}$ is submitted to semipreparative polyacrylamide gel electrophoresis (7.5%) in Tris-HCl buffer, pH 8.9, 0.2 M. Five components are isolated and recovered by this method, from the anode to the cathode: RTF$_{38a,b,c,d,e}$. RTF$_{38c}$ is biologically active, migrates as a single band in sodium dodecyl sulfate (SDS) polyacrylamide gel electrophoresis (R_f 0.51), is homogeneous in high-performance liquid chromatography and gives a simple band when submitted to immunoelectrophoresis with an anti-RTF$_{38}$ serum.

III. Detection and Measurement of Inhibin

The study of inhibin was held up for a long time by the lack of biological tests suitable for its detection and measurement. Now, bioassays of inhibin activity are available *in vivo* and *in vitro*. Radioimmunoassays and radioreceptor assays are being developed.

Methods of measuring inhibin must obviously meet criteria of specificity, sensitivity, precision, and reproducibility. These criteria have been evaluated very little to judge from the literature, and to date most methods have been concerned with detection rather than quantitative measurement.

Furthermore, a reference preparation has been sadly lacking until quite recently, when Hudson *et al.* (1979) distributed a lyophilized preparation of ovine testicular lymph given an arbitrary biological potency of 1 U/mg.

In bioassays, both *in vivo* and *in vitro*, specificity is ascertained in three ways. First, inhibin activity is defined by its preferential action on FSH secretion; the threshold dose that affects the level of FSH is less than the one that affects LH secretion. The experimental condi-

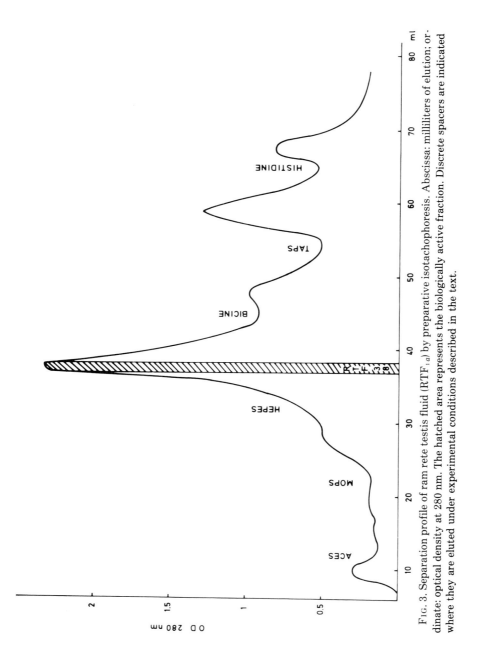

FIG. 3. Separation profile of ram rete testis fluid (RTF$_{1a}$) by preparative isotachophoresis. Abscissa: milliliters of elution; ordinate: optical density at 280 nm. The hatched area represents the biologically active fraction. Discrete spacers are indicated where they are eluted under experimental conditions described in the text.

tions *in vivo* are often chosen to ensure this selective or specific response on FSH levels. Second, the secretion of other pituitary hormones, such as prolactin and TSH, should not be affected by inhibin. Last, the test preparation should not contain any substance known to be capable of interfering in the assay for example, sex steroids, fractions of gonadotropins, and enzymes.

A. *In Vivo* TESTS

1. *Selective Reduction of Serum FSH Levels by Inhibin*

Reduction occurs in intact rats or rats castrated a few hours or several days previously (Fig. 4; Table I). The age and the sex of the rat affect this test (see review of Setchell *et al.*, 1977).

Many authors now use 35-day-old rats; at this age serum levels of FSH have risen sharply (Nandini *et al.*, 1976). Recently, castrated adult mice have also been used (Lee *et al.*, 1977). Other animals were used in earlier attempts to identify inhibin; these included castrated rams (Lee *et al.*, 1974; Baker *et al.*, 1976) and castrated rabbits (Franchimont *et al.*, 1977). The inhibin preparations were injected intravenously.

The duration, frequency, and routes of injection have varied from one study to another. One or several injections have been given over 24 hours or several days intravenously, subcutaneously, or intraperitoneally. It is worth stressing that the results are more consistent when injections are given twice daily for 72 hours, starting immediately after castration.

Finally, Hopkinson *et al.* (1977a) give dihydrotestosterone for 48 hours, in doses ranging from 20 to 120 µg per/100 gm body weight per day, at the same time as the test material to male and female rats (weighing 320–350 gm) that have just been castrated. This maintains LH at precastration levels whereas the rise in FSH after castration is unaffected.

These methods are useful for the detection of inhibin in biological fluids, but their lack of precision and reproducibility limit their application (Table I).

2. *Inhibition of Human Chorionic Gonadotropin (HCG)- Induced Ovarian and Uterine Weight Increase*

Another *in vivo* assay method measures the inhibition of the (HCG)-induced ovarian or uterine weight increase in immature rats or mice following the administration of preparations containing in-

TABLE I

SOME CHARACTERISTICS OF INHIBIN ASSAYS[a]

Parameters	In vivo		In vitro	Radioimmunoassay
	Inhibition of FSH levels 24 hours after castration[b]	Inhibition of HCG-augmented uterine weight increase[c]	Inhibition of LH-RH-induced FSH release	RTF homogeneous system, RTF_c as tracer and reference anti-RTF$_{38}$ serum
Number of dose levels of any (standard or unknown) preparations	4	4	> 4	At least 10
Measured responses	Absolute FSH levels	Mouse uterus weight	Absolute FSH levels or % of FSH reduction	$B_x/B_o \times 100$
Slope (a)	−125.8	23.9	−46.5	−31.6
Index of precision (λ)	0.25–0.84	0.1	0.04–0.15	0.01–0.1
Coefficient of intraassay variation	12.3–21%	8.3%	3.2–6%	$< 5\%$
Coefficient of interassay variation	32%	11.7%	17%	$< 12\%$

[a] FSH, follicle-stimulating hormone; HCG, human chorionic gonadotropin; LH-RH, luteinizing hormone-releasing hormone; RTF, ram rete testis fluid.
[b] Franchimont et al. (1977).
[c] Ramasharma et al. (1979).

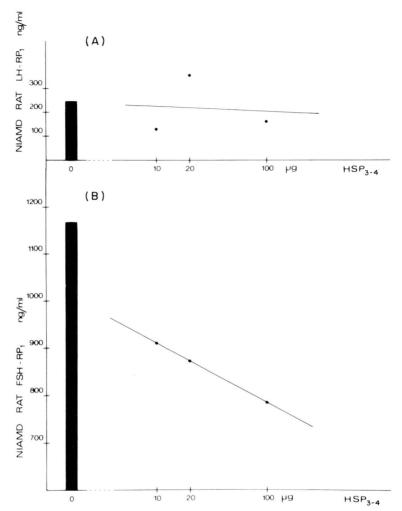

FIG. 4. Effect of several doses of human seminal plasma (HSP$_{3-4}$) on follicle-stimulating hormone (FSH) (panel B) and luteinizing hormone (LH) (panel A) levels in castrated rats. Male Wistar rats weighing 120 ± 10 gm were castrated at time 0. Twenty-two hours later, they received by tail vein either 0.5 ml of physiological saline (control group) or the material to be tested, diluted in 0.5 ml of 0.9% NaCl. Two hours later (24 hours after castration) the animals were anesthetized with ether and blood was removed by cardiac puncture for assay of FSH and LH. Each fraction was assayed in 6 rats, and the control group consisted of 10 animals. Black columns represent the control value of castrated rats treated with NaCl 0.9%. Formulas of regression lines and their significance are as follows. Panel A (LH): $Y = -22.2 \log X + 246.6$, $t = 0.094$ (NS), $r = 0.093$; panel B (FSH): $Y = -125.8 \log X + 1035.9$, $t = 55.1$, $r = 0.999$. There is a dose-response relationship for FSH levels only. Reproduced from Franchimont (1979a), with permission of the publisher.

hibin. Chari *et al.* (1976) have used ovarian weights in rats, and Setchell and Sirinathsinghji (1972) and Ramasharma *et al.* (1979) measured uterine weights in mice.

The explanation of this test rests on the fact that the increase in weight induced by HCG is possible only in the presence of endogenous FSH, which HCG liberates approximately 1 hour after administration (Ramasharma *et al.*, 1979) (Fig. 5). The inhibin preparations act by reducing endogenous FSH secretion. Although the results of individual experiments appear to be interesting, we agree with Setchell *et al.* (1977) that this type of test is often unreliable. The uterine and ovarian response, although simple to evaluate, is not reproducible from one assay to another presumably because of variability in response of the animals. It is also sensitive to slight variations in the dose of HCG. If too high a dose of HCG is given, the uterine and ovarian responses are reduced and the effect of inhibin is lost. Aspects of this method used by Ramasharma *et al.* (1979) are summarized in Table I.

B. *In Vitro* ASSAYS

1. *Pituitary Cell Culture*

The monolayer pituitary cell culture to assay inhibin was first developed by Baker *et al.* (1976) in Melbourne. Dispersed anterior pituitary cells from mature rats in short-term culture are used according to the method of Hopkins and Farquhar (1973).

The cells are cultured for 2 days in the absence of test material, which is then added for the next 3 days. The culture medium is then removed for the assay of FSH and LH (Fig. 6). The cells are further cultured over a 6-hour period in semisynthetic medium, Dulbecco Modified Eagle's Minimum Essential Medium (DHEM), with or without the addition of a dose ($10^{-8}M$) of LH-RH. The culture medium is collected for the assay of FSH and LH under basal conditions or after stimulation by LH-RH.

At the end of this culture period, the cells are recovered, then destroyed by the addition of distilled water, and the gonadotropin content of the cells is determined.

There is a relationship between the logarithm of the dose of inhibin added to the culture, on the one hand, and, on the other, the secretion of FSH into the medium after 3 days of culture without LH-RH, after 6 hours of incubation with LH-RH, and the FSH content of the cells (Fig. 6.).

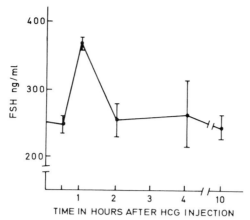

Fɪɢ. 5. Effect of human chorionic gonadotropin (HCG) injection on serum follicle-stimulating hormone (FSH) levels. HCG was administered at time 0, and serum samples were collected at different time intervals thereafter ($N = 5$). FSH in serum (ng/ml mean ± SD) was assayed using rat FSH radioimmunoassay provided by NIAMD. Reproduced from Ramasharma *et al.* (1979), with permission of the authors and publisher.

The selective effect of inhibin on FSH secretion is evident. In fact, the liberation of LH is affected only in response to LH-RH and by a much higher dose of inhibin than that required to impair FSH secretion. Furthermore, basal LH secretion after 3 days' incubation and intracellular LH content are not altered by increasing amounts of inhibin.

The slope of the reduction curve of FSH is steepest when FSH secretion is stimulated by LH-RH (Fig. 6). This condition forms the best *in vitro* bioassay for measuring inhibin (Table I).

In order to ensure the specificity of the observed response, we also measure the levels of prolactin and thyrotropin-stimulating hormone (TSH). Normally, these levels remain unchanged by the addition of LH-RH, irrespective of the presence or the absence of inhibin. The levels of thesé hormones fall if there is any nonspecific toxic effect on the pituitary cell culture.

2. *Incubated Pituitary Halves*

A second *in vitro* assay has been described by Setchell *et al.* (1977). Pituitary halves from adult rats, incubated in a suitable medium, retain a reasonable histological appearance for some hours and release FSH and LH into the medium. This release can be stimulated by LH-

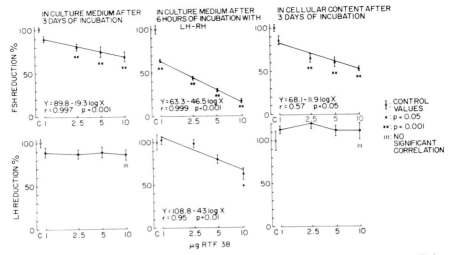

F$_{IG}$. 6. Effect of increasing amounts of a preparation of inhibin (RTF$_{38}$) on follicle-stimulating hormone (FSH) (upper panels) and luteinizing hormone (LH) (lower panels) secretion by dispersed pituitary cells in culture medium after 3 days of incubation under basal condition (left) or after 6 hours of incubation with 10^{-8} M LH-releasing hormone (LH-RH) (center). The right-hand panels correspond to the intracellular FSH and LH contents in basal conditions after 3 days of incubation. Ordinate: reduction of FSH and LH secretion or intracellular content expressed as percentage of the control value (100%).

RH. Inhibin slightly reduces the basal production of FSH but has a marked effect on the LH-RH-stimulated release (Fig. 7). Release of LH is unaffected or may even be slightly increased. In our hands, this assay has been found to be less sensitive, precise, and reproducible, but much shorter and simpler, than the dispersed cell culture assay.

C. R$_{ADIOLIGAND}$ A$_{SSAYS}$

Two preliminary methods for radioimmunoassay (Sheth *et al.*, 1978) and radioreceptor assay (Sairam *et al.*, 1978) have now been described. The published data are still too provisional to allow judging their quality or usefulness.

We have set up a radioimmunoassay for ovine inhibin with a molecular weight greater than 10,000.

The purified preparation of RTF$_{38c}$ (see Fig. 3) was used as a tracer and reference preparation. This preparation was labeled according to the method of Greenwood *et al.* (1963). Labeled hormone was separated from radioactive salts by Sephadex G-25 filtration. One of

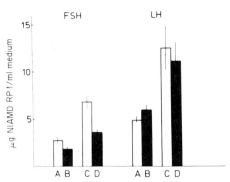

FIG. 7. Effect of Amicon-treated ram rete testis fluid (RTF) on the response to luteinizing hormone-releasing hormone (LH-RH) of incubated rat pituitary (RP) halves.
Two pituitary halves were incubated for 4 hours at 37°C in an atmosphere of 95% O_2,
5% CO_2. LH-RH was added to a concentration of 4 ng/ml. All pituitary halves were
preincubated for 30 minutes in medium alone. A, medium alone; B, medium + RTF; C,
medium + LH-RH; D, medium + RTF + LH-RH. RTF produced a slightly lower basal
follicle-stimulating hormone (FSH) release and markedly inhibited the effect of LH-RH
on FSH with no significant effect on LH. Reproduced from Setchell *et al.* (1977), with
permission of the authors and publisher.

the antisera obtained in rabbits with a semipurified inhibin preparation (RTF$_{38}$) was used as a final dilution of 1:200,000. A double antibody system allowed the separation of free labeled inhibin from
labeled inhibin bound to antibody.

Figure 8 illustrates inhibin curves obtained with the successive
preparations of RTF obtained during the purification procedure. They
are parallel. The ratios of the amount of RTF$_{38c}$ to the quantities of
crude RTF, RTF$_{1a}$, and RTF$_{38}$ capable of displacing 50% of bound
labeled RTF$_{38c}$ were, respectively, 0.017, 0.1, and 0.32. A complete
cross-reaction was observed between RTF preparations, on the one
hand, and, on the other hand, HSP$_{3-4}$, bovine testicular extract, and
bovine follicular fluid (BFF). In contrast, there was no cross-reaction
with LH-RH, somatostatin, pituitary hormones, and RTF$_3$, the low
molecular weight inhibin fraction of RTF. Table I describes some
characteristics of this inhibin radioimmunoassay.

D. PRESENT POSITION OF INHIBIN ASSAYS AND OUTLOOK
FOR THE FUTURE

There is no doubt that assays for inhibin have been improved since
1972, when the first work establishing the existence of this hormone
was based on *in vivo* bioassays. These tests were poorly sensitive, not

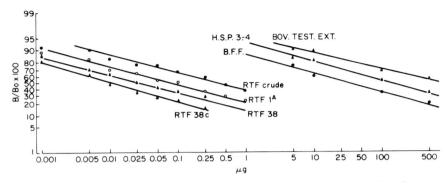

F<small>IG</small>. 8. Inhibition curves of several inhibin preparations expressed in logit-log in a radioimmunoassay for ram rete testis fluid (RTF) inhibin. Preparations of high molecular weight inhibin obtained at each step of purification from RTF gave parallel curves. Three other inhibin preparations from human seminal plasma (HSP_{3-4}), aqueous extract of bovine testis (Bov. Test Ext) and bovine follicular fluid (BFF) also displayed parallel inhibition curves, although with a much lower immunological potency.

precise, and barely adequate to detect inhibin in several biological fluids. The improvement has consisted in using an *in vitro* assay, the reduction of basal and/or LH-RH-induced FSH secretion by isolated pituitary cells. Its sensitivity and precision allow this technique to be used to follow the yield and specific activity of inhibin during the successive steps of purification. But this *in vitro* assay is still not adequate for measuring inhibin levels in biological fluids in order to establish the secretion of the hormone in normal and pathological conditions. Such physiopathological investigations require more sensitive assays, such as radioimmunoassay or radioreceptor assays. These ligand assays are still underdeveloped and not yet fully validated.

In future research on inhibin, the assays used should meet criteria for reliability, and the respective merits and limitations of the *in vitro* and *in vivo* assays need to be borne in mind. *In vivo* methods will still be of interest to confirm the inhibition of FSH secretion observed *in vitro*. Observation of an inhibitory effect *in vivo* also serves to demonstrate absorption of the active substance from the injection site and its transport to and action on the hypothalamohypophysial axis. Lack of biological effect *in vivo*, even though observed *in vitro*, could be explained by failure of absorption, by elevated metabolic clearance, by a homeostatic reaction masking the inhibitory effect of inhibin, or by inadequate experimental conditions.

The *in vitro*, assay is very attractive for several reasons already discussed—sensitivity, precision, broad linear log dose-effect relationship, and low requirement of active material. But some experimental conditions are critical. First, pituitary cells, once attached to the dishes, must be incubated with and without inhibin preparations for the optimal time for a highly significant and dose-related effect; 3 days appears to be the optimal duration for incubation (Eddie *et al.*, 1978, 1979; de Jong *et al.*, 1979). Furthermore, the choice of sex and age of the pituitary donor animals may affect assay responsiveness. Many authors use adult male rats (Steinberger and Steinberger, 1976; Eddie *et al.*, 1978, 1979; de Jong *et al.*, 1979), although Lagace *et al.* (1979) use adult female rats. A preliminary experiment, however, has suggested to us that prepubertal male rats may be the best donors. Thus, 10^{-6} pituitary cells from immature male rats released identical amounts of FSH and LH under basal conditions and twice as much FSH as LH when gonadotropin secretion was stimulated by LH-RH. In contrast, the same number of cells from adult male rats secreted four times as much LH as FSH under basal conditions and two to six times as much LH as FSH when LH-RH was added to the culture medium. Under basal conditions and with LH-RH stimulation, the total amount of FSH secreted into the culture medium by 10^{-6} pituitary cells was three to four times higher when the donor animals were prepubertal than when they were adult. The specificity of *in vitro* assays must be assessed carefully. Absence of nonspecific factors capable of destroying cells, added LH-RH, and secreted gonadotropins are prerequisites. Furthermore, one should take into consideration the presence of substances, such as steroids (Labrie *et al.*, 1978) or possible unidentified factors (de Jong *et al.* 1979), capable of modifying the secretion of gonadotropins by the cells separately from the action of inhibin. These interferences may explain the lack of parallelism of inhibition curves and even stimulatory effects on gonadotropin secretion when crude extracts are used instead of purified preparations.

Finally, a model should be chosen that gives the widest range between the threshold doses acting on FSH and LH secretion. For that objective, the basal secretion of gonadotropins is the most appropriate condition, since basal LH levels are unaffected by doses of inhibin that produce significant suppression of the basal secretion of FSH (Fig. 6) (Steinberger and Steinberger, 1976; Labrie *et al.*, 1978; de Jong *et al.*, 1979). In contrast, inhibin reduces LH-RH-induced secretion of both gonadotropins, the secretion of FSH being affected more than that of LH (Fig. 6).

An internationally acceptable reference preparation should be provided that does not contain nonspecific factors that affect the assay or steroids and other substances that act on pituitary cells. It must give an inhibition curve that is parallel to those obtained with inhibin preparations from several sources (see Fig. 25). Ovine testicular lymph, proposed by Baker *et al.* (1978), seems to be a good candidate. A control medium devoid of inhibin, such as the lymph collected from castrated rams (Eddie *et al.*, 1979), is also useful to serve as a "blank" in the evaluation of the assay data.

A radioimmunoassay (RIA) will permit investigators to follow purification procedures and to define inhibin secretion in health and disease. But to carry out a valid RIA, classic criteria must be met: purity of the tracer devoid of labeled contaminants and of damaged forms; specific antibody production; efficient technique for separating free labeled inhibin and labeled inhibin bound to antibody; absence of partial or complete cross-reaction with other substances and of non-specific interferences by constituents of biological fluids (i.e., proteins, enzymes, and ions); complete immunological identity between the standard preparation and inhibin to be assayed; adequate sensitivity, precision, reproducibility, and accuracy. All these criteria should be assessed before applying the RIA to the measurement of immunoreactive inhibin in preparative samples and biological fluids.

IV. PHYSICOCHEMICAL AND IMMUNOLOGICAL CHARACTERISTICS OF INHIBIN

1. *Inhibin Is Not a Steroid*

The sex steroids testosterone, 17β-estradiol, dihydrotestosterone, and progesterone have been measured in semipurified inhibin preparations after appropriate extractions. The preparations were found not to contain sufficient quantities of these sex steroids to explain the inhibiting effect on FSH secretion either *in vivo* or *in vitro* (Franchimont *et al.*, 1975b, 1979a; Hopkinson *et al.*, 1977a).

Furthermore, the biological fluids containing inhibin and used without solvent extraction, such as the culture medium of Sertoli cells (Steinberger and Steinberger, 1976), granulosa cells (Erickson and Hsueh, 1978), follicular fluid (Welschen *et al.*, 1977; de Jong *et al.*, 1978), and rete testis fluid (Setchell *et al.*, 1977), remained active even though they had been pretreated with charcoal alone or charcoal dextran for the purpose of removing most of the sex steroids.

It is also known that steroids such as 17β-estradiol and the androgens (testosterone and dihydrotestosterone) stimulate the secretion of FSH by pituitary cells in culture (Labrie *et al.*, 1978; Lagace *et al.*, 1979), and when an inhibitory effect appears, as is the case with estrogens, it is primarily more marked on the synthesis and on the release of LH both *in vivo* and *in vitro* than on FSH (see review by Setchell *et al.*, 1977; de Jong *et al.*, 1979).

2. *Inhibin Is Not the Androgen-Binding Protein*

French and Ritzen (1973) have shown that Sertoli cells under the influence of FSH secrete a protein that has the property of binding testosterone and 5α-dihydrotestosterone. Different preparations of inhibin extracted from human and bull seminal plasma and rete testis fluid have been tested for the presence of androgen-binding protein. None of them bind either testosterone, dihydrotestosterone, or tritiated 17β-estradiol (Franchimont *et al.*, 1975b,c, 1977, 1978).

3. *Inhibin Does Not Cross-react with Gonadotropins*

Active fractions of inhibin show no cross-reaction with FSH or LH of human, ovine, murine, or other origin. It is therefore not a modified gonadotropin (Franchimont *et al.*, 1975b, 1977).

4. *Molecular Weight and Amino Acid Composition*

There are inconsistencies in the estimates of the molecular weight of inhibin. These result from the fact that few of the studies have been performed with completely purified inhibin (Chari *et al.*, 1978; Sairam *et al.*, 1978). Inhibin also appears to be biochemically heterogeneous (Davies *et al.*, 1976; Franchimont *et al.*, 1978; Baker *et al.*, 1978).

Dialysis experiments using Amicon membranes and electrophoretic migration in sodium dodecyl sulfate (SDS) show that inhibin activity resides in fractions with molecular weights greater than 10,000 in most biological fluids studied: bull seminal plasma (BSP) (Chari *et al.*, 1978; Sairam *et al.*, 1978), ram rete testis fluid (Davies *et al.*, 1976; Franchimont *et al.*, 1977), porcine follicular fluid (Channing *et al.*, 1978), and the culture medium of Sertoli cells (Steinberger and Steinberger, 1976) and of granulosa cells (Anderson *et al.*, 1979).

The assigned molecular weight usually lies between 10,000 and 30,000. Inhibin from BSP has been obtained in a pure state by Chari *et al.* (1978), by acetone precipitation followed by filtration on Sephadex G-100, using 4 *M* urea–0.05 *M* sodium acetate buffer, pH 4, as eluent, then by straight elution analysis using carboxymethyl cellulose.

On the basis of gel filtration studies, SDS electrophoresis, and amino acid analysis, the molecular weight was estimated to be 19,000.

The amino acid composition was as follows: (Trp, Met, Arg)$_1$ His$_2$ Val$_4$ (Ile, Pro)$_5$ Ala$_6$ Thr$_7$ Phe$_8$ (Gly, Leu)$_9$ (Glu, Ser)$_{10}$ Tyr$_{11}$ Lys$_{13}$ Cys$_{14}$ Asp$_{21}$.

Sairam *et al.* (1978) have also managed to purify and characterize inhibin (which they call follitropin-suppressing principle) from bull ejaculate by ethanol precipitation, pH fractionation, then a series of chromatographic steps with Sephadex G-100, sulfopropyl Sephadex G-50 at pH 4.5, and DEAE-cellulose at pH 9. They obtained a protein with a molecular weight of approximately 15,000, active *in vivo* at doses of 5–10 μg in reducing the levels of FSH in castrated immature rats and inhibiting the uterine weight increase produced by 10 IU of HCG in 27-day-old female mice.

Some biological activity has also been found in protein fractions of much greater molecular weight, in the region of 90,000 (Davies *et al.* 1976, 1978; Baker *et al.*, 1976). Cahoreau *et al.* (1979) found the active fraction of RTF extracted by ethanol to have a molecular weight greater than 160,000 on the basis of Sephadex filtration and more than 100,000 on the basis of ultrafiltration on XM100 membranes.

On the other hand, inhibin-like biological activity has been found in peptide fractions of low molecular weight (< 5,000) extracted from ram testes by Moodbidri *et al.* (1976) and from human seminal fluid by Franchimont *et al.* (1978).

There are two fractions of RTF extract that show inhibin activity, one of high molecular weight (> 10,000), the other of low molecular weight (< 5,000). Only 3–6% of the total inhibin activity is located in the low molecular weight elution zone. The high molecular weight form gives rise to the low molecular weight form each time the former is subjected to chromatography on Sephadex G-200 (Fig. 9) (Franchimont *et al.*, 1978) or G-100 (Davies *et al.*, 1978). Moreover, when the large molecular weight fraction was submitted to gel filtration in 4 *M* urea, all the "inhibin" activity shifted to a fraction with a molecular weight less than 5000 (Davies *et al.*, 1978).

The high molecular weight form could be a polymer of low molecular weight forms, or a combination of natural inhibin with a carrier, or even a unique precursor that can liberate the active fragment under appropriate conditions. It could equally well be an agglomeration of two different substances in which the low molecular weight fragment might be absorbed on the larger protein. In our RIA, there is no cross-reaction between high and low molecular weight forms of inhibin.

As shown in Table II, there is no relationship between the several sources of inhibin and their molecular weights.

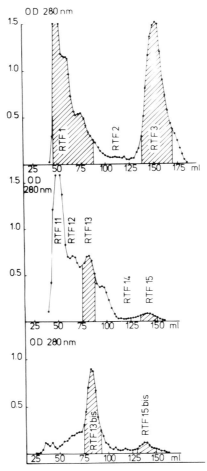

FIG. 9. Serial separation of ram rete testis fluid (RTF). *Upper panel:* After lyophilization, RTF (750 mg) was submitted to gel chromatography on Sephadex G-100 (88 × 1.6 cm column; PO$_4$ buffer 0.05 M, pH 7.5). Biological activity was located in RTF$_1$ and RTF$_3$ fractions. *Middle panel:* When RTF$_1$ (50 mg of protein) was further chromatographed on Sephadex G-200 (88 × 1.6 column; NH$_4$HCO$_3$ buffer, 0.05 M, pH 7), the resulting elution pattern consisted of five peaks: RTF$_{11}$, RTF$_{12}$, RTF$_{13}$, RTF$_{14}$, and RTF$_{15}$. RTF$_{15}$ was eluted in the same position as RTF$_3$ when it was chromatographed on Sephadex G-200. *Lower panel:* When RTF$_{13}$ (20 mg of protein) was submitted to further gel filtration on Sephadex G-200 (87 × 1.6 cm column; NH$_4$HCO$_3$ buffer 0.05 M, pH 7), the biological activity was again recovered in two peaks in the areas of high (RTF$_{13}$ bis) and low (RTF$_{15}$ bis) molecular weight. Hatched areas were biologically active.

TABLE II
Molecular Weight of Inhibin According to Source

Sources of inhibin preparations	Approximative molecular weight	Method of determination	Authors
Rete testis fluid	10,000–20,000	Sephadex G-100[a]	Baker et al., 1976
	15,000–25,000 and 80,000	Sephadex G-100	Davies et al., 1976
	< 5,000, 20,000, 90,000	Sephadex G-100	Davies et al., 1978
	1500	Sephadex G-75	Moodbidri et al., 1976
	> 10,000 and < 5000	Sephadex G-100	Franchimont et al., 1978
	≥ 160,000	Sephadex G-200	Cahoreau et al., 1979
	> 100,000	Ultrafiltration	Cahoreau et al., 1979
Human seminal plasma	19,000	SDS PAGE[b]	Sheth et al., 1978
	<5,000	Sephadex G-100	Franchimont et al., 1978
Bovine seminal plasma	18,800	Sephadex G-100	Chari et al., 1978
	21,500	SDS PAGE	
	15,000	Gel filtration	Sairam et al., 1978
Ovine testicular extract	10,000–70,000	Sephadex G-100	Baker et al., 1976
Human follicular fluid	23,000	SDS PAGE	Chari et al., 1979
Bovine follicular fluid	> 10,000	Ultrafiltration	de Jong and Sharpe, 1976
Rat inhibin			
Sertoli cell factor	> 12,000	Dialysis	Steinberger and Steinberger, 1976
Seminiferous tubule culture	Not fractionated	Sephadex G-100	Eddie et al., 1978

[a] According to their elution zone.
[b] SDS PAGE, sodium dodecyl sulfate polyacrylamide gel electrophoresis.

5. *Alteration of Biological Activity*

The active material with a molecular weight greater than 10,000 loses its activity when digested by trypsin, pepsin, or papain (Fig. 10). It is also thermolabile; boiling testicular extract (Nandini *et al.,* 1976) or culture medium from Sertoli cells (Steinberger and Steinberger, 1976) destroys the biological activity. Furthermore, heating RTF to 80°C for 30 minutes destroys its inhibin activity (Setchell *et al.,* 1977). We have also observed reduction of inhibin activity when the high molecular weight (> 10,000) extract of RTF is heated to 60°C for 30 minutes (Franchimont *et al.,* 1978).

6. *Lack of a Carbohydrate Moiety*

It is not clear whether inhibin possesses a carbohydrate moiety. Chari (1977) looked for possible carbohydrate components in extracts of inhibin from bull seminal plasma, using specific colorimetric techniques, but they found no evidence for carbohydrate. Furthermore, an extract of hamster ovaries obtained by Chappel *et al.* (1979) that

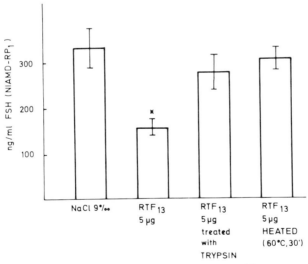

Fig. 10. Effect of an inhibin preparation (RTF_{13}) extracted from ram rete testis fluid (RTF) on luteinizing hormone-releasing hormone (LH-RH)-stimulated follicle-stimulating hormone (FSH) release in dispersed rat pituitary cell (RP) (10^5 cells) culture. Each column represents the FSH release (± 1 standard deviation) after 6 hours of incubation with LH-RH (10^{-8} *M*), when to the culture medium was added NaCl, 0.9% or 5 μg of RTF_{13} untreated, submitted to trypsin digestion, or heated at 60°C for 30 minutes. Only untreated RTF_{13} significantly (* = $p < 0.01$) reduced FSH release.

possessed inhibin-like activity did not contain any carbohydrate capable of being fixed on a column of concanavalin A.

7. *Immunochemical Behavior*

Beginning in 1975, we immunized rabbits with active fractions of HSP, BSP, and RTF. Antisera prepared in the rabbit and subsequently administered to rats led to an increase in endogenous FSH levels. We interpreted this to be the result of immunological neutralization of endogenous inhibin (Franchimont *et al.*, 1975c). The rabbits submitted to immunization under these conditions showed higher FSH levels than nonimmunized rabbits, whereas the levels of LH were identical to the control values (Table III).

Moreover, when 0.25 ml of antiserum raised against the active fraction (Ac_{II}) of BSP was injected daily into adult rats for 4 days a highly significant increase in endogenous FSH levels resulted, whereas the increase in levels of LH was barely significant. The concentration of testosterone in the rats treated with antiserum was no different from that in rats given normal rabbit serum (Fig. 11). This increase in endogenous FSH levels was significant because the nonspecific effect of rabbit immunoglobulins in the second antibody precipitation phase of the radioimmunoassays for FSH and LH had been carefully controlled.

By use of the RIA of ovine inhibin $(RTF_{38\,c})$ described in Fig. 8, cross-reactions between several preparations from different sources were established.

TABLE III

FSH AND LH LEVELS IN RABBITS IMMUNIZED WITH INHIBIN PREPARATIONS[a]

Female Rabbits immunized with	FSH[b] (ng/ml)	LH[b] (ng/ml)
Control $(N = 4)$	$468 \pm 47SD$	$202 \pm 101SD$
RTF_{38}	1100	160
BSP Ac_{II}	1290	280
BFF	770	256

[a] FSH, follicle-stimulating hormone; LH, luteinizing hormone; RTF, ram rete testis fluid; BSP AC_{II}, active fraction of bull seminal plasma; BFF, bovine follicular fluid; SD, standard deviation.

[b] Assayed according to Dufy-Barbe *et al.* (1973) and expressed as nanograms of rabbit pituitary FSH and LH reference preparation.

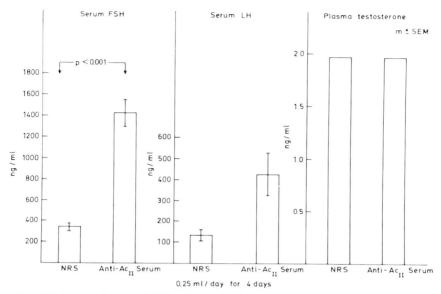

Fig. 11. Levels of serum follicle-stimulating hormone (FSH) and luteinizing hormone (LH) and of plasma testosterone in adult rats treated for 4 days with a normal rabbit serum (NRS) and with an anti-inhibin serum (anti-Ac_{II} serum). Anti-inhibin serum significantly increases FSH levels. The augmentation of LH was not significant. There was no change in plasma testosterone levels.

V. Biological Properties of Inhibin

Inhibin selectively impairs the secretion of FSH as much *in vivo* as *in vitro*. It also can cause a reduction in the secretion of LH, but much larger doses are required. This biological activity of inhibin occurs regardless of the species from which it originates. Inhibin from different species is active in monkeys, rats, mice, and rabbits.

A. Sites of Action of Inhibin

1. *Pituitary Action*

Inhibin certainly acts on the pituitary. No matter whether it is extracted from human seminal plasma or RTF (Setchell *et al.*, 1977; Baker *et al.*, 1976; Franchimont *et al.*, 1978), ram testicular lymph (Baker *et al.*, 1978), the culture medium of Sertoli cells (Steinberger and Steinberger, 1976; Lagace *et al.*, 1979; de Jong *et al.*, 1978), or follicular fluid (de Jong *et al.*, 1978; Shander *et al.*, 1979), inhibin exerts an effect on basal FSH levels and on the FSH response to LH-RH in isolated cultured pituitary cells (Fig. 6). It is also true that an effect can be observed on the LH response to LH-RH but consistently much larger doses of the inhibin preparation are required and the inhibition curve is different from that for FSH. In Fig. 6, it is clear that a significant inhibition of LH-RH-induced FSH release was obtained with 1 μg of RTF_{38} per milliliter whereas 10 μg of RTF_{38} were needed to produce a significant reduction of LH levels under the same conditions.

The degree of inhibitory activity is quantitatively and temporally cumulative, since an increase both in the dose and length of exposure resulted in an increased degree of inhibition of pituitary release of FSH both in the presence and in the absence of LH-RH.

In vivo in male rats (Franchimont *et al.*, 1975b) and in female rats under precisely controlled conditions [preestrous rat in which preovulatory LH and FSH surges were blocked with phenobarbital (Wise *et al.*, 1979)], inhibin preparations inhibit the response of the gonadotroph to injection or perfusion of exogenous LH-RH (Fig. 12). With variation of experimental conditions (quantities of LH-RH and inhibin, route of injection of LH-RH, interval between pretreatment with inhibin and injection of LH-RH, etc.), the effect can be made more or less specific on FSH release (Wise *et al.*, 1979) or less discriminately on both FSH and LH secretion (Franchimont *et al.*, 1975b).

2. *Hypothalamic Action*

The data of Lugaro *et al.* (1974) suggested an action of inhibin at the level of the hypothalamus. These investigators injected their active extract (100 ng) prepared from bull spermatozoa into the third ventricle and observed a reduction in the levels of FSH. In contrast, no effect on LH was determined.

In vitro, we have shown that inhibin preparations extracted from HSP and RTF decrease the endogenous LH-RH content of isolated hypothalami of rats after short-term incubation with several concentrations of inhibin (Demoulin *et al.*, 1979b).

The entire hypothalami were dissected from the preoptic area to the mammillary bodies in adult male rats. The fragments were kept cold during the collection. The hypothalami were then incubated for 1 hour at 37°C in an atmosphere of air/CO_2 (95/5 v/V). Each tube contained an equivalent of 1 or 2 hypothalami in 1 ml of phosphate-buffered

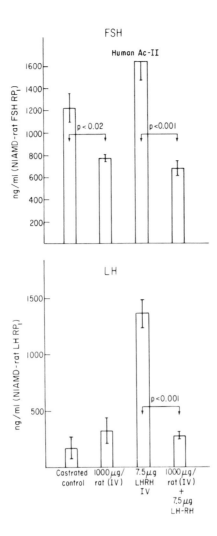

FIG. 12. Effect of a crude extract of human seminal plasma (HSP) (AC_{II}) on basal follicle-stimulating hormone (FSH) and luteinizing hormone (LH) levels and their response to LH-releasing hormone (LH-RH). Adult male rats (250 gm) were used 4 days after castration. They received intravenously either 0.5 ml of NaCl 0.9% alone or 1000 µg of the crude preparation of HSP dissolved in the same volume of diluent. Three hours later, some rats were injected intravenously (IV) with 7.5 µg of LH-RH. Twenty minutes later, they were killed and serum FSH and LH were measured. The columns represent the mean values ($N = 6$) ± SEM. Inhibin preparations significantly decreased basal FSH levels without affecting basal LH levels and also inhibited the FSH and LH responses to LH-RH.

saline supplemented with glucose ($1.5 \times 10^{-2} M$) and bacitracin ($2 \times 10^{-5} M$) (Rotsztejn et al., 1976). The hypothalami were incubated in triplicate with several concentrations of inhibin fractions obtained from human seminal plasma (HSP_3) or ram rete testis fluid (RTF_{38}). After the incubation, the hypothalami were removed and homogenized by ultrasonication in 2 ml of 2 N acetic acid. After centrifugation at 3000 g for 10 minutes at $4°C$, the supernatants were collected and stored at $-20°C$ until assayed.

LH-RH (GnRH)-specific radioimmunoassays (Bourguignon et al., 1979) were performed in aliquots of hypothalamic extracts previously neutralized with ammonium hydroxide.

The amounts of immunoreactive GnRH found in isolated hypothalami after incubation with increasing concentrations of inhibin are shown in Fig. 13. Using HSP_3, a small molecular weight fraction obtained from human seminal plasma, a dose-related decrease of intrahypothalamic GnRH was observed. This decrease was statistically significant when as much as 2.5 μg of HSP_3 were added per hypothalamus ($p < 0.001$). Using RTF_{38}, a high molecular weight fraction obtained from RTF, a dose-related decrease of GnRH content was also found. In the presence of 10 μg of RTF_{38} added per hypothalamus, the GnRH contained in the hypothalamus was significantly decreased ($p < 0.05$).

These observations demonstrate a dose-dependent effect of inhibin on hypothalamic structures synthesizing and storing GnRH. These data might be interpreted either as reduced synthesis or increased enzymatic degradation of GnRH. Measurements of GnRH peptidases, studies of GnRH contained in and released from nerve endings of mediobasal hypothalamus, and identification of GnRH metabolites are in progress in our laboratory.

3. Direct Action on the Gonad

As described in Section V,D,2, the incorporation of tritiated thymidine into testicular DNA was studied *in vivo* and *in vitro* in normal rats during puberty, aged 42 days, weighing 150 gm, and showing spermatozoa and/or spermatids from stage 12 in 40% of seminiferous tubules (Franchimont et al., 1979b). *In vitro* fragments of the testis of these animals were incubated for 3 hours with different inhibin preparations in the presence of tritiated thymidine (1 μCi per milliliter of culture medium). Two inhibin preparations showed a powerful inhibitory effect on the incorporation of tritiated thymidine. These were

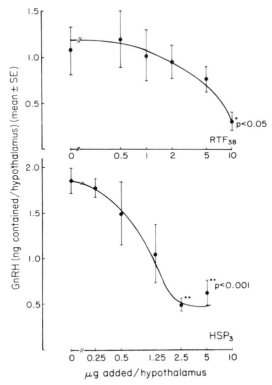

FIG. 13. Effect of increasing amounts of semipurified inhibin preparations extracted from ram rete testis fluid (RTF_{38}) and human seminal plasma (HSP_3) on hypothalamic luteinizing hormone-releasing hormone (LH-RH, GnRH) content. Ordinate: LH-RH (GnRH) content in nanograms per hypothalamus ± SEM. Abscissa: amount of inhibin preparations added per hypothalamus.

the active fractions from human seminal plasma (HSP_{3-4}) and RTF_3 that contained the substances of molecular weight less than 5000 (Table IV).

In contrast, under these experimental conditions the effect of the high molecular weight (> 10,000) fraction of RTF on the incorporation of tritiated thymidine into testis fragments maintained in organ culture was not statistically significant (Table IV). A comparison of RTF_3 (MW < 5000) and RTF_{38} (MW > 10,000) on an equimolar basis is needed before concluding that RTF_{38} has no gonadal action.

These preliminary findings suggest that certain inhibin preparations exert a direct inhibitory effect on the synthesis of DNA by actively dividing spermatogonia at the beginning of spermatogenesis.

TABLE IV

TRITIATED THYMIDINE INCORPORATION INTO TESTICULAR DNA *in Vitro*

Treatment[a]	Culture medium[b]	Dpm/mg DNA ($\times 10^{-3}$)	SD ($\times 10^{-3}$)	p
NaCL, 0.9%	5	63.4	11.6	
RTF$_{38}$, 20 μg	5	47.6	10	NS
RTF$_3$, 20 μg	5	34.6	6.8	< 0.005
HSP$_{3-4}$, 20 μg	5	38.7	9.4	< 0.002

[a] RTF, ram rete testis fluid; HSP, human seminal plasma.
[b] Each culture consisted of at least 20 testicular explants of 1 mm^3 volume.

B. MECHANISM OF ACTION OF INHIBIN AT THE PITUITARY LEVEL

1. *Specificity of Action on the Gonadotroph*

Inhibin, whether it be an extract of RTF or of bovine or human seminal fluid, specifically acts on gonadotropin secretion and has no effect whatsoever on TSH, prolactin, or growth hormone either *in vivo* or *in vitro* (Franchimont *et al.*, 1975b, 1978).

2. *Selective Action on FSH Secretion*

In vitro, inhibin exerts an effect not only on FSH, but also on LH release induced by LH-RH. Nevertheless, its action is more selective on FSH secretion. In fact, the minimum dose required to lower FSH levels significantly is much less than the dose that reduces LH levels. This selective action is even more apparent in experiments *in vitro*, in which basal levels of LH and LH cell contents are not lowered in the range of doses of inhibin used (Fig. 6).

In vivo the action of inhibin is the result of direct effects on the pituitary and on the hypothalamus, as will be shown.

3. *Action on the Synthesis and Release of the Gonadotropins*

In vitro, various preparations of inhibin (extract of RTF, follicular fluid, etc.) lead to a concomitant reduction of the quantity of FSH in the culture medium and within the cells after 72 hours of incubation in the absence of LH-RH (Fig. 14). This action is more marked on the cell content than on the quantities of FSH released into the culture medium. Under our chosen experimental conditions, no effect was

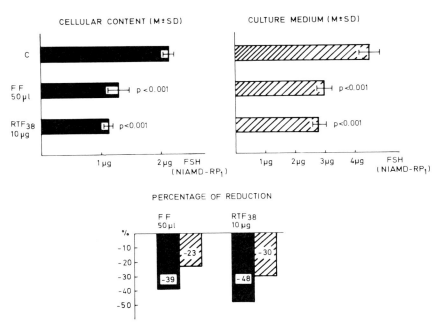

FIG. 14. Effect of 50 μl of steroid-free bovine follicular fluid (FF) and 10 μg of ram rete testis fluid (RTF$_{38}$) on amounts of follicle-stimulating hormone (FSH) cell content and in culture medium after 3 days of incubation. Bar C: Control values observed in the absence of inhibin preparations. The upper part of the graph indicates absolute FSH amounts $\pm$ SD, and the lower part represents the reduction of FSH amounts in cellular content (black columns) and in culture medium (hatched columns) expressed as percentage, the control values representing 0%. Under these experimental conditions, no effect was observed on luteinizing hormone intracellular and culture medium contents.

observed on the quantities of LH present in either the culture medium or the cells. These actions on the quantities of FSH in the two compartments show that the inhibin preparations tested have an effect on FSH synthesis under basal conditions. In fact, if the actions were limited to an inhibition of FSH release, the level of FSH would be reduced in the culture medium whereas the quantities of FSH in the cells would remain the same or be even greater than in the control cells (Franchimont *et al.*, 1978).

Convincing evidence of the action of inhibin on FSH synthesis has been provided by the experiments of Chowdhury *et al.* (1978). These authors studied the incorporation of [³H]leucine into FSH and LH produced by organ cultures of rat anterior pituitaries cultured in a medium previously used for 2–5 days to culture Sertoli cells. The Sertoli cell factor present in the culture medium selectively reduced the incorporation of labeled leucine into immunoprecipitable FSH without decreasing its incorporation into LH.

As both these experiments were performed *in vitro* in the absence of LH-RH, it is clear that the observed effect was caused by a direct inhibin-like action on FSH synthesis by the gonadotroph.

4. *Receptors to Inhibin in the Gonadotrophs*

Sairam *et al.* (1978) studied the binding of ^{125}I-labeled bovine inhibin by a crude membrane preparation from frozen ovine pituitary glands. Unlabeled preparations of inhibin from several species inhibited this binding, and LH-RH, ovine LH, bovine serum proteins, and rat liver extract failed to displace any of the isotope bound to the receptors.

It is evident from this experiment that the receptor for inhibin is different from that for LH-RH and that the action of the testicular hormone is not due to competition for LH-RH receptors.

C. Kinetics of the Action of Inhibin on Gonadotropin Secretion *in Vivo*

Experiments in which rats are given various inhibin preparations have been very useful for showing inhibin action, but the "one point" response to pulses of injected material does not allow the assessment of the effect of inhibin on the secretion of the gonadotrophs over a long period. The limited nature of these experiments is evident from the inconsistent results, often a specific inhibition of FSH, rarely on LH alone (Hodgen *et al.*, 1974), more frequently on both gonadotropins.

To overcome this difficulty, several studies were undertaken in animals in order to determine the kinetics of the action of different inhibin preparations. They all showed that a delay of several hours was necessary for inhibin to exert an inhibitory effect on FSH levels that would persist beyond the period of administration of the test material. Furthermore, these experiments revealed differences in the kinetics of the reduction of FSH and LH concentrations.

The first studies of the kinetics of inhibin action were made by Lee *et al.* (1974), Keogh *et al.* (1976), and Baker *et al.* (1976).

Crude testicular extracts equivalent to between 1.0 and 3.0 kg net weight of bovine testes were infused into five castrated rams over a period of 10–24 hours. Blood samples were collected before, during, and after the infusion either continuously (samples of 3–8 hours duration) or intermittently (three blood samples at 15-minute intervals every 3–8 hours). Under these conditions, extracts of bull testes infused into castrated sheep will lower plasma FSH levels after a lag period of about 12 hours. These decreases, which have ranged from 15 to 58% of preinfusion levels, persist for at least 24 hours after the infusion has been stopped. The levels of LH frequently showed a small decline within 3–5 hours of the beginning of the infusion but subsequently rose at 24 hours either with saline or testis extracts. Testosterone levels were unaffected.

More recently, Cahoreau *et al.* (1979) and Blanc *et al.* (1978) have clearly demonstrated that a nonsteroidal factor from RTF suppresses the secretion of both FSH and LH, but with different kinetics. Castrated or cryptorchid animals were bled every 15 or 30 minutes for 25 hours. Twenty milliliters of charcoal-treated RTF were injected at the fifth and at the sixth hour after the beginning of sampling. Human serum albumin or γ-globulins were injected similarly in controls. In all cases, the LH secretion pattern was altered first; plasma FSH levels were lowered much later, at a time when the LH secretion pattern had returned to normal. RTF injections resulted in the suppression of LH peaks for 3–5 hours starting in the first hours after treatment. FSH was progressively lowered after the first injection, and the maximum FSH inhibition was observed about 8 hours after the first injection and lasted for about 7 hours.

We have perfused rabbits, castrated at least 15 days earlier, with 0.9% saline solution followed 3 days later with an active fraction, P_{II}, of RTF obtained after precipitation with alcohol, washing with acetone, filtration on Sephadex G-200, and chromatography on DEAE-cellulose (Franchimont *et al.*, 1977). This is in the high molecular weight (> 10,000) category (Franchimont *et al.*, 1978). Blood samples were taken every 20 minutes for 8 hours, then at longer intervals. The test material was perfused for 6 hours from the end of hour 1 to the end of hour 7. As shown in Fig. 15, the level of FSH fluctuated widely during the control perfusion. When the active preparation was infused, one saw a marked reduction in FSH that appeared only 4–5 hours after the beginning of perfusion. From that time FSH values were stable, and they remained low for 24 hours after the start of the perfusion. The level of LH also fluctuated widely during the control perfusion and in the hour preceding the infusion of the active fraction. When the infusion was begun, the pulses of LH were lost and the levels of LH also fell. This effect was transitory, for at the end of the perfusion the LH values were similar to those seen during the control period (Fig. 16).

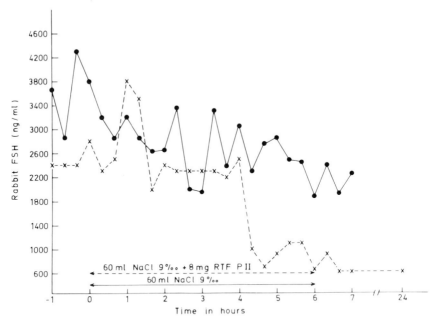

Fɪɢ. 15. Serum follicle-stimulating hormone (FSH) levels before, during, and after a 6-hour perfusion of 60 ml of NaCl, 0.9% (●—●) and 60 ml of NaCl, 0.9%, containing 8 mg of active fraction (PII) extracted from RTF in a castrated male rabbit (X---X). A significant decrease of FSH levels appeared after 4 hours of infusion and persisted for 24 hours after the beginning of the perfusion.

Kinetic studies are practically impossible to perform in rats because of the difficulty of taking frequent blood samples. It is interesting to know that the injection of inhibin preparations into rats castrated 2 or 3 weeks earlier leads to a simultaneous reduction of FSH and LH and, in some cases, to a reduction of LH without altering FSH levels (Hodgen *et al.*, 1974). Using intact adult rats injected every 8 hours for 24, 48, or 72 hours and with the blood sampled 4 hours after the last injection, Lee *et al.* (1977) found that at 28 hours LH levels were significantly suppressed but FSH levels were not. In contrast, at 52 hours and 76 hours LH secretion was unaltered and FSH was significantly suppressed.

In monkeys, the injection or perfusion of inhibin appears to have little effect on LH, but, characteristically, after a latent period there is a prolonged reduction of FSH levels.

Keogh (1978) showed that a preparation of ovine testicular lymph, when infused over a period of 24 hours, caused a 50% fall in the level

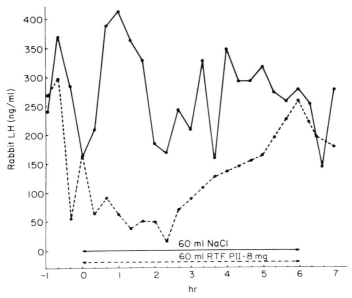

FIG. 16. Serum luteinizing hormone (LH) levels before, during, and after a perfusion of 60 ml of NaCl, 0.9% (● — ●) and 60 ml of NaCl, 0.9%, containing 8 mg of active fraction (PII) extracted from ram rete testis fluid (RTF) in a castrated male rabbit (● --- ●). LH pulses disappeared with the beginning of the perfusion, and LH levels decreased for the first 3 hours. During the last 3 hours of perfusion, basal LH levels progressively increased to reach control values at the end of the perfusion.

of FSH that persisted for up to 48 hours. A control animal received an equivalent amount of protein prepared from the thoracic duct lymph of a castrated animal. No modification of LH levels was observed.

Channing *et al.* (1979) treated four long-term castrated adult female monkeys. The porcine follicular fluid (PFF) (15 or 5 ml) was administered subcutaneously in two doses 6 hours apart. Blood was sampled every 6 hours, 18 hours before and 3 days after the injections. The PFF administration led to a progressive decline of serum FSH that started within 18 hours and was maintained for about 3 days (Fig. 17).

These concordant kinetic studies show that the action of inhibin on pituitary secretion of gonadotropins *in vivo* is complex and clearly involves direct effects on the pituitary and the hypothalamus, as previously discussed. Species differences in the gonadotropin response are possible, in particular in monkeys, in which no action on LH was detected (Shashidhara-Murthy *et al.*, 1979; Keogh, 1978; Channing *et al.*, 1979).

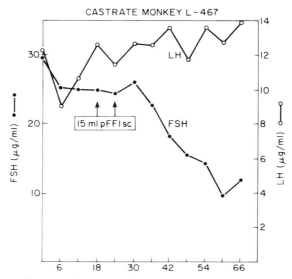

Fig. 17. Temporal course (abscissa, in hours) of inhibitory action of porcine follicular fluid (PFFl) upon serum luteinizing hormone (LH) (right ordinate) and follicle-stimulating hormone (FSH) (left ordinate) in a castrated monkey. The fluid was given subcutaneously in two 5-ml doses 6 hours apart followed by blood sampling every 6 hours thereafter for 3 days. A long-term castrated female monkey was used for this study. Serum LH and FSH levels were measured in each blood sample. Reproduced from Channing *et al.* (1979), with permission of the authors and publisher.

The brief reduction in LH secretion observed after administration of inhibin may be caused by one or both of the following mechanisms: reduced production and release of LH-RH by the hypothalamus (see Section V,A,2), or inhibition of pituitary LH release under LH-RH control (see Section V,A,1).

The existence of a latent phase before the inhibitory effect on FSH levels is observed, and the persistence of this effect well beyond the period of inhibin administration argues for a major action on pituitary synthesis of FSH.

The latent period and prolonged effect after administration of inhibin preparations cannot be explained by the half-life of FSH. The latent period is of the order of 4–12 hours in a variety of experiments whereas the half-life of FSH calculated from the slope of its disappearance curve in the absence of pituitary secretion is approximately 4.5 hours (Franchimont and Burger, 1975; Lincoln, 1978). Moreover, the inhibitory effect on FSH secretion lasts for 24 hours after the administration of inhibin. This time course favors an action of inhibin on FSH synthesis.

D. INTERACTIONS BETWEEN INHIBIN, ANDROGENS,
    AND ESTROGENS

Little work has been done on the problem of the interaction between the sex steroids and inhibin. Nevertheless, this problem is fundamental, as inhibin is not the sole factor regulating FSH secretion. Thus, 21 days after complete destruction of germ cells either by efferent duct ligation or by severe heating, the increase of FSH levels is only 30% of that observed 21 days after castration (Main *et al.,* 1978).

Some synergistic effects have been observed in *in vivo* experiments.

Serum FSH is only partially suppressible by estradiol in ovariectomized female mouse, even when estradiol is given in larger than physiological amounts. In these maximally estrogenized ovariectomized mice, ovarian transplantation, on the one hand, and administration of porcine follicular fluid, on the other hand, result in FSH blood levels that are within the range shown during the estrous cycle in intact females (Bronson and Channing, 1978).

Hopkinson *et al.* (1977b) studied the effects of testosterone alone; of an active inhibin preparation extracted from human seminal plasma, prepared by cold ethanol precipitation, acetone drying, and chromatography on Sephadex G-50; and of both substances together on the FSH and LH levels in adult male rats castrated 40 hours before sacrifice. Testosterone alone given subcutaneously in a dose of 50 μg/100 gm body weight had no effect on FSH levels whereas LH returned to precastration levels. The inhibin extract given alone had a limited effect on FSH levels. In contrast, testosterone and the extract given together led to a marked reduction of FSH to levels similar to those seen in intact adult animals. The levels of testosterone were the same in both groups of rats given testosterone either alone or with the extract of human seminal plasma. This experiment demonstrated a synergistic effect of testosterone and inhibin on the reduction of FSH levels and also a lack of any effect of inhibin on the absorption or clearance of testosterone.

In the same year, Marder *et al.* (1977) treated fluid from medium and large follicles of pigs with charcoal to remove steroids. The follicular fluid thus treated significantly reduced in a dose-dependent manner FSH levels in both ovariectomized and sham-ovariectomized rats. However, there was a lower threshold to porcine follicular fluid in the sham-ovariectomized rats with higher estradiol levels than in ovariectomized animals, which suggests a synergistic effect of estradiol and ovarian inhibin on FSH negative feedback control.

In contrast, inhibin opposes the stimulating effects of androgens and estrogens on gonadotropin secretion induced by LH-RH *in vitro*. Lagace *et al.* (1979) studied the direct pituitary site for feedback action of sex steroids and inhibin and their interaction with LH-RH in the control of FSH and LH secretion in dispersed pituitary cell cultures. Estrogens stimulated both the LH and the FSH response to LH-RH, whereas androgens (testosterone and dihydrotestosterone) inhibited LH and stimulated FSH secretion. Porcine follicular fluid or granulosa cell culture medium as well as Sertoli cell culture medium, treated with dextran-coated charcoal to remove endogenous steroids, exerted an inhibitory effect on the LH-RH-induced release of both gonadotropins although the effect on FSH secretion occurred earlier and with lower concentrations than the effect on LH secretion. Furthermore, inhibin-containing media completely reversed the stimulatory effect of estrogens on LH-RH-induced LH and FSH secretion (Fig. 18) and of androgens on LH-RH-induced FSH secretion. An additive effect of dihydrotestosterone and inhibin present in bovine follicular fluid has been observed on LH release induced by LH-RH in dispersed pituitary cell culture (Fig. 18).

E. EFFECTS OF INHIBIN ON GONADAL FUNCTION

1. *Effect on Spermatogenesis*

Few experiments have been undertaken to study the effects of inhibin on spermatogenesis. De Jong *et al.* (1978) gave bovine follicular fluid, devoid of steroids, for 12 days to 21-day-old male rats and were able to show a delay in pubertal development of the testes compared with control animals, reduction of testicular weight, retardation of spermatogenesis, and decrease in the number of pachytene spermatocytes. These effects were produced even though the levels of FSH were reduced only during the first 4 days of treatment and the levels of LH were significantly increased.

We have given different inhibin preparations, extracts of human seminal fluid of low molecular weight (HSP_{3-4}) and of RTF with a molecular weight greater than 10,000 (RTF_{13}) and with a molecular weight less than 5000 (RTF_3), in doses totaling 160 μl/100 gm body weight administered as four injections intraperitoneally over 36 hours to rats of different ages. We measured the incorporation of

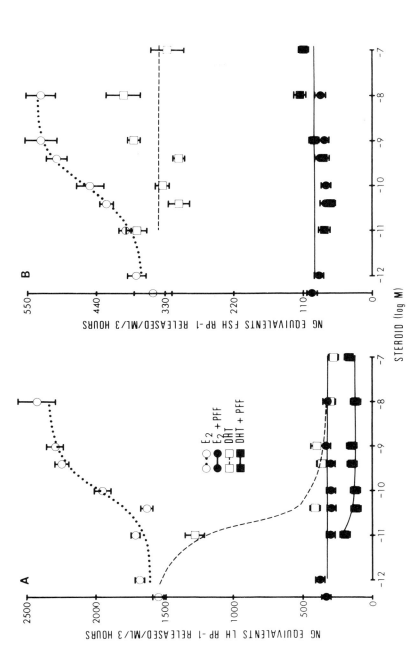

FIG. 18. Effect of increasing concentrations of estradiol (E_2) and dihydrotestosterone (DHT) in the presence (filled symbols) or the absence (open symbols) of porcine follicular fluid (PFF) on (A) the luteinizing hormone (LH) and (B) the follicle-stimulating hormone (FSH) responses to $0.1 \, nM$ LH-releasing hormone (LH-RH). LH-RH was present during a 3-hour incubation period after a 40-hour preincubation with the indicated steroids or porcine follicular fluid. Reproduced from Lagace *et al.* (1979) with permission of the authors and publisher.

tritiated thymidine injected 3 hours before sacrifice into testicular DNA and the labeling of germinal cells by autohistoradiography. The inhibin preparations markedly reduced the incorporation of tritiated thymidine into testicular DNA and the uptake by type B spermatogonia compared with the same preparation previously degraded by trypsin and heated to 60°C for 1 hour (Fig. 19). This effect was apparent in 42- to 49-day-old rats in which spermatogenesis commences and progresses at the same time as a significant incorporation of thymidine into testicular DNA is observed (Table V). In contrast, in adult rats, no effect was observed on the incorporation of [³H] thymidine, which is ten times less than that seen in pubertal rats (Franchimont et al., 1979b). Inhibin preparations specifically act on testicular DNA synthesis since they induce no modification of thymidine incorporation into hepatic DNA (Table V).

Inhibin thus appears to inhibit the synthesis of DNA implicated in the mitoses of germinal cells (particularly, spermatogonia type B) in pubertal animals. These cells, as they divide, signify the beginning of spermatogenesis. This effect is doubtless mediated by the reduction of the secretion of FSH. It is known, in fact, that after FSH withdrawal by injecting specific anti-FSH serum, there is also an inhibition of [³H]thymidine incorporation into DNA (Murty et al., 1979). But a direct effect of inhibin on the multiplication of germinal cells disclosed by the incorporation of tritiated thymidine in the testicular DNA has been observed in vitro with the low molecular weight preparations of inhibin: HSP₃₋₄ and RTF₃ (see Table IV). The action of these inhibin preparations, as much in vivo as in vitro, resembles that of testicular chalones described by Clermont and Mauger (1974). These substances extracted from testes exert an inhibitory effect on germ cells, particularly on the multiplication of spermatogonia type A.

In adults, inhibin has no detectable effect either because the frequency of mitoses is insufficient for an effect to be observed, or because cell multiplication ceases to be dependent on FSH and secondarily on inhibin. Steinberger (1971) showed that in adult rats spermatogenesis can be maintained by testosterone alone.

2. Effect on Gonadotropin Secretion during the Estrous Cycle and on Follicular Maturation

Schwartz and Channing (1977) showed that the pattern of FSH secretion was modified during the estrous cycle of the rat by the injection of porcine follicular fluid previously treated with charcoal. Thus, the elevation of blood FSH levels that appears between proestrus and estrus in response to the natural preovulation peak of LH or an ar-

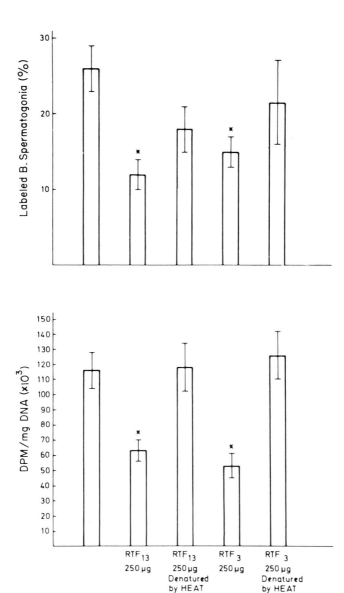

Fig. 19. Effect of NaCl, 0.9%, and two inhibin preparations from ram rete testis fluid (RTF$_{13}$ and RTF$_3$) either untreated or denatured by heating and trypsin digestion on (upper part) the percentage of spermatogonia type B labeled with tritiated thymidine and detected by autohistoradiography; and on (lower part) incorporation of labeled thymidine into testicular DNA expressed as dpm/mg DNA ($\times$ 10^4). RTF$_{13}$ and RTF$_3$ significantly reduce ($* = p < 0.01$) the percentage of labeled spermatogonia and the thymidine incorporation into DNA compared with control animals treated with NaCl, 0.9% (first column) or with animals treated with denatured preparations.

TABLE V

Incorporation of Tritiated Thymidine into Testicular and Hepatic DNA in Rats at Different Stages of Spermatogenesis Maturation: Influence of Inhibin Treatment (160 μG/100 gm Body Weight)

Incorporation into	Age (days)	Percentage of seminiferous tubules containing spermatozoa and/or spermatids from stage 12[a]	N	Thymidine incorporation (dpm/mg DNA ($\times 10^{-3}$) $\pm$ SEM)			
				NaCl, 0.9%	RTF$_{13}$	RTF$_3$	HSP$_{3-4}$
Testicular DNA	42	40%	10	117 $\pm$ 5.0	64.3 $\pm$ 4.8[b]	53 $\pm$ 5.7[b]	67.1 $\pm$ 4.2[b]
	49	91%	6	43 $\pm$ 3.5	ND[c]	20 $\pm$ 1.7[b]	ND
	56	100%	6	23 $\pm$ 1.7	ND	23 $\pm$ 1.5	ND
Hepatic DNA	42	40%	5	184 $\pm$ 10.6	ND	196 $\pm$ 6.5	ND

[a] Seminiferous tubules (200–300) were examined by optical microscopy.

[b] $p < 0.01$ compared to animals of the same age treated with NaCl, 0.9%.

[c] ND, not determined.

tificial peak of LH (induced by the inhibition of the natural preovulation peak of LH by pentobarbital and replaced by exogenous LH) can be suppressed by the steroid-free fluid given intraperitoneally in two doses of 0.5 ml each (Fig. 20). This inhibitory factor does not alter the LH levels or modify estradiol and progesterone secretion rates and does not affect rupture of the follicle. Under these experimental conditions, treatment by steroid free porcine follicular fluid inhibited the second elevation of FSH, which may recruit follicles for the next cycle (Schwartz, 1969; Schwartz *et al.*, 1973).

De Jong *et al.* (1978) obtained somewhat different results in long-term experiments with much smaller doses of follicular fluid. These investigators injected adult female rats with charcoal-treated bovine follicular fluid daily over five estrous cycles. The dose was 0.25 ml/100 gm body weight for the first 17 days, subsequently 1 ml/100 gm. Under these conditions, the authors did not observe any changes in vaginal smears. Furthermore, the number of ova in the tubes from the second to the fifth estrous cycle was no different from controls treated

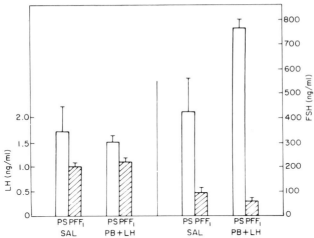

FIG. 20. Effect of porcine follicular fluid (PFF) and porcine serum (PS) on (LH) (left) and (FSH) (right) serum levels in rats at 4 A.M. on the day of estrus. Rats were treated with either saline (SAL) or pentobarbital (PB) at 1:30 P.M. and 3 P.M. on the day of proestrus; the pentobarbital-treated rats also received 8 μg of LH at 3:30 P.M. Porcine serum or porcine follicular fluid was injected at 3:45 P.M. (0.5 ml) and at 6:30 (0.5 ml). Rats exhibiting 4-day cycles were used. Standard error of the mean is indicated above each bar. The PFF led to a significant decrease of serum FSH levels in both experimental conditions, whereas serum LH was not significantly different as a result of the two pretreatments or in serum versus follicular fluid treatments. Reproduced from Schwartz and Channing (1977), with permission of the authors and publisher.

with bovine plasma. FSH levels fell 8 hours after the first injection, then there was an increase in FSH and LH levels as compared with control values. The blood levels are, nevertheless, difficult to interpret because they were not taken systematically during the five estrous cycles but at very wide intervals.

A most interesting experiment was performed by Channing *et al.* (1979), who demonstrated that inhibin inhibits follicular maturation and can modify the midcycle FSH peak in monkeys.

Porcine follicular fluid (PFF) from small and medium follicles was pooled, charcoal-treated, and injected intraperitoneally in 4-ml doses every 8 hours between days 1 and 4 of the menstrual cycle of 4 rhesus monkeys. Treatment was followed by laparotomy on day 12 to 14 of the cycle, with recovery of the preovulatory follicle. Serum FSH levels were measured in daily blood samples for one control menstrual cycle prior to treatment and throughout one treatment cycle. The PFF

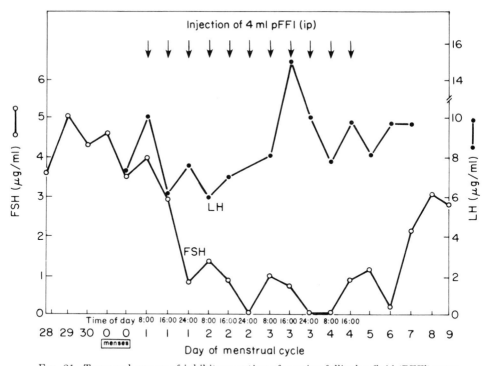

F<small>IG</small>. 21. Temporal course of inhibitory action of porcine follicular fluid (PFFl) upon serum (FSH) in a rhesus monkey given porcine follicular fluid every 8 hours for 4 days during the early follicular phase of the menstrual cycle. Reproduced from Channing *et al.* (1979), with permission of the authors and publisher.

caused a significant decrease in serum FSH levels within 24–36 hours of the start of the treatment in the 4 animals. FSH levels returned to preinjection control levels within 1–3 days after cessation of treatment (Fig. 21). There was a decline of less than 5% in serum LH levels. The follicle present on days 12–14 of the treatment cycle was smaller than normal and contained few granulosa cells (0.1×10^6 cells) compared to control preovulatory follicles, which contained 2 to 50×10^6 cells, i.e., less than 10% of the normal number of granulosa cells. The action of inhibin on follicular maturation is certainly mediated by FSH, but a direct effect of inhibin on the follicle is not excluded.

Two monkeys were given PFF for 4 days at midcycle. In one case in which the treatment was started 1 day prior to the expected midcycle surge of FSH, the midcycle FSH surge was delayed until after cessation of PFF treatment. In the other monkey, in which treatment was started 8 hours after the start of the FSH surge, the surge was shortened to about one-third of normal.

VI. ORIGIN AND TRANSPORT OF INHIBIN

A. TESTICULAR ORIGIN

The testis is the source of inhibin, as shown by its presence in testicular extracts. The site of production appears to be the seminiferous tubules because large quantities of the hormone are found in the rete testis, where the secretion of the seminiferous tubules accumulates. Eddie *et al.* (1978) have also identified a substance produced by cultures of rat seminiferous tubules that suppressed the LH-RH-induced secretion of FSH by pituitary cell cultures and inhibited the secretion of LH to a lesser extent.

The experiments of Steinberger and Steinberger (1976) have shown unequivocally that the Sertoli cell is directly involved in the synthesis and secretion of inhibin, called for this reason Sertoli cell factor. In fact, pituitary cells cocultured with isolated Sertoli cells consistently released significantly less FSH than pituitary cells grown alone or cultured with spleen or kidney cells. In contrast, the LH levels in the control and coculture were similar. Furthermore, the culture medium of viable Sertoli cells alone inhibited the spontaneous and LH-RH-induced FSH release in dispersed pituitary cell culture. Since only minimum or no inhibition of FSH release was caused by ruptured Sertoli cells, the inhibin appears to be synthesized by Sertoli cells *in vitro*.

Other evidence for the role of the Sertoli cell in the secretion of inhibin has been provided by Demoulin *et al.* (1979a). Mice testes were maintained in organ culture, and after 4 days the culture medium was removed and placed on dispersed rat pituitary cells. When the testes were cultured at 37°C, spermatogenesis was greatly altered by day 4, whereas the Sertoli cells maintained their normal light microscopic appearance. This medium depressed the LH-RH-induced FSH release without affecting LH release. After 8 days of culture, Sertoli cells were also affected and the inhibitory effect on FSH secretion disappeared (Figs. 22 and 23).

When testis was cultured at 31°C, spermatogenesis was altered histologically at day 8 whereas Sertoli cells remained in good condition for 20 days. The culture medium maintained its inhibin effect for the 20 days of the experiment. Thus, there was a relationship between the histological appearance of the Sertoli cells and inhibiting potency of the culture medium. In contrast, alteration of gametogenesis did not have any effect on the inhibin activity of the culture medium.

Although there is no doubt that the Sertoli cells are responsible for the secretion of inhibin, the possible role of spermatogenesis in the in-

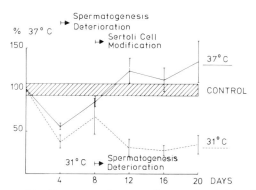

FIG. 22. Influence of testis organ culture medium on luteinizing hormone-releasing hormone (LH-RH)-induced follicle-stimulating hormone (FSH) release (expressed as percentage of the control release representing 100% ± SD = hatched area) by dispersed pituitary cells in culture. When the testis organ culture is performed at 37°C, spermatogenesis is deeply altered after 4 days and Sertoli cells are damaged after 8 days of culture. Release of FSH is significantly reduced by the testis organ culture medium collected on day 4 of culture, but not by the samples of culture medium collected later. When testis organ culture is performed at 31°C, spermatogenesis is altered after 8 days of culture, but no histological modification of Sertoli cells appears for the 20 days of culture. Testis organ culture medium collected on days 4, 8, 12, 16, and 20 of culture significantly depresses the LH-RH-induced FSH secretion, Reproduced from Demoulin *et al.* (1979a), with permission of the authors and publisher.

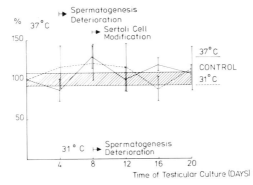

FIG. 23. Influence of testis organ culture medium on luteinizing hormone-releasing hormone (LH-RH)-induced LH release (expressed as percentage of the control release representing 100% ± SD = hatched area) by dispersed pituitary cells in culture. No significant modification of LH release was induced by any of the testis organ culture (at 31°C and 37°C) medium collected every 4 days.

duction of this secretion remains doubtful. Indeed, in some studies there was an inverse linear relationship between the level of FSH, and the qualitative (Franchimont *et al.*, 1972) and quantitative (De Kretser *et al.*, 1972) aspects of spermatogenesis observed in testicular biopsies. On the other hand, in many other studies, serum FSH levels were exceptionally high when late spermatid numbers were normal (Borsch *et al.*, 1973; De Kretser *et al.*,1974; Christiansen, 1975). Furthermore, inhibin activity was observed in extracts of human seminal plasma coming from oligospermic as well as normal subjects, but not from azoospermic patients (Franchimont, 1972). Moreover, it is known that Sertoli cells alone are not capable of reducing FSH levels in the absence of spermatogenesis. Such is the case in the Sertoli cell-only syndrome patients (De Kretser *et al.*, 1972). Finally, Hopkinson *et al.* (1978) studied the modification of germinal epithelium and the changes of gonadotropin levels in rats submitted to irradiation of the scrotum. In their experiments, gonadotropin levels were strongly negatively correlated with both tubular cytoplasm (mainly Sertoli cells) and the spermatid counts. Levels of FSH and LH were significantly higher on day 39 after irradiation as compared to day 26, and this increase coincided with an 85% decrease in the spermatid count. Over the same time interval, the spermatocyte and basal cell counts did not change significantly.

This possible relationship between spermatogenesis and the Sertoli cell resulting in the secretion of inhibin is not excluded by the experiments of Steinberger and Steinberger (1976). As a matter of fact, cultures of Sertoli cells still contain germinal cells (less than 20%) and the rate of release of FSH-inhibiting substance into the medium declines after 7 days.

Cells of the germinal type might be able to release more or less specific factors that could modulate the secretion of inhibin. These germinal cell factors could persist for some time in spite of the disappearance or alteration of the gametogenic cells or exert a prolonged effect on the secretion of inhibin by Sertoli cells. Careful studies are needed to confirm or refute the hypothesis of this possible relationship between Sertoli cells producing inhibin and germinal cells (spermatids?) that provide the signal or the material for inhibin production.

B. FOLLICULAR ORIGIN

In several animal species inhibin activity has been found in follicular fluid pretreated with charcoal to remove the sex steroids.

The models that are used to show this inhibin activity vary from one study to another. Thus, de Jong and Sharpe (1976) and Welschen et al. (1977) studied the reduction of FSH levels in adult male rats castrated less than 24 hours before sacrifice. Welschen et al. (1977) also studied the inhibition of FSH in unilaterally ovariectomized rats. Schwartz and Channing (1977) observed inhibition of the natural or induced FSH peak during preestrus in adult rats. Last, Marder et al. (1977) observed significant falls of FSH levels both in rats ovariectomized precisely in metestrus and in sham-operated animals. Under these various conditions, the levels of LH were little if at all modified. Data from the literature are contradictory concerning the levels of ovarian inhibin during follicular development. According to Lorenzen et al. (1978), the concentration of inhibin (which they call folliculostatin) diminishes with the growth of the follicle in the pig. In contrast, Welschen et al. (1977) found inhibin in small bovine follicles (5–10 mm in diameter), and maximum concentrations were reached in medium and large (11–20 mm in diameter) follicles. Very little inhibin was found in follicular cysts (diameter greater than 20 mm).

Inhibin, or folliculostatin, found in the follicular fluid of different animals appears to be produced by granulosa cells.

Erickson and Hsueh (1978) showed that the granulosa cells in culture secrete a substance that acts directly on pituitary cell cultures and preferentially suppresses FSH secretion. The inhibitory effect on FSH levels by the culture medium is greater the more numerous the granulosa cells in the culture. A slight reduction of LH release is observed when the inhibitory effect of FSH reaches its maximum of approximately 60% (Fig. 24).

Granulosa cells acquire the ability to produce inhibin early in follicular development.

The inhibin-like substance secreted by porcine granulosa cells *in vitro* appears to have a molecular weight greater than 10,000 (Anderson *et al.*, 1979).

C. SIMILARITY OF OVARIAN AND TESTICULAR INHIBIN

Several arguments favor the identity of inhibin in extracts from biological fluids of males and females.

1. *Similarity of the Inhibitory Effects on Cultured Dispersed Pituitary Cells*

When different quantities of inhibin preparations extracted from human seminal fluid, RTF, and the follicular fluid of mares and women are incubated with pituitary cell cultures in the presence or the absence of LH-RH, the curves of reduction of FSH release into the culture medium, expressed as a percentage of the initial value, are parallel for the various preparations (Fig. 25).

Similar results were obtained by de Jong *et al.* (1978) and by Lagace

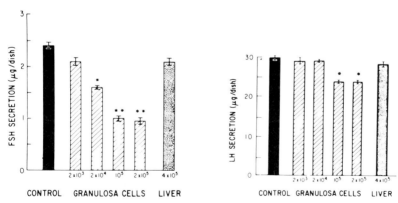

FIG. 24. Release of follicle-stimulating hormone (FSH) and luteinizing hormone (LH) by pituitary cells incubated with spent media (800 μl) from increasing numbers of rat granulosa cells obtained from preovulatory follicles and maintained in culture for 3 days (mean ± SE of the mean of duplicate determinations of four separate dishes) (* = $p < 0.01$; ** = $p < 0.001$). Reproduced by Erickson and Hsueh (1978), with permission of the authors and publisher.

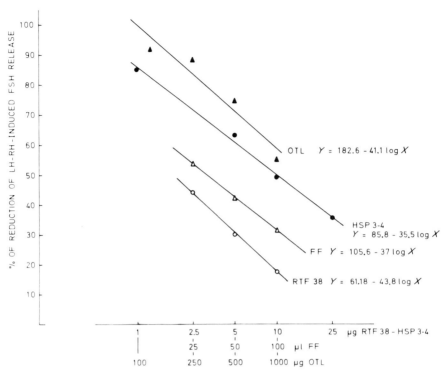

F$_{IG}$. 25. Reduction of luteinizing hormone-releasing hormone (LH-RH)-induced follicle-stimulating hormone (FSH) release by progressive amounts of several preparations of inhibin. The curves are parallel. OTL, ovine testicular lymph, $a = 41.1$; HSP$_{3-4}$, fraction 3–4 of human seminal plasma (Fig. 1), $a = 35.5$; FF, mare follicular fluid, $a = 37$; RTF$_{38}$, semipurified fraction of ram rete testis fluid (Fig. 3), $a = 43.8$.

et al. (1979), who compared the biological activity of inhibin in porcine follicular fluid and Sertoli cell culture medium. In the experiments of both these groups of investigators, the effect of porcine follicular fluid on basal as well as LH-RH-induced LH and FSH release in anterior pituitary cells in culture was indistinguishable from the results obtained with Sertoli cell culture medium.

2. *Efficacy of Inhibin in Animals of Both Sexes*

The active material extracted from biological fluids from males. HSP, BSP, and RTF, reduces FSH levels in normal and castrated, adult and prepubertal, rats of both sexes.

Active preparations obtained from bovine or porcine extracts of ovaries or follicular fluid reduce FSH levels in normal or castrated animals, as much in males as in females.

3. *Immune Reactions*

Anti-inhibin antisera have been obtained by immunizing rabbits with active preparations of BSP and RTF (Franchimont *et al.*, 1975c, 1977).

Injecting adult rats with these antisera (0.25 ml/100 gm body weight daily for 4 days) resulted in a rise of FSH levels toward the end of treatment in both male and female rats. This effect is attributed to the neutralization of endogenous inhibin. In contrast, LH levels did not increase significantly, and testosterone concentrations remained unchanged (Fig. 11).

Radioimmunological studies of the different preparations show complete cross-reaction between inhibin extracted from BFF and RTF. Inhibin extracts from BFF and RTF completely inhibited the binding of tracer to the antibody. The inhibition curves are parallel (Fig. 8).

D. Transport of Inhibin to the Hypothalamopituitary Axis

There are no data available that enable us to understand how inhibin leaves the ovary or testis and reaches the hypothalamus and pituitary.

In males, there are several possibilities. As the hormone appears to be produced within Sertoli cells, it could leave these cells from their basal surface directly into the lymph or the blood or from their luminal surfaces into the rete testis fluid or from both surfaces. It must not be forgotten that almost all the rete testis fluid is reabsorbed in the head of the epididymis (Setchell, 1970), and this results in a modification of the ionic and protein composition of seminal fluid.

VII. Possible Roles of Inhibin

Inhibin seems to be the feedback agent for quantitative information on rate of sperm production and on follicular maturation. Its first role is to modulate the hormones involved in the regulation of gametogenesis.

A. Negative Feedback on FSH Secretion

All inhibin preparations share the property of selective reduction of FSH secretion. This inhibition is rarely complete, and experiments to date do not permit an assessment of the intensity of FSH suppression under physiological conditions. The experiments are usually set up under circumstances in which FSH secretion is high (castrated animals), do not take account of the biological half-life of inhibin, which is still unknown, and use very impure preparations containing truly minute quantities of the active ingredient. Furthermore, inhibin is doubtless not the only factor that regulates FSH secretion (see Section V,D). Apart from a probable direct action of inhibin (discussed in Section VII,C), this gonadal hormone acts via the reduction of FSH secretion and its consequences.

1. *In Female Animals*

Follicle-stimulating hormone intervenes in the multiplication and functional differentiation of granulosa cells (secretion of FSH at the beginning of the cycle) and in the development of new follicles for the subsequent cycle (preovulatory peak of FSH). At present, one can say on the basis of studies in monkeys (Channing *et al.*, 1979) that early follicular deprivation of FSH induced by active fractions from follicular fluid is deleterious to the later growth of the follicle and of the granulosa cells. Furthermore, in rats (de Jong *et al.*, 1978) unilateral ovariectomy increases FSH levels without modifying the circulating estradiol concentration. Levels of FSH return to normal 28 hours after operation, when the remaining ovary contains twice as many large follicles as an ovary in an intact animal. Follicular fluid prevents this specific rise in FSH without affecting LH levels. One can guess that inhibin has a role in the short-term regulation of the number of developing follicles in the ovary.

In contrast, the fact that there can be ovulation in follicular fluid-treated rats who do not have a preovulatory FSH surge demonstrates the lack of requirement of preovulatory FSH for follicular rupture and oocyte maturation (Schwartz and Channing, 1977).

The role of FSH in the morphological changes of luteinization has been little studied. The effects of inhibin on this process remain unknown.

2. *In Male Animals*

The role of FSH in the initiation and maintenance of spermatogenesis remains in dispute.

During the pubertal period, FSH increases testicular weight and the diameter of the seminiferous tubules (Greep *et al.*, 1942; Simpson *et al.*, 1951). It further intervenes in the multiplication and differentiations of spermatogonia A_0 and A_1 and increases the number of pachytene spermatocytes. It restores the number of spermatogonia type A reduced by hypophysectomy in rats or lambs when testosterone is equally essential (Hochereau de Reviers and Courot, 1978). Treatment of immature male rats (25 days old) with specific anti-FSH serum for a period of 15 days brought about an arrest of spermatogenesis without having any adverse effects on accessory organs and their functions (Shivashanker *et al.*, 1977). Thus, germinal cells—but particularly type A spermatogonia, pachytene spermatocytes, and spermatids—are markedly reduced. All these data show that FSH is needed for the maintenance of different cells in seminiferous epithelium during the completion of the first wave of spermatogenesis.

Our experiments (see Section V,E,1) on the incorporation of tritiated thymidine into testicular DNA show that inhibin preparations reduce the synthesis of DNA *in vivo* and subsequently the mitotic activity of type B spermatogonias during puberty (in 42-day-old rats weighing 150 gm). In 53-day-old animals whose scrota were irradiated 11 days earlier, inhibin similarly reduced the incorporation of tritiated thymidine into DNA (Franchimont *et al.*, 1979b). This incorporation must occur in type A spermatogonia during regeneration (Clermont and Mauger, 1974).

In adult rats, rams, or bulls (Greep *et al.*, 1942; Simpson *et al.*, 1951), there is a positive correlation between the total number of Sertoli cells in the testis and of spermatogonia. Hypophysectomy does not affect the number of Sertoli cells, but it diminishes the stock of spermatogonia and the efficacy of spermatogenesis. In adult rats, FSH maintains the stock of spermatogonia and restores their divisions, whereas meiosis and spermiogenesis are better maintained by LH (Hochereau de Reviers and Courot, 1978). This action of FSH on the early phases of spermatogenesis confirms the earlier work of Means (1975). These authors show that FSH increases the mitotic rate and reduces degeneration among the spermatogonia. Furthermore, Orth and Christensen (1978) have shown by autoradiography that FSH binding sites occur over the surface of spermatogonia in concentrations similar to those of Sertoli cells in the basal compartment of the seminiferous tubules. Other authors believe that it is spermiogenesis that is dependent on FSH (Steinberger, 1971: Gemzell and Kjessler, 1964).

The work of Murty *et al.* (1979) similarly shows that FSH is needed for the maintenance of spermatogenesis in adults. Thus, chronic FSH withdrawal in subhuman primates affects the fertility of the adult male. The administration of antisera specifically directed against FSH reduces the fertility rate to zero and reduces the number of spermatozoa to 44% of those found in control animals and the number of living spermatozoa is no more than 7.4%.

It seems logical to think that spermatogenesis is under the control of FSH as well as other hormones. FSH acts particularly on the multiplication of spermatogonia. Inhibin could depress this action. Conversely, a lack of inhibin when spermatogenesis fails would increase FSH with recruitment of spermatogonia in order to restore spermatogenesis.

B. NEGATIVE FEEDBACK ON LH SECRETION

Inhibin also exerts an effect on LH secretion. This hormone is less sensitive to inhibin, probably because the mechanisms of inhibition of FSH and LH are different. Thus, inhibin has no inhibiting effect on the synthesis of LH by the gonadotroph *in vitro* unlike that of FSH (see Fig. 6). In contrast, the effect on secretion of endogenous LH-RH *in vitro* and on gonadotropin secretion by exogenous LH-RH, as much *in vitro* as *in vivo*, leads us to think that inhibin essentially acts on the release of LH (see Section V,B). It results in an inhibition of the secretion of LH that is more limited and much weaker than that on FSH, while tonic secretion of LH is maintained.

The physiological importance of the action of inhibin on the secretion of LH and its peripheral effects has not yet been seriously studied.

C. IS INHIBIN A CYBERNINE?

Since 1976, various studies have shown that the ovary produces substances that modify its response to gonadotropins and prevent different stages of the reproductive cycle from developing. These substances may be included among the cybernines, which are products formed in a tissue that regulate locally the function of this parenchyma (Guillemin, 1978). Channing and co-workers showed that the granulosa cell produces a peptide factor, molecular weight approximating 2000, that inhibits the spontaneous maturation of isolated oocytes (Tsafriri *et al.*, 1976). This factor also opposes the production of progesterone by the cumulus surrounding the oocyte *in vitro* (Channing *et al.*, 1978).

Ledwitz-Rigby *et al.* (1977) have also demonstrated the presence of an inhibitor of luteinization in follicular fluid. It is present in large quantities in the fluid of small follicles and prevents the granulosa cells from luteinizing, i.e., from assuming the typical morphology and increasing progesterone production. It also reduces the formation of LH receptors and the production of cyclic AMP (cAMP) in response to exogenous LH (Channing *et al.*, 1978).

Other factors less well characterized biologically have also been found, on the one hand, in follicular fluid, an inhibitor of the effect of FSH that depresses cAMP production induced by FSH in granulosa cells of small follicles (Channing *et al.*, 1978) and, on the other hand, in the corpus luteum, LH receptor-binding inhibitor (LHRBI), which reduces binding of LH to the receptors on luteinized cells and on granulosa cells (Sakai *et al.*, 1977). LHRBI increases in the corpus luteum of the pig in proportion to its age and may play a role in the decline of luteal function. The secretion of progesterone under the influence of LH is also inhibited by this factor.

In aqueous testicular extracts, Reichert and Abou-Issa (1977) have provided evidence for a polypeptide factor, molecular weight approximately 1400, that inhibits the binding of FSH to freshly prepared testicular receptors.

In males, it nevertheless seems that some inhibin preparations exert a direct effect on spermatogenesis independent of FSH. In fact, one can observe an inhibition of the incorporation of tritiated thymidine into testicular DNA in the presence of inhibin compared with the values obtained in its absence. This action *in vitro* of inhibin makes it comparable to the testicular chalone described by Clermont and Mauger (1974, 1976) and defined as "an internal secretion produced by a tissue for the purpose of controlling, by inhibition, the mitotic activity of the same tissue" (Bullough, 1967). These authors think, though without definite proof, that chalones come from spermatogonia, and it is known that inhibin is secreted by Sertoli cells. Inhibin, produced by Sertoli cells and modifying the mitotic activity of germinal cells within the same seminiferous tubules, also meets the definition of a cybernine.

To say either that there is a common origin or structure of these ovarian and testicular factors and inhibin, or the opposite, would not be justified at this time. None of these factors have yet been tested to assess their effect on FSH secretion. Conversely, the possible action of inhibin on the maturation of the oocyte, on luteinization, and on LH binding to its receptors has yet to be studied.

As for the spermatogonial chalones described by Clermont and

Mauger (1974, 1976), it could be speculated that inhibin is implicated in the control of the numerical growth of spermatogonial stem cells. In adults, it would maintain the spermatogonial stem cell population in a steady state and, as a result, arrest the growth of seminiferous tubules. This action of inhibin could occur directly and/or via FSH secretion.

VIII. Summary and Conclusions

There is now convincing evidence for the existence of inhibin. This hormone is formed in the seminiferous tubules by Sertoli cells in males and by granulosa cells in the follicles of females.

Inhibin is not a steroid but is peptidic in nature. Its biological action is destroyed by digestion with trypsin or pepsin and by heat. It induces antibodies capable of neutralizing endogenous inhibin in adult male or female animals into which they are injected. The peptide is not identical to androgen-binding protein, nor is it a fragment of gonadotropins. Its molecular weight is not exactly defined, and it may exist in two forms. The relationships between these two forms have not yet been elucidated.

Inhibin exerts preferential inhibition on the synthesis and release of FSH by pituitary gonadotrophs maintained in culture. The dose required to exert an effect on LH is much higher. It reduces the amount of endogenous LH-RH in the hypothalamus maintained in culture. In the intact animals, the observed effect on gonadotropin levels is the result of the action of inhibin at both sites. Inhibin has no effect on the secretion of TSH, prolactin, or growth hormone either *in vivo* or *in vitro*. It undoubtedly has an effect on gonadal function in males and females via a reduction of FSH secretion, but a direct action on the gonad also is suspected.

Acknowledgments

This work was supported by Grant 74039 from the World Health Organization, Geneva.

We are indebted to Dr. A. Parlow and the National Institute of Arthritis, Metabolism, and Digestive Diseases, for a very generous supply of the material, which enabled us to perform our radioimmunoassays of rat FSH, LH, TSH, and prolactin. We are very grateful also to Dr. W. M. G. Tunbridge, from Newcastle General Hospital, who very kindly reviewed this manuscript; to Dr. J. Walton and Professor Waites (University of Reading, United Kingdom), and Professor Amann (Pennsylvania State

University), who provided us with ram rete testis fluid; and to Dr. A. Mattei (University of Aix, Marseilles, France), who provided us with human seminal plasma. This manuscript was typed with great care and patience by Françoise Renard, whom we thank most warmly.

REFERENCES

Anderson, L. D., Shander, D., Barraclough, C. A., and Channing, C. P. (1979). Unpublished observations cited by Shander, D., Anderson, L. D., Barraclough, C. A., and Channing, C. P. (1979). *Proc. Workshop on Ovarian Follicular and Corpus Luteum Function 1978* (C. P. Channing, J. Marsh and W. Sadler, eds.). Plenum, New York. In press.

Baker, H. W. G., Bremner, W. J., Burger, H. G., De Kretser, D. M., Dulmanis, A., Eddie, L. W., Hudson, B., Keogh, E. J., Lee, V. W. K., and Rennie, G. C. (1976). *Recent Prog. Horm. Res.* **32**, 429.

Baker, H. W. G., Burger, H. G., De Kretser, D. M., Eddie, L. W., Higginson, R. E., Hudson, B., and Lee, V. W. K. (1978). *Int. J. Androl. Suppl.* **2**, 115.

Blanc, M. R., Cahoreau, C., Courot, M., Dacheux, J. L., Hochereau-De-Reviers, M. T., and Pisselet, C. (1978). *Int. J. Androl. Suppl.* **2**, 139.

Borsch, G., Hett, M., Mauss, J., Schach, H., and Scheidt, J. (1973). *Andrologie* **5**, 317.

Bourguignon, J. P., Hoyoux, Cl., Reuter, A., and Franchimont, P. (1979). *J. Clin. Endocrinol. Metab.* **48**, 78.

Bronson, F. H., and Channing, C. P. (1978). *Endocrinology* **103**, 1894.

Bullough, W. S. (1967). "The Evolution of Differentiation." Academic Press, New York.

Cahoreau, C., Blanc, M. R., Dacheux, J. L., Pisselet, C., and Courot, M. (1979). *J. Reprod. Fertil. Suppl.* **26**, 97.

Channing, C. P., Hillensjo, F., and Schaerf, F. W. (1978). *Clin. Endocrinol. Metab.* **7**, 601.

Channing, C. P., Anderson, L. D., and Hodgen, G. D. (1979). *Proc. Workshop on Ovarian Follicular and Corpus Luteum Function 1978*, (C. P. Channing, J. Marsh, and W. Sadler, eds.). Plenum, New York. In press.

Chappel, S. C., Acott, T., and Spies, H. G. (1979). *Proc. Workshop on Ovarian Follicular and Corpus Luteum Function 1978*, (C. P. Channing, J. Marsh, and W. Sadler, eds.). Plenum, New York. In press.

Chari, S. (1977). *Endokrinologie* **70**, 99.

Chari, S., Duraiswami, S., and Franchimont, P. (1976). *Horm. Res.* **7**, 129.

Chari, S., Duraiswami, S., and Franchimont, P. (1978). *Acta Endocrinol. (Copenhagen)* **87**, 434.

Chari, S., Hopkinson, C. R. N., Daume, E., and Sturm, G. (1979). *Acta Endocrinol. (Copenhagen)* **90**, 157.

Chowdhury, M., Steinberger, A., and Steinberger, E. (1978). *Endocrinology* **103**, 644.

Christiansen, P. (1975). *Acta Endocrinol. (Copenhagen)* **78**, 192.

Clermont, Y., and Mauger, A. (1974). *Cell. Tissue Kinet.* **7**, 165.

Clermont, Y., and Mauger, A. (1976). *Cell. Tissue Kinet.* **9**, 99.

Davies, R. V., Main, S. J., Young, M. G. W. L., and Setchell, B. P. (1976). *J. Endocrinol.* **68**, 26.

Davies, R. V., Main, S. J., and Setchell, B. P. (1978). *Int. J. Androl. Suppl.* **2**, 102.

de Jong, F. H., and Sharpe, R. M. (1976). *Nature (London)* **263**, 71.

de Jong, F. H., Welschen, R., Hermans, W. P., Smith, S. D., and Van der Molen, H. J. (1978). *Int. J. Androl. Suppl.* **2**, 125.

de Jong, F. H., Smith, S. D., and Van der Molen, H. J. (1979). *J. Endocrinol.* **80**, 91.

De Kretser, D. M., Burger, H. G., Fortune, D., Hudson, B., Long, A. R., Paulsen, C. A., and Taft, H. P. (1972). *J. Clin. Endocrinol. Metab.* **35**, 392.

De Kretser, D. M., Burger, H. G., and Hudson, B. (1974). *J. Clin. Endocrinol. Metab.* **38**, 787.

Demoulin, A., Koulischer, L., Hustin, J., Hazee-Hagelstein, M. T., Lambotte, R., and Franchimont, P. (1979a). *Horm. Res.* **10**, 177.

Demoulin, A., Bourguignon, J. P., and Franchimont, P. (1979). *Acta Endocrinol. (Copenhagen) Suppl.* **225**, 227.

Dufy-Barbe, L., Faure, J. M. A., and Franchimont, P. (1973). *Endocrinology* **92**, 1318.

Eddie, L. W., Baker, H. W. G., Dulmanis, A., Higginson, R. E., and Hudson, B. (1978). *J. Endocrinol.* **78**, 217.

Eddie, L. W., Baker, H. W. G., Higginson, R. E., and Hudson, B. (1979). *J. Endocrinol.* **81**, 49.

Erickson, G. F., and Hsueh, A. J. W. (1978). *Endocrinology* **193**, 1960.

Franchimont, P. (1968). *Ann. Endocrinol.* **29**, 403.

Franchimont, P. (1972). *J. R. Coll. Physicians, London,* **6**, 283.

Franchimont, P., and Burger, H. G. (1975). "Human Growth Hormone and Gonadotrophins in Health and Diseases." Elsevier/North-Holland, Amsterdam.

Franchimont, P., Millet, D., Vendrely, E., Letawe, J., Legros, J. J., and Netter, A. (1972). *J. Clin. Endocrinol. Metab.* **34**, 1003.

Franchimont, P., Demoulin, A., and Bourguignon, J. P. (1975a). *Horm. Res.* **6**, 177.

Franchimont, P., Chari, S., and Demoulin, A. (1975b). *J. Reprod. Fertil.* **44**, 335.

Franchimont, P., Chari, S., Hagelstein, M. T., and Duraiswami, S. (1975c). *Nature (London)* **257**, 402.

Franchimont, P., Chari, S., Hazee-Hagelstein, M. T., Debruche, M. L., and Duraiswami, S. (1977). *In* "The Testis in Normal and Infertile Men" (P. Troen and H. R. Nankin, eds.), p. 253. Raven, New York.

Franchimont, P., Demoulin, A., Verstraelen-Proyard, J., Hazee-Hagelstein, M. T., Walton, J. S., and Waites, G. M. H. (1978). *J. Int. Androl. Suppl.* **2**, 69.

Franchimont, P., Demoulin, A., Verstraelen-Proyard, J., Hazee-Hagelstein, M. T., and Tunbridge, W. M. G. (1979a). *J. Reprod. Fertil. Suppl.* **26**, 123.

Franchimont, P., Bologne, R., Demoulin, A., Hustin, J., Verstraelen-Proyard, J., and Gysen, P. (1979b). *C. R. Soc. Biol. (Paris)* **173**, 654.

French, F. S., and Ritzen, E. M. (1973). *J. Reprod. Fertil.* **32**, 479.

Gemzell, C., and Kjessler, B. (1964). *Lancet* **1**, 644.

Greenwood, F., Hunter, W., and Glover, J. (1963). *Biochem. J.* **89**, 114.

Greep, R. O., Van Dyke, H. B., and Chow, B. F. (1942). *Endocrinology* **30**, 635.

Guillemin, R. (1978). *Science* **202**, 390.

Hochereau-de-Reviers, M. T., and Courot, M. (1978). *Ann. Biol. Anim. Biochim. Biophys.* **18**, 573.

Hodgen, G. D., Nixon, W. E., and Turner, C. K. (1974). *I.R.C.S. Med. Sci.* **2**, 1233.

Hopkins, C. R., and Farquhar, M. G. (1973). *J. Cell. Biol.* **59**, 276.

Hopkinson, C. R. N., Sturm, G., Daume, E., Fritze, E., and Hirschhauser, C. (1975). *I.R.C.S. Med. Sci.* **3**, 588.

Hopkinson, C. R. N., Daume, E., Sturm, G., Fritze, E., Kaiser, S., and Hirschhauser, C. (1977a). *J. Reprod. Fertil.* **50**, 93.

Hopkinson, C. R. N., Fritze, E., Chari, S., Sturm, G., and Hirschhauser, C. (1977b). *I.R.C.S. Med. Sci.* **5**, 83.

Hopkinson, C. R. N., Dulisch, B., Gauss, G., Hilscher, C., and Hirschhauser, C. (1978). *Acta Endocrinol. (Copenhagen)* **87**, 413.

Hudson, B., Baker, H. W. G., Eddie, L. W., Higginson, R. E., Burger, H. G., de Kretser, D. M., Dobos, M., and Lee, V. W. K. (1979). *J. Reprod. Fertil. Suppl.* **26**, 17.

Johnsen, S. G. (1970). *Acta Endocrinol. (Copenhagen)* **64**, 193.

Keogh, E. J. (1978). Personal communication.

Keogh, E. J., Lee, V. W. K., Rennie, G. C., Burger, H. G., Hudson, B., and De Kretser, D. M. (1976). *Endocrinology* **98**, 997.

Klinefelter, H. F., Reifenstein, E. C., and Albright, F. (1942). *J. Clin. Endocrinol.* **2**, 615.

Korenman, S. G., and Sherman, B. M. (1976). *In* "Endocrine Function of the Human Ovary" (V. H. T. James, M. Serio, and G. Giusti, eds.), p. 359 (Sereno Symp. No. 7). Academic Press, New York.

Labrie, F., Lagace, L., Ferland, L., Kelly, P. A., Drouin, J., Massicotte, J., Bonne, C. Raynaud, J. P., and Dorrington, J. H. (1978). *Int. J. Androl. Suppl.* **2**, 81.

Lagace, L., Massicotte, J., Drouin, J., Giguere, V., Dupont, A., and Labrie, F. (1979). *In* "Recent Advances in Reproduction and Regulation of Fertility" (G. P. Talwar, ed.), p. 82. Elsevier/North-Holland, Amsterdam.

Ledwitz-Rigby, F., Rigby, B. W., Gay, V. L., Stetson, M. Young, J., and Channing, C. P. (1977). *J. Endocrinol.* **74**, 175.

Lee, V. W. K., Keogh, E. J., De Kretser, D. M., and Hudson, B. (1974). *I.R.C.S. Med. Sci.* **2**, 1406.

Lee, V. W. K., Pearce, P. T., and De Kretser, D. M. (1977). *In* "The Testis in Normal and Infertile Men" (P. Troen and H. R. Nankin, eds.), p. 293. Raven, New York.

Lincoln, G. A. (1978). *J. Reprod. Fertil.* **53**, 31.

Lorenzen, J. R., Schwartz, N. B., and Channing, C. P. (1978). *60th Ann. Meeting Endocrine Soc. Abst.* 46.

Lugaro, G., Cassellato, M. M., Mazzola, G., Fachini, G., and Carrea, G. (1974). *Neuroendocrinology* **15**, 62.

McCullagh, D. D. (1932). *Science* **76**, 19.

Main, S. J., Davies, R. V., and Setchell, B. P. (1978). *J. Endocrinol.* **79**, 255.

Marder, M. L., Channing, C. P., and Schwartz, N. B. (1977). *Endocrinology* **101**, 1639.

Martins, T., and Rocha, A. (1931). *Mem. Inst. Oswaldo Cruz* **25**, 73.

Means, A. R. (1975). *Endocrinology* **5**, 203.

Moodbidri, S. B., Joshi, L. R., and Sheth, A. R. (1976). *I.R.C.S. Med. Sci.* **4**, 217.

Murty, G. S. R. C., Sheela-Rani, C. S., Mougdal, N. R., and Prasad, M. R. N. (1979). *J. Reprod. Fertil. Suppl.* **26**.

Nandini, S. G., Lidner, H., and Mougdal, N. R. (1976). *Endocrinology* **98**, 1460.

Orth, J., and Christensen, A. K. (1978). *Endocrinology* **103**, 1944.

Paulsen, C. A., Leonard, J. M., De Kretser, D. M., and Leach, R. B. (1972). *In* Gonadotropins" (B. B. Saxena, C. G. Beling, and H. M. Gandy, eds.), p. 628. Wiley (Interscience), New York.

Ramasharma, K., Shashidhara-Murthy, H. M., and Mougdal, N. R. (1979). *Biol. Reprod.* **20**, 831.

Reichert, L. E., Jr., and Abou-Issa, H. (1977). *Biol. Reprod.* **17**, 614.

Rotsztejn, W. H., Charli, J. L., Pattou, E., Epelbaum, J., and Kordon, C. (1976). *Endocrinology* **99**, 1663.

Sairam, M. R., Ranganatham, M. R., and Lamothe, P. (1978). *Biol. Reprod.* **18**, 58.

Sakai, C., Engel, B., and Channing, C. P. (1977). *Proc. Soc. Exp. Biol. Med.* **155**, 373.

Schwartz, N. B. (1969). *Recent Prog. Horm. Res.* **25**, 1.

Schwartz, N. B., and Channing, C. P. (1977). *Proc. Natl. Acad. Sci. U.S.A.* **74**, 5721.

Schwartz, N. B., Krone, K., Talley, W. L., and Ely, C. A. (1973). *Endocrinology* **92**, 1165.

Setchell, B. P. (1970). *In* "The Testis" (A. D. Johnson, W. R. Gomes, and N. L. Van Demark, eds.), Vol. 1, p. 109. Academic Press, New York.

Setchell, B. P., and Jacks, F. (1974). *J. Endocrinol* **62**, 675.

Setchell, B. P., and Main, S. J. (1974). *Biol. Reprod.* **24**, 245, 361.

Setchell, B. P., and Sirinathsinghji, D. J. (1972). *J. Endocrinol.* **53**, LX.

Setchell, B. P., Davies, R. V., and Main, S. J. (1977). *In* "The Testis" (A. D. Johnson, W. R. Gomes, and N. L. Van Demark, eds.), Vol. 6, p. 189. Academic Press, New York.

Shashidhara-Murthy, H. M., Ramasharma, K., and Mougdal, N. R. (1979). *J. Reprod. Fertil. Suppl.* **26**, 61.

Shander, D., Anderson, L. D., Barraclough, A., and Channing, C. P. (1979). *Proc. Workshop on Ovarian Follicular and Corpus Luteum Function, 1978* (C. P. Channing, J. Marsh, and W. Sadler, eds.). Plenum, New York. In press.

Sheth, A. R., Vaze, A. Y., and Thakur, A. N. (1978). *Indian J. Exp. Biol.* **16**, 1025.

Simpson, M. E., Li, C. H., and Evans, H. M. (1951). *Endocrinology* **48**, 370.

Shivashanker, S., Prasad, M. R. N., Thampan, T. N. R. V., Sheela Rani, C. S., and Mougdal, N. R. (1977). *Indian J. Exp. Biol.* **15**, 845.

Steinberger, A., and Steinberger, E. (1976). *Endocrinology* **99**, 918.

Steinberger, E. (1971). *Physiol. Rev.* **52**, 1.

Swerdloff, R. S., Walsh, P. C., Jacobs, H. S., and Odell, W. D. (1971). *Endocrinology* **88**, 120.

Tsafriri, A., Pomerantz, S. H., and Channing, C. P. (1976). *Biol. Reprod.* **14**, 511.

Welschen, R., Hermans, W. P., Dullaart, J., and de Jong, F. H. (1977). *J. Reprod. Fertil.* **50**, 129.

Wise, P. M., De Paolo, L. V., Anderson, L. D., Channing, C. P., and Barraclough, C. A. (1979). *Proc. Workshop on Ovarian Follicular and Corpus Luteum Function, 1978* (C. P. Channing, J. Marsh, and W. Sadler, eds.). Plenum, New York. In press.

VITAMINS AND HORMONES, VOL. 37

Hormonal Control of Calcium Metabolism in Lactation

SVEIN U. TOVERUD AND AGNA BOASS

*Department of Pharmacology, School of Medicine, and
Dental Research Center,
University of North Carolina at Chapel Hill,
Chapel Hill, North Carolina*

I.   Introduction 303
II. Regulation of the Serum Calcium Concentration in Lactation 305
     A. Parathyroid Hormone 305
     B. Calcitonin 309
     C. Vitamin D 316
     D. Summary 320
III. Intestinal Calcium Absorption 321
     A. Structural and Functional Changes in the Intestine during Lactation .. 321
     B. Regulation of Calcium Absorption 323
     C. Calcium Absorption in Lactating Rats 324
     D. Calcium Absorption in Lactating Ruminants 328
     E. Calcium Absorption in Lactating Women 329
IV. Urinary Calcium Excretion in Lactation 331
V.   Calcium and Vitamin D in Milk 335
     A. Calcium 335
     B. Vitamin D 335
VI. Skeletal Calcium Content 338
     A. Lactating Rats 338
     B. Lactating Women 338
VII. Conclusions and Hypotheses 341
     References 343

I. Introduction

The increased need for calcium to satisfy the demands of milk production and at the same time to maintain the blood calcium concentration at an adequate level makes the normal physiological condition of lactation of special interest to endocrinologists concerned with the calcemic hormones and calcium homeostasis. The rat is an especially advantageous animal for study of lactation because the much higher rate of calcium excretion in milk in the rat than in the human, relative to body size, puts greater stress on homeostatic mechanisms in the rat and accentuates hormonal changes that may be only subtle in human lactation. Findings in the rat may help to focus attention on factors and interactions that could profitably be objects of clinical investigation.

The daily loss of calcium in the milk of the lactating rat usually exceeds 100 mg, 100 times more than the daily urine calcium. Over a 21-day period the lactating rat transfers to her litter approximately 2.5 gm of calcium, equal to 60% of the calcium content of her skeleton. Nevertheless, the lactating rat loses only 5–10% of her skeletal calcium stores during the 3-week lactation period. Adaptive changes must of necessity take place in calcium intake and in the efficiency of intestinal calcium absorption to replenish calcium lost in the milk. Adjustments that prevent wide fluctuations in the serum calcium on the low side with ensuing tetany or on the high side with excessive urinary calcium and possible ectopic calcification also take place.

In this review evidence will be presented, largely from the authors' laboratory, that indicates that the adaptive mechanisms in the rat involve elevated blood levels of calcitonin and 1,25-dihydroxycholecalciferol [1,25-$(OH)_2D_3$]. There is indirect evidence that parathyroid hormone also is increased. Briefly, the serum calcium level is maintained at a level 10% lower than that of nonlactating rats, in part by an action of calcitonin. Parathyroid hormone and 1,25-$(OH)_2D_3$, in concert, prevent further reduction in the serum calcium level. There is marked elevation of intestinal calcium absorption, which may involve 1,25-$(OH)_2D_3$ as well as other factors. Continued intake of vitamin D during lactation is required not only to prevent marked hypocalcemia in the mother, but also to prevent true vitamin D-deficiency rickets in the suckling pups.

Calcium metabolism in lactating women will also be reviewed and contrasted with that in the rat. Lactation in ruminants will be discussed only briefly, mainly for purposes of species comparison. Several reviews contain a detailed discussion of special problems in ruminant lactation, such as parturient paresis (Simkiss, 1967; Mayer et al., 1969b; Braithwaite, 1976).

Hormones other than the calcemic hormones, such as glucocorticoids, will not be discussed further, because there is no information on their role in calcium metabolism in lactation. However, it is quite possible that future studies may uncover such a role because excess glucocorticoids may lead to alterations in bone and calcium metabolism (Nelson, 1979) and because serum levels of glucocorticoids are elevated in lactating rats (Kamoun and Haberey, 1969; Ota et al., 1974; Smotherman et al., 1976) and cows (Wagner and Oxenreider, 1972; Shayanfar et al., 1975).

II. Regulation of the Serum Calcium Concentration in Lactation

A. Parathyroid Hormone

The parathyroid gland is a major factor in the maintenance of the serum calcium level within a narrow range. It secretes the parathyroid hormone (PTH), which acts directly on bone and kidney and indirectly on the intestine to increase the serum calcium concentration. The rate of secretion of PTH is inhibited by a high concentration of the serum ionized calcium, and when the ionized calcium level falls this inhibition is relieved and more PTH is secreted. These relationships constitute a negative feedback system for the regulation of the circulating level both of PTH and of calcium (see review by Munson et al., 1963; Sherwood et al., 1966; Blum et al., 1974).

Removal of the parathyroid glands is typically followed by a gradual fall in serum calcium to levels that vary according to the dietary calcium intake. In rats fed a diet very low in calcium (0.02% calcium and 0.4% phosphorus), the serum calcium may drop rapidly to as low as 5–6 mg/dl after parathyroidectomy.

Lactating rats are even more dependent on PTH for maintenance of a normal serum calcium level than nonlactating rats, as indicated by the more rapid fall in serum calcium after parathyroidectomy in lactating rats fed a diet that contained adequate amounts of calcium, phosphorus, and vitamin D than in nonlactating rats fed the same diet. Three hours after the operation the lactating rats showed a decrease in serum calcium of 2 mg/dl, whereas in the parathyroidectomized nonlactating rats there had been no change at this time (Toverud et al., 1978b).

While these results are consistent with the conclusion that the rate of PTH secretion and the serum PTH are elevated in lactating rats, direct evidence such as assay for PTH in serum is not yet available. However, there is some additional evidence for a state of functional hyperparathyroidism during lactation in the rat, namely, that the weight of the parathyroid glands is significantly higher (17%, $p < 0.05$) relative to body weight than in nonlactating female rats (Toverud et al., 1978a). In lactating cows, Sherwood et al. (1966) reported elevated circulating levels of immunoreactive PTH. The data in lactating women are scanty and conflicting. Cushard et al. (1972) found increased levels of plasma PTH in pregnant women, but not during lactation. On the other hand, Retallack *et al.* (1977) reported elevated levels in lactating women beginning at the sixth week of lactation, not easily explained because they had found, during the 3 preceding weeks, an increase rather than a decrease in serum ionized calcium. In further studies of PTH in relation to serum calcium in lactating women it will be desirable to relate changes in serum calcium to dietary intake of calcium and loss of calcium in the milk.

The important role of PTH in the regulation of serum calcium during lactation is well illustrated by the inversely correlated variations in the serum levels of calcium and immunoreactive PTH in lactating cows reported by Littledike (1976). When milking was stopped for 2–3 days, the serum calcium rose above control levels and serum PTH fell; when milking was again resumed, serum calcium fell rapidly to levels below 8–9 mg/dl concomitantly with a rise in serum PTH. These changes were reversed after 2 days' milking (and lactation). The author's interpretation was that resumption of lactation involved a large drain of calcium from the body that resulted in a fall in serum calcium before PTH-related mechanisms had time to mobilize enough calcium to compensate for the loss. When milking and lactation were stopped, the rise in serum calcium above the control level was thought to reflect a rebound phenomenon of continued mobilization of calcium before the PTH-stimulated processes could slow to reduced rates. Recently, we have described a similar rebound phenomenon in the rat (Pike *et al.*, 1979). We found that lactating rats, 2 days after their litters had been weaned, showed a temporary marked rise in serum calcium from 9.6 to 13 mg/dl, even though the diet contained only 0.4% calcium. This change coincided with a decrease in the serum level of 1,25-dihydroxyvitamin D_3 (see Section II,C on vitamin D and Table IV). Although it is likely that PTH is the mediator of this rebound phenomenon in rats, as it appears to be in cows, this interpretation will remain uncertain until serum levels of PTH can be measured before and after weaning in the rat.

The consequences for lactation in general of removal of the parathyroid glands depend on the time of removal of the glands. If the operation is carried out 8 weeks before conception, to allow time for adaptation to the aparathyroid state, the litter weight at weaning is only moderately reduced (Fry *et al.*, 1979). However, if rats are parathyroidectomized immediately before pregnancy or during lactation, growth of the litters is impaired to a greater extent (G. Toverud, 1926; Cowie and Folley, 1945; S. U. Toverud, 1963; Fairney and Weir, 1970). In the study of Toverud (1963) rat pups with parathyroidectomized lactating mothers did not gain weight (and also did not lose weight) over a 6-day period after the operation, which confirmed the observation of Cowie and Folley (1945) that parathyroidectomy can seriously impair milk secretion but does not stop it. The underlying cause of the reduced milk secretion may be the marked and sudden fall in serum calcium. Many rats will show spontaneous or elicited hypocalcemic tetany when parathyroidectomy is carried out during lactation. The hypocalcemia can be completely prevented by maintaining the parathyroidectomized lactating rats on a high-calcium diet (Boass *et al.*, 1980).

In addition to the generally debilitating effects of tetany, hypocalcemia can lead to a decrease in the water content of milk (Toverud, 1963; Neuenschwander and Talmage, 1963). Regardless of the cause of hypocalcemia, whether parathyroidectomy or vitamin D deprivation, the total solids content of the milk was found to be inversely correlated with the serum calcium level (Toverud, 1963) (see Section V,A and Table II). The cause of the failure of growth of the pups of the parathyroidectomized mothers could therefore be twofold: deficiency of calories because of reduced milk supply and dehydration from impairment of water transport into the milk. The failure of Fry *et al.* (1979) to confirm this relationship between serum calcium level and milk solids in their experiments, in which parathyroidectomy had been performed 10 weeks earlier, may have been because milk secretion in their rats had adapted in some manner to long-standing hypocalcemia.

If the secretion rate of PTH is elevated during lactation in the rat as well as in the cow, as we assume, the most likely basis for the hypersecretion is persistent or intermittent hypocalcemia, as in other examples of secondary hyperparathyroidism. There is ample evidence for such hypocalcemia in the cow, particularly at the time of initiation of lacation. The prevalent condition of parturient paresis (milk fever) is caused by a profound drop in serum calcium, which leads to hypocalcemic tetany and death if left untreated. The cause of the inability of certain susceptible cows to maintain the serum calcium within normal limits at the time of parturition remains elusive. It has been suggested that an inadequate potential for rapid, marked increase in parathyroid gland activity may be the cause of parturient paresis (see reviews by Ramberg *et al.*, 1975; Braithwaite, 1976). Other causes that have been suggested, not specifically supported by the available data, are an inadequate increase in serum 1,25-dihydroxyvitamin D_3 (Horst *et al.*, 1977) and excessive secretion of calcitonin (Braithwaite, 1976).

That lactating rats fed a normal diet maintain a serum calcium that is significantly lower (by 1 mg/dl) than that maintained by nonlactating control rats was shown as early as 1932 by Kletzien *et al.* We confirmed this observation in rats fed Purina Laboratory Chow, which contains 1.1% calcium, 0.8% phosphorus, and 5 IU of vitamin D_3 per gram of diet (Toverud *et al.*, 1976), as well as in rats on a diet with 0.4% calcium and 0.4% phosphorus (Boass *et al.*, 1977). This mild hypocalcemia must be related in part to the rapid rate of transfer of calcium from blood to milk because the serum calcium level returned to that of nonlactating rats within 15–20 hours after removal of the litters; there was no change in the serum protein level (Toverud *et al.*, 1978b). Calculations based on estimates of daily milk yield (Toverud *et al.*, 1976) indicate that the amount of calcium transferred to the mammary gland each minute is approximately 0.2 mg, or 15% of the total calcium content of the blood. This rate of loss of calcium into the milk is 100 times greater than the rate of loss of calcium into the urine. It should therefore not be surprising that a lactating rat maintains a lower "normal" serum calcium level than a nonlactating rat.

We investigated the possibility that an insufficiency of PTH relative to need might be a cause of the low serum calcium in lactating rats by giving both lactating and nonlactating intact rats injections of PTH in doses from 40 to 460 units/100 gm body weight, doses that raise serum calcium considerably in parathyroidectomized rats. No increase in serum calcium was observed in either group (Toverud *et al.*, 1978b). The lack of increase in the nonlactating rats had been predicted from previous experiments; intact rats are resistant to a single injection of even a large dose of PTH. However, in the lactating rats, with a low serum calcium at the beginning and suspected PTH insufficiency, it seemed conceivable that additional PTH might at least have raised the serum calcium to the level of the nonlactating controls. This did not occur.

However, in an extension of this experiment, after the thyroid glands had been removed (by thyroparathyroidectomy) from both lactating and nonlactating rats, injection of 40 units of PTH raised the serum calcium markedly in both groups and to the same level (Fig. 1) (Toverud *et al.*, 1978b). The increase was larger in the lactating rats; they began at a lower level. Thus, it appears that once the inhibitory influence of the thyroid gland (i.e., calcitonin) is removed, PTH is as active or even more active in lactating rats than it is in nonlactating rats. We suggest, therefore, that PTH insufficiency or lack of responsiveness to PTH is not responsible for the moderate hypocalcemia of

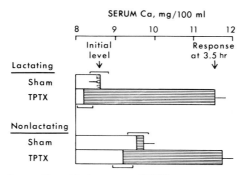

FIG. 1. Effect of parathyroid hormone (PTH) on serum calcium in acutely thyroparathyroidectomized (TPTX) and intact lactating and nonlactating rats. Nonlactating rats deprived of their litters 1 week earlier and lactating rats on days 14–16 of lactation were fasted overnight. After an initial blood sample was obtained from the tail, thyroparathyroidectomy or a sham operation (SHAM) was performed, followed immediately by a subcutaneous injection of Lilly parathyroid extract (PTE) (40 U/100 gm body weight). A second blood sample was obtained from the heart 3.5 hours later. □, Mean initial serum levels. The end of the shaded area represents the final serum levels. The brackets represent ± SE for the initial serum levels, and the horizontal lines represent ± SE of the mean change in serum levels (▤). There were seven or eight rats in each group, and mean body weights were 409 and 366 gm for lactating and nonlactating rats, respectively. The effect of PTH was significant ($p < 0.01$) only in the TPTX rats. From Toverud et $al.$ (1978b).

lactating rats. It is likely that, as discussed in Section II,B, calcitonin is a more important factor here than lack of PTH.

If the Ca:P ratio of the diet is unusually high (> 2:1), the serum calcium level of lactating rats may be as high or higher than that of nonlactating controls (Kamárková et $al.$, 1967; Blahosova et $al.$, 1974).

B. CALCITONIN

Gray and Munson (1969) and Munson and Gray (1970) demonstrated in acutely thyroidectomized young male rats that intragastric administration of a calcium salt or ingestion of a calcium-containing meal resulted in marked hypercalcemia, whereas after the same treatment in thyroid-intact rats or in thyroidectomized rats given calcitonin the serum calcium rose only slightly or not at all. They concluded that in normal rats calcitonin protects against postprandial hypercalcemia; their results were confirmed by others (Harper and Toverud, 1973: Perault-Staub et $al.$, 1974; Talmage et $al.$,

1975). These findings suggested to us that this protective function of calcitonin might be of special importance during lactation, when intestinal absorption of calcium is greatly increased. Furthermore, Lewis *et al.* (1971) and Taylor *et al.* (1975) reported greater loss of bone mineral during lactation in thyroxine-treated thyroidectomized rats than in intact rats and attributed the difference to the action of calcitonin. (These experiments were rather preliminary in nature and deserve repetition with varied experimental conditions, for example, different levels of dietary calcium and vitamin D and of thyroxine replacement dose.) Additional suggestive evidence for a role of calcitonin in lactation was provided by Garel *et al.* (1974), who found elevated levels of serum calcitonin in lactating as well as pregnant ewes.

Subsequently, we (Toverud *et al.*, 1976) showed that calcitonin, whether released endogenously or injected, was even more effective in preventing hypercalcemia in lactating than in nonlactating rats. In these experiments, lactating and nonlactating rats, with or without the thyroid gland, were given a standard dose of calcium chloride by gavage (10 mg of calcium per 100 gm body weight) (Fig. 2). In rats deprived of the thyroid (thyroparathyroidectomized) the oral calcium

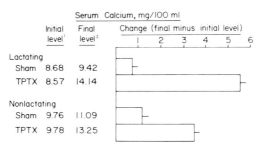

FIG. 2. Thyroid protection against hypercalcemia in lactating and nonlactating rats. The numbers in the columns represent the mean serum calcium levels before (initial level) and 2 hours after (final level) sham operation or thyroparathyroidectomy (TPTX) and calcium gavage. Each horizontal bar represents the mean change in serum calcium over the 2-hour period for a separate group of 6–8 rats. In all figures, the horizontal line represents the standard error. Lactating rats (mean body weight 290 gm) and nonlactating rats, which had their litters removed 1 week earlier (mean body weight 324 gm), were fasted overnight, bled, and operated on just before calcium administration. Calcium was given by gavage as 0.18 M $CaCl_2$ in a total dose of 10 mg of calcium per 100 gm body weight. Blood was again obtained 2 hours after the initial sample. In this figure as well as in Figs. 3 and 4, the initial level of the lactating rats was significantly different from that of the nonlactating rats at $p < 0.01$. The effects of TPTX and of lactation as well as the effect of the interaction (TPTX × lactation) were significant (1,28 DF) at $p < 0.01$. [1]SE = 0.14–0.16. [2]SE = 0.31–0.36. From Toverud *et al.* (1976).

was followed by a marked rise in serum calcium 2 hours later in both the lactating and nonlactating groups. However, the rise was much greater in the lactating than in the nonlactating rats (5.5 vs 3.5 mg/dl), presumably because of more efficient intestinal absorption of calcium during lactation. In thyroid-intact rats (sham-operated) the response to oral calcium was much smaller than in the thyroidectomized rats and the same (1 mg/dl) for both lactating and nonlactating rats. It was therefore clear that the thyroid gland of the lactating rat could prevent a greater potential rise in serum calcium than the gland of the nonlactating rat. In thyroidectomized lactating rats a small intravenous dose of porcine calcitonin (5 MRC mU/100 gm body weight) prevented hypercalcemia at 2 hours (Fig. 3) just as endogenous calcitonin did in thyroid-intact rats. In contrast, the same small dose of calcitonin did not affect significantly the hypercalcemia in thyroidectomized nonlactating rats, although no doubt a larger dose would have done so. Thus, calcitonin is a more potent antihypercalcemic agent in lactating than in nonlactating rats.

We also found that calcitonin is a more potent antihyperphosphatemic agent in lactating than in nonlactating rats. Hyperphosphatemia, which occurs in thyroparathyroidectomized rats after calcium gavage, is effectively prevented in lactating rats with intact

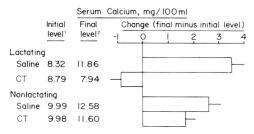

FIG. 3. Prevention of hypercalcemia by intravenous calcitonin (CT) in thyroparathyroidectomized (TPTX) lactating rats. The numbers in the columns represent the mean serum calcium levels before (initial level) and 2 hours after (final level) TPTX and intravenous injection of CT or saline. Each horizontal bar represents the mean change over the 2-hour period for a group of 5-7 rats. Lactating rats (mean body weight 340 gm) and nonlactating rats, which had their litters removed 1 week earlier (mean body weight 352 gm), were fasted overnight, bled, and thyroparathyroidectomized just before calcium gavage and intravenous injection of CT or saline. Calcium was administered by gavage as 0.18 M CaCl$_2$ in a total dose of 10 mg of calcium per 100 gm body weight. Saline or porcine CT (5 MRC mU/100 gm body weight) was injected intravenously immediately after the administration of calcium. Blood was again obtained 2 hours after the initial sample. The effects of CT and of the interaction (CT × lactation) were significant (1,20 DF) at $p < 0.01$. [1]SE = 0.22-0.26. [2]SE = 0.48-0.57. From Toverud et al. (1976).

thyroid glands. In thyroparathyroidectomized rats given calcium by gavage, a small dose of calcitonin intravenously not only prevented the rise in serum inorganic phosphorus, but actually caused a fall in this level. In contrast, the same dose of calcitonin was without effect in similarly treated nonlactating rats (Toverud *et al.*, 1976).

We measured serum calcitonin in fasted and fed lactating rats in comparison with control nonlactating rats of the same age (6 months) (Toverud *et al.*, 1978b) by use of a radioimmunoassay for rat calcitonin (Cooper *et al.*, 1976). The mean values were the same in lactating and nonlactating rats after a 20-hour fast, but after the rats had been fed for 2 hours serum calcitonin rose two- to threefold in the lactating rats; there was no detectable increase in the nonlactating rats after feeding (Fig. 4). The importance of feeding for the maintenance of a high blood level of calcitonin in lactating rats was also shown in another study (Cooper *et al.*, 1977), in which circulating calcitonin was more than 10-fold higher in fed than in fasted rats. Since Peng and Garner (1978) have shown that serum calcitonin rises in nonlactating female rats of the same age after feeding, it would be desirable to repeat the experiment illustrated in Fig. 4 with lactating rats of the strain used by them (CDF strain descended from Fischer 344). We predict that the rise will be even higher in lactating rats. In the experiment shown in Fig. 4, serum calcium did not increase in either group

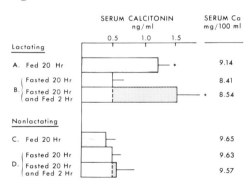

FIG. 4. Serum calcitonin (CT) in fed and fasted rats. Groups of five to seven lactating and nonlactating rats were fed Purina Chow either ad libitum overnight (groups A and C) or fasted overnight for 20 hours (groups B and D). An initial blood sample was taken from each group at the end of this period; the mean serum CT levels are indicated by the two sets of bars labeled *Fed 20 Hr* and *Fasted 20 Hr*. Groups B and D were given food ad libitum for 2 hours, after which a second blood sample was taken. ▨, Change in serum CT over the 2-hour period for groups B and D. The horizontal lines represent the standard error (SE). The mean serum calcium level is given opposite the appropriate bar; SE ranged from ± 0.14 to ± 0.20 mg/100 ml. *Significantly greater than the level for group B *Fasted 20 Hr* at $p < 0.01$. From Toverud *et al.* (1978b).

after eating; it remained at the low level of 8.5 mg/dl in the lactating rats even though the calcium content of the food consumed during the 2-hour period was approximately 100 mg. Presumably, the extra calcitonin released in response to eating prevented a postprandial rise in serum calcium. (One may only speculate about the factors responsible for the lack of rise in serum calcitonin in the nonlactating rats after they had eaten the same amount of food as the lactating rats and in the face of no demonstrated increase in serum calcium.)

The conclusion that secretion of calcitonin is more sensitive to stimuli in lactating than in nonlactating rats is supported by two other lines of evidence. First, intragastric administration of calcium (10 mg/100 gm body weight) as calcium chloride was found to cause a significant increase in serum calcitonin 30 minutes later in lactating rats but not in nonlactating rats, even though the serum calcium did not exceed 10 mg/dl in the lactating rats (Toverud et al., 1978b). Second, thyroid glands from lactating rats released three times as much calcitonin during incubation in vitro in medium with 1 mM calcium as did glands from nonlactating rats (Toverud et al., 1978a). Thyroid glands from lactating rats contained no more calcitonin than those from nonlactating rats (Toverud et al., 1978b); when glands from both types of rats were incubated in medium with 2.5 mM calcium, essentially the same amount of calcitonin was released into the medium by both sets of glands (Toverud et al., 1978a). It thus appears that in lactating rats the calcitonin-secreting mechanism in the thyroid C cells has an increased sensitivity to low concentrations of calcium. This would be consistent with increased release of calcitonin during lactation while the serum calcium tends to be about 1 mg/dl lower than in nonlactating rats. It is not meant to suggest that the release of calcitonin after feeding is mediated by calcium. The mediator in the rat is thought to be an unknown gastrointestinal principle that is increased in response to food constituents, glucose (Cooper and Obie, 1978), and triglycerides (Garel and Besnard, 1979) as well as calcium.

We observed (Fig. 4) that at the end of 2 hours of feeding the serum calcium of lactating rats (previously fasted for 20 hours) was essentially the same as at the beginning of the meal and that over the same time interval serum calcitonin had increased threefold. It is logical to conclude that the added calcitonin was responsible for preventing a postprandial rise in serum calcium and that calcitonin participates in the regulation of serum calcium in the lactating rat. Additional evidence for this view was obtained in a related experiment (Fig. 5) in which we attempted to accentuate a feeding-induced rise in serum calcium by temporarily halting milk secretion by separation of the lit-

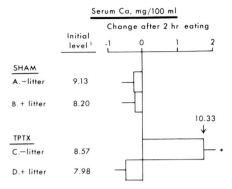

FIG. 5. Effect of the thyroid gland on serum calcium in fed lactating rats. Groups of five or six lactating rats (14–16 days of lactation) were fasted overnight (18–20 hours). The litters of groups A and C were kept away from the mothers overnight and for the remainder of the experiment, whereas the litters of groups B and D were kept with the mothers the entire time. At the end of the fasting period, an initial blood sample was taken immediately before the rats were subjected to thyroparathyroidectomy (TPTX) or a sham operation (SHAM). All rats were then given food ad libitum for 2 hours. A second blood sample was taken at the end of this period. The mean initial serum calcium levels are given in the column to the left (SE = ± 0.20), and the mean change in serum calcium from the initial to the second blood sample is indicated by the bar. The horizontal lines represent the standard error. *The change is significant at $p < 0.01$. From Toverud *et al.* (1978b).

ters from the mothers overnight. When these mother rats were thyroparathyroidectomized and allowed to eat for 2 hours, a rise in serum calcium of 1.8 mg/dl ($p < 0.01$) was observed at the end of the feeding period, whereas in their nonthyroidectomized counterparts the serum calcium had not changed significantly. This demonstration depended on the separation of the mother from the litters; the serum calcium did not rise after feeding in the thyroidectomized rats with suckling litters. Therefore, the results of the experiments in Figs. 4 and 5 show that both calcitonin and the drain of calcium into the milk are factors that protect the lactating rat against hypercalcemia after feeding.

Recent observations by Kalu indicate that a rise in serum calcium immediately after (30–120 minutes) thyroparathyroidectomy can be observed in both young and old rats in the fed as well as fasted state (Kalu, 1978). Our observations in the lactating rat discussed above should therefore be interpreted as illustrations of a general role of calcitonin that becomes especially important during lactation in the rat, when rapid and prolonged intestinal calcium absorption can easily cause hypercalcemia.

The possibility that serum calcitonin may be elevated in lactating women as well as in rats was investigated by Becker and co-workers in a study carried out in the Clinical Research Unit of North Carolina Memorial Hospital (Toverud *et al.*, 1978a; Becker *et al.*, 1979). Some of the results from this study, given in Table I, show that of the 16 nonlactating women serving as a control group (group I) none had detectable serum levels of calcitonin in blood samples obtained approximately 1 hour after breakfast. When 18 lactating women of the same age were examined, two women had detectable levels of calcitonin and all had serum calcium levels within the normal range (9.5–10.5 mg/dl). Six women who had breastfed for many months, and who likewise were normocalcemic, were admitted to the Clinical Research Unit for 3 days; during this time blood samples were obtained after fasting overnight, as well as after administration of calcium and pentagastrin according to a standard procedure (Hennessy *et al.*, 1974). All six women had a detectable serum calcitonin level in at least one blood sample; only one woman failed to show an elevated fasting calcitonin level, and all but one responded to a calcium infusion. Thus, in contrast to nonlactating women and other healthy people who do not show detectable calcitonin levels with our assay, one-third of the lactating women in this study had measurable serum levels of calcitonin. Even so, the effect of lactation on serum calcitonin is not as great in women as it is in rats, which is not surprising if one considers the relatively greater calcium stress in rats. Future studies might well be carried out with women secreting large quantities of milk and with blood samples taken at noon when the calcitonin blood level appears to be at its peak in nonlactating women, according to a recent study (Hilliard *et al.*, 1977). These conditions may accentuate differences in calcitonin blood levels between lactating and nonlactating women.

TABLE I

BLOOD LEVELS OF CALCITONIN IN LACTATING WOMEN[a]

Patient group	Age (years)	Duration of lactation (months)	Frequency of detectable levels	Range (pg/ml)
I. Nonlactating women	27	—	0/16	< 60
II. Lactating women	28	2	2/18	215–1837
III. Lactating women	31	32	6/6	60–1800

[a] From Becker *et al.* (1979).

C. Vitamin D

Nelson and Evans (1961) suggested that the need for vitamin D by the lactating rat is small or nonexistent if diets adequate in calcium and phosphorus are given. However, experiments carried out by Toverud (1963) in Ragnar Nicolaysen's laboratory at the University of Oslo with a colony of rats maintained on a diet that contained minimal amounts of vitamin D led us to the contrary conclusion; a continual supply of vitamin D is needed during lactation. These experiments showed that lactating rats developed significant hypocalcemia (7.1 mg/dl) compared to vitamin D-fed controls (9.7 mg/dl) when completely deprived of vitamin D for only 1 week during lactation, even though the diet contained 1.1% calcium and 0.8% phosphorus (Toverud, 1963) (Table II). When the calcium content of the diet was decreased to 0.24%, a greater degree of hypocalcemia (5.7 mg/dl) developed, and when deprived of vitamin D for several months, lactating rats had serum calcium levels as low as 3.5 mg/dl.

Recently we (Boass *et al.*, 1977) and Halloran and DeLuca (1979) have confirmed the marked sensitivity of the serum calcium level of lactating rats to lack of dietary vitamin D. In addition, a collaborative study with Haussler and associates at the University of Arizona has allowed us to relate the hypocalcemia of D-deprived lactating rats to changes in the serum levels of $1,25\text{-}(OH)_2D_3$, the hormonal metabolite of vitamin D (Boass *et al.*, 1977). Vitamin D-fed lactating rats had significantly lower serum calcium and significantly higher serum levels of $1,25\text{-}(OH)_2D_3$ than nonlactating rats consuming the same diet (Table III). The serum calcium level and the serum level of $1,25\text{-}(OH)_2D_3$ of lactating rats on a vitamin D-free ($-$D) diet were both markedly lower than in vitamin D-fed ($+$D) lactating rats. Thus, the elevated level of $1,25\text{-}(OH)_2D_3$ seen in the lactating rats fed the complete diet appears to be essential for maintenance of the normal levels of serum calcium during lactation. This study (Boass *et al.*, 1977) was the first to demonstrate elevated levels of $1,25\text{-}(OH)_2D_3$ during lactation. Horst *et al.* (1977) and Barton *et al.* (1977) found higher serum levels of $1,25\text{-}(OH)_2D$ during the first 2 days of lactation in cows compared to 1 and 2 days before parturition, which were the only periods examined. Kumar *et al.* (1979) have now reported high serum levels of $1,25\text{-}(OH)_2D_3$ in lactating women (2- to 4-weeks postpartum) as well as in pregnant women. High levels of this metabolite have also been found in children, in young rats, and in the laying hen, all of which are representative of physiological states in which there is also a need for an increased amount of calcium (Haussler and McCain, 1977).

TABLE II

SERUM CALCIUM AND MILK COMPOSITION IN CALCIUM- AND
VITAMIN D-DEPRIVED RATS[a,b]

| Expt. No. and group | No. of rats | Diet | | | Serum Ca (mg/dl) | Milk | |
		Ca (%)	P (%)	Vit. D (D.U./day)		Total solid (%)	Ca/total solid (mg/gm)
27 A	10	1.11	0.8	40	9.7 ± 0.2	29.2 ± 0.7	8.1 ± 0.3
B	11	1.11	0.8	0	7.1 ± 0.4	30.5 ± 0.9	8.6 ± 0.3
22 C	12	0.24	0.4	70	9.3 ± 0.1	30.3 ± 0.9	8.7 ± 0.3
D	12	0.24	0.4	0	5.7 ± 0.5	34.4 ± 0.9	9.0 ± 0.2
23 E	12	0.57	0.5	0	5.9 ± 0.2	34.5 ± 0.8	9.1 ± 0.3
	14	0.02	0.5	0	5.2 ± 0.3	37.4 ± 1.4	9.1 ± 0.5
32 G	8	0.53	0.5	0	3.5 ± 0.1	37.7 ± 1.3	8.7 ± 0.7

[a] From Toverud (1963).

[b] The numbers are means ± SE. Rats in experiments 27, 22, and 23 were kept on a stock diet (containing minimal amounts of vitamin D but adequate amounts of calcium and phosphorus) until day 7 of lactation, at which time a basic vitamin D-free diet containing the stated amounts of calcium and phosphorus was given. The basic diet consisted of 73% whole wheat flour, 15% casein, 10% arachis oil, 2% salt mixture (calcium- and phosphorus-free), and a vitamin D-free vitamin mixture. When vitamin D was given, it was administered in oil by mouth every other day. Milk and blood samples were obtained 7 or 8 days later. Rats in experiment 32 were maintained on the basic vitamin D-free diet for 26 weeks before they were milked and bled on day 12 or 13 of lactation. A group of nonlactating females of comparable age and weight maintained on the same vitamin D-free diet for 26 weeks had an average serum calcium level of 8.5 mg/dl. The litters of the rats in experiment 32 weighed on day 7 essentially the same as litters from mothers consuming a complete diet, in spite of the extremely low serum Ca level. Analysis of correlation between serum calcium and total milk solid revealed a correlation coefficient of -0.61 ($N = 43$) for all rats in groups B, D, E, and G and -0.48 ($N = 79$) for all rats in all groups; both coefficients were significant at $p < 0.05$.

TABLE III

SERUM CALCIUM, PHOSPHATE, AND 1,25-(OH)$_2$D$_3$ LEVELS
IN LACTATING AND NONLACTATING RATS[a,b]

Groups	Diet	Ca (mg/dl)	P (mg/dl)	1,25-(OH)$_2$D$_3$ (pg/ml)
Lactating	+D	9.4 ± 0.2*	5.4 ± 0.2*	267 ± 6*
Lactating	−D	7.6 ± 0.2	3.7 ± 0.2	76 ± 6
Nonlactating	+D	10.1 ± 0.2	4.6 ± 0.2	72 ± 6

*Significantly different from values for lactating − and nonlactating +D ($p < 0.01$).
[a] Modified from Boass et al. (1977).
[b] The +D diet contained 5 IU of vitamin D$_3$ per gram of diet, and both +D and −D diets contained 0.4% Ca and 0.4% P. Blood samples were obtained on day 20 of lactation after the rats had been fed the diets for 13 days. Rats were from the Holtzman Co. (Madison, Wisconsin). Each value is mean ± SE of 7–11 rats.

1,25-(OH)$_2$D$_3$ is considered to be the hormonal form of vitamin D because (a) it is the most potent of the D metabolites; (b) it is formed in and secreted by an endocrine gland, the kidney; (c) it is carried in the circulation to distant sites, where it exerts its actions; and (d) its circulating level is stringently controlled. Evidence for such control is the absence of an increase in the blood level of 1,25-(OH)$_2$D$_3$ in the face of a manyfold increase in the blood level of the precursor, 25-(OH)D$_3$, during chronic administration of excess vitamin D (Hughes et al., 1976, 1977). Regulation of the blood level of 1,25-(OH)$_2$D$_3$ may involve negative feedback by the hormone itself on its synthesis in the kidney. Factors that, on the other hand, can stimulate renal 1α-hydroxylation of 25-hydroxyvitamin D$_3$ and cause an elevation of the 1,25-(OH)$_2$D$_3$ level in the blood are hypophosphatemia and increased circulating PTH, as well as hypocalcemia independent of PTH (Haussler and Mc-Cain, 1977).

The elevation of the 1,25-(OH)$_2$D$_3$ blood level in the vitamin D-fed lactating rats could not have been due to hypophosphatemia, since the serum phosphate values for the vitamin D-fed lactating rats were actually higher than those for the nonlactating controls (Table III). Increased 1,25-(OH)$_2$D level could have been due to the relative hypocalcemia, which was clearly demonstrated, or to increased secretion of PTH, which is a usual consequence of hypocalcemia. In fact, we have recently shown that PTH is indeed required for the maintenance of the high 1,25-(OH)$_2$D$_3$ blood level in the lactating rat (Pike et. al., 1979). Parathyroidectomy of rats on day 13 of lactation caused a marked drop in serum calcium and a decrease in the blood level of 1,25-(OH)$_2$D$_3$ to a level 30% that of sham-operated lactating rats. The level of the latter rats (with intact parathyroid glands) was 5 times higher than that of nonlactating control rats. Since the serum level of 1,25-(OH)$_2$D$_3$ in the parathyroidectomized lactating rats was still twice that of the nonlactating controls, it is possible that other hormones, such as prolactin, also may contribute to elevation of the 1,25-(OH)$_2$D$_3$ blood level in lactating rats. In fact, prolactin administration to chicks has been shown to enhance both the activity of the renal 1-hydroxylase and the circulating concentration of 1,25-(OH)$_2$D$_3$ (Spanos et al., 1976). Furthermore, inhibition of prolactin secretion by bromocriptine administration can markedly reduce the blood level of 1,25-(OH)$_2$D$_3$ in lactating rats, an effect that can be reversed by administration of prolactin (MacIntyre et al., 1977). However, since treatment with bromocriptine reduced litter survival by 80% (MacIntyre et al., 1977), and therefore must have impaired milk secretion markedly, the reduction in serum 1,25-(OH)$_2$D$_3$ could have been due to the absence of several other factors associated with full lactation, such as reduced serum calcium and elevated serum PTH.

The finding of elevated blood levels of 1,25-$(OH)_2D_3$ in mid and late lactation in rats prompted a study of the time of onset and duration of the elevation of 1,25-$(OH)_2D_3$. Blood samples were therefore obtained at different times between late pregnancy and 1 week after lactation. As shown in Table IV, the blood level of 1,25-$(OH)_2D_3$ was elevated during the last days of pregnancy, as it is also in women (Pike et al., 1977). By 1–2 days postpartum, 1,25-$(OH)_2D_3$ had fallen to control levels. It then increased again, so that by day 8 of lactation the level was almost as high as during pregnancy. It remained high throughout the rest of lactation, and then, 1–2 days after weaning, it fell precipitously to a level far below that of the controls. The drop in 1,25-$(OH)_2D_3$ coincided with a rebound increase in the serum calcium level. Presumably the rising serum calcium inhibited secretion of PTH and thus eliminated the signal for synthesis of 1,25-$(OH)_2D_3$. Finally, by day 7 after weaning, serum 1,25-$(OH)_2D_3$ and calcium had returned to control levels. Whatever mechanisms are involved, the fluctuations in the blood level of 1,25-$(OH)_2D_3$ reflect the varying requirements for vitamin D during late pregnancy, lactation, and weaning (Pike et al., 1979).

The data described above also allowed determination of the correlation between levels of serum calcium and 1,25-$(OH)_2D_3$. A linear

TABLE IV

SERUM LEVELS OF 1α,25-$(OH)_2D_3$ AND CALCIUM IN PREGNANT, LACTATING, AND WEANED RATS[a,b]

Reproductive stage	Number of rats	Serum levels	
		1α,25-$(OH)_2D_3$ (pg/ml)	Ca (mg/dl)
Controls	8	99	10.2
Day 21 of pregnancy	7	179*	10.2
Days 1–2 of lactation	8	110	10.4
Days 7–8 of lactation	8	172*	10.1
Days 13–16 of lactation	8	160*	9.6*
Day 2 after weaning	8	43*	13.0*
Day 7 after weaning	8	102	10.4
		SE:± 13	± 0.2

[a] Modified from Pike et al. (1979).

[b] Control rats were nonlactating, nonpregnant, age-matched female animals. All serum levels are the average of triplicate determinations of each of 6–8 individual rat serum samples ± SE. Values designated with an asterisk are significantly different from the control, $p < 0.01$. All rats were fed a complete diet containing 0.4% Ca, 0.4% P, and 5 IU of D_3 per gram of diet (Boass et al., 1977).

regression analysis of individual $1,25\text{-}(OH)_2D_3$ values on the corresponding calcium levels ($N = 55$) revealed a correlation coefficient of -0.61 ($p < 0.001$). Barton *et al.* (1977) reported in preliminary form a similar correlation ($r = -0.58$) between serum calcium and $1,25\text{-}(OH)_2D_3$ in cows with and without parturient paresis over a 5-day period around the time of parturition. The strong correlation with calcium over a wide, physiological range of serum calcium values in our study suggests that this ion modulates the biosynthesis of $1,25\text{-}(OH)_2D_3$, presumably through regulation of PTH secretion rate (Pike *et al.*, 1979). The small lowering of the serum calcium during the first week of lactation, which has been well documented in other experiments (Toverud *et al.*, 1976), is not apparent from the data in Table IV, presumably because comparison was not made to a comparable group of nonlactating rats sampled at the same time.

The physiological role of the elevated serum level of $1,25\text{-}(OH)_2D_3$ in lactating rats is probably related more to maintenance of serum calcium and phosphorus levels than to intestinal calcium absorption, since vitamin D-deprived rats with no elevation of $1,25\text{-}(OH)_2D_3$ have severe hypocalcemia and hypophosphatemia, but near normal net absorption of calcium (to be discussed in Section III,C).

In their preliminary report on the role of calcitonin in lactation, Taylor *et al.* (1975) also presented data on rats deprived of dietary vitamin D for 2 weeks before mating and throughout pregnancy and lactation. Their failure to find a significant decrease in serum calcium on day 24 of lactation, as evidence of vitamin D deficiency, may have been because extensive vitamin D reserves had accumulated prior to the experiment. The importance of prior vitamin D intake was illustrated by our failure to achieve hypocalcemia after vitamin D deprivation during lactation when the rats had previously been fed Purina Chow (5 IU of D_3 per gram) in contrast to rats on a low vitamin D diet (0.02 IU/gm) (Boass *et al.*, 1980). Alternatively, the failure of Taylor *et al.* (1975) to detect hypocalcemia may have been because blood samples were taken at 24 days rather than at the time of peak lactation (days 16–18), and because of the use of 8 rather than 10 young in a litter.

D. Summary

In summary, all three calcium-regulating hormones—PTH, calcitonin, and $1,25\text{-}(OH)_2D_3$—appear to be of special importance for regulation of serum calcium in lactation. The evidence is particularly strong in the rat that removal of the source of these hormones (including dietary vitamin D deprivation) leads to greater impairment in serum calcium regulation during lactation than during nonlactation, as the following changes in lactating rats indicate: (a) hypocalcemia develops more rapidly both after parathyroidectomy and after vitamin D deprivation; (b) a greater degree of hypercalcemia occurs after thyroidectomy and intragastric calcium administration during lactation. Our studies have also shown that the blood levels of calcitonin and 1,25-(OH)$_2$D$_3$ are elevated during lactation, that calcitonin secretion is related to eating, and that the elevated blood level of 1,25-(OH)$_2$D$_3$ is essential for normal calcium homeostasis. We propose that calcitonin helps to maintain a low normal serum calcium level during lactation. Elevated blood levels of calcitonin have also been found in some lactating women, although their serum calcium level was not different from that of nonlactating women. Elevated blood levels of PTH have been found in lactating cows; presumably they are in response to the frequently occurring decrease in serum calcium during early lactation.

III. Intestinal Calcium Absorption

A. Structural and Functional Changes in the Intestine during Lactation

The caloric needs of lactating rats, goats, and cows are increased approximately fourfold at the time when maximal milk production is achieved (Payne and Wheeler, 1968). Food intake increases gradually during lactation in the rat so that at peak lactation food consumption is almost four times as high as in nonlactating rats, as shown by Cripps and Williams (1975) (Fig. 6), Fell et al. (1963), and our own studies (Toverud et al., 1976; Boass et al., 1980). Similar increases in food intake have also been observed in lactating mice (Harding and Cairnie, 1975). Lactating women, on the other hand, have relatively smaller increases in caloric demands (Filer, 1975; Pitkin, 1976). It appears that the increased appetite is in part caused by the stimulus of suckling rather than just by the metabolic drain of milk production, since Cotes and Cross (1954) observed increased food intake in lactating rats with sectioned galactophores, which prevented the pups from obtaining milk.

Lactation in rats, mice, and sheep leads to both structural and functional changes in the small intestine (Cripps and Williams, 1975; Elias and Dowling, 1976; Campbell and Fell, 1964; Harding and Cairnie, 1975). Among the changes in the rat jejunum are increases (in the range 25–50%) in villus height, crypt depth, and weight of both wet and dry defatted tissue. There are relatively smaller increases in the ileum. Increases in the weight of the stomach, cecum, and colon and in total length of small intestine were also observed. We have con-

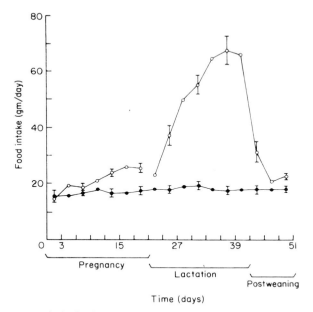

Fɪɢ. 6. Changes in daily food intake (grams per day) in control (virgin) albino rats and in mated albino rats during pregnancy, lactation, and postweaning. ○, Experimental group ($N = 4$); ●, control group ($N = 5$). Mean values with their standard errors, are indicated by vertical bars, for every second mean value. From Cripps and Williams (1975).

firmed the increased intestinal length (Toverud *et al.*, 1978b) and also found increased weight of the liver (unpublished experiments), as Kennedy *et al.* (1958) also had observed. Perfusion studies *in vivo* revealed a 50% increase in glucose absorption in the jejunum (mg/cm per hour), while a two- to threefold increase was seen in the ileum (Elias and Dowling, 1976). Cripps and Williams (1975) found increased absorption of glucose and leucine whether absorption was expressed as moles per hour or as moles per hour per millimeter of intestinal length.

Development of intestinal hypertrophy in lactation requires the presence of an increased amount of food in the intestine at least at one time during the day, Campbell and Fell (1964) produced partial hypertrophy of the alimentary canal by feeding lactating rats a restricted amount of food only once daily. This food was consumed rapidly. When the same amount of food was fed in three portions during the day, alimentary hypertrophy did not develop.

The mechanism of the intestinal adaptive changes most likely involves a systemic factor rather than a local one, since Thiry-Vella intestinal segments, from which food and duodenal secretions were excluded, showed the same mucosal hyperplasia and increased absorption as similar segments from control lactating rats (Elias and Dowling, 1976). Of the various hormones that could be the unknown systemic factor, enteroglucagon appears to be the most likely candidate, according to Elias and Dowling (1976), partly because the intestinal tissue content of this hormone increases in lactation (Jacobs et al., 1976).

B. Regulation of Calcium Absorption

Calcium absorption takes place along the entire small intestine. Absorption by active transport occurs primarily in the proximal small intestine and to a lesser extent in the ileum of young animals (Schachter and Rosen, 1959). Most of the calcium absorbed by the intact animal is absorbed by the ileum, presumably by diffusion, because of its great length and slow passage of the intestinal contents (Marcus and Lengemann, 1962; Cramer, 1972). The biochemical mechanism of absorption of calcium is not known, although it is believed that calcium entry into the intestinal mucosal cells is mediated by transport proteins acting at the brush border, and that movement within the cells involves packaging of calcium in membrane vesicles or mitochondrial binding of calcium (see reviews by Norman, 1978; DeLuca, 1978). One of the proteins implicated is a specific calcium binding protein synthesized in mucosal cells in response to vitamin D administration (see review by Wasserman et al., 1978).

Factors that influence the efficiency of calcium absorption include vitamin D, age, and the extent of skeletal mineralization. Vitamin D is essential for calcium absorption in humans and dogs and it enhances calcium absorption in rats. Recent evidence indicates that vitamin D exerts its effect through an interaction of $1,25\text{-}(OH)_2D_3$ with the genetic mechanism in mucosal cells that results in enhanced synthesis of one or more of the transport proteins that are believed to be involved in calcium entry into the cells (see reviews by Haussler and McCain, 1977; DeLuca, 1978; and Lawson, 1978). Long before the discovery of $1,25\text{-}(OH)_2D_3$ as the hormonal form of vitamin D, Nicolaysen and co-workers (Haavaldsen et al., 1956) showed that the efficiency of calcium absorption in rats was dependent on the degree of mineralization of the skeleton, provided vitamin D was present. Since dietary calcium deprivation resulted in decreased skeletal mineral stores, Nicolaysen postulated that the decrease in mineral stores caused the release of an "endogenous factor," which then mediated increased calcium absorption in the presence of vitamin D. The identity of the "endogenous factor" is not yet certain, although some evidence suggests that enhancement of $1,25\text{-}(OH)_2D_3$ synthesis by PTH is the essence of the "endogenous factor" (DeLuca, 1978). This presupposes that a decrease in skeletal mineral content results in a decrease in serum calcium as a signal for increased PTH secretion. Since only a small serum calcium decrease of short duration would be required to trigger increased PTH secretion, and, since this is difficult to document experimentally, it has not yet been possible to verify the postulated sequence of events as an explanation of the "endogenous factor" as mediator of the adaptation phenomenon. The increase in calcium absorbed after calcium deprivation declines with increasing age as does also the calcium absorption response to a given dose of $1,25\text{-}(OH)_2D_3$ (Horst *et al.*, 1978). The same authors pointed to parallel decreases in the blood level and intestinal content of $1,25\text{-}(OH)_2D_3$ as a probable explanation for the decreases in calcium absorption with age.

C. Calcium Absorption in Lactating Rats

The best illustration of the marked increase in calcium absorption that occurs in lactating rats is provided by the data of Fournier and Susbielle (1952) summarized in Table V. When rats were limited to a calcium intake of 100 mg/day, net absorption of calcium was in most cases less than one-tenth this amount both before and during pregnancy. During lactation there was a gradual increase to a value approximately fivefold higher. After weaning, calcium absorption decreased slowly over the next 5 days, after which time the prepregnancy level was reached. Even more profound changes were seen when the calcium intake was restricted to 27 mg/day. During the second and third weeks of lactation the rats absorbed almost 100% of the ingested calcium, and this high rate was maintained for at least 6 days after weaning. The persistence of the elevated absorption after weaning is consistent with the hypothesis of Nicolaysen that calcium absorption is regulated according to the degree of sufficiency of the skeletal mineral stores. In the rats restricted to a daily intake of 27 mg of calcium, lactation must have caused a relatively greater loss of skeletal mineral, which then required a longer time to replenish compared to those allowed a daily intake of 100 mg of calcium. Because of the magnitude of the increase in calcium absorption during lactation (fivefold in rats ingesting 100 mg of Ca per day) and because the high rate persisted for several days after weaning, it is clear that there is a specific mechanism that regulates calcium absorption in addition to that responsible for the small (20–40%) increase in absorption of other nutrients, such as glucose and amino acids, as referred to in Section III,A.

TABLE V
NET CALCIUM ABSORPTION AND URINARY CALCIUM
EXCRETION BEFORE, DURING, AND AFTER LACTATION
IN VITAMIN D-FED RATS[a]

	Intake of calcium (mg/day)[b]			
	100 mg/day		27 mg/day	
Time	Ca absorbed	Ca in urine	Ca absorbed	Ca in urine
Before pregnancy	4–12	0.9–4	5–13	1–4
During pregnancy	4–12	0.6–4	5–11	1–3
During lactation				
Days 9–12	22–45	0.1–2	20–27	0–0.3
Days 18–21	38–58	0.1–0.5	22–26	0
After lactation				
Day 1	35–47	0.7–2	19–26	0–0.4
Day 2	31–40	1–10	15–26	1–3
Day 3	20–24	9–15	21–24	0.6–1
Day 4	14–19	6–16	24–25	0.5–1
Day 6	7–11	2–4	21–26	2–3
Day 20	—	—	15–17	2–3

[a] Modified from Fournier and Susbielle (1952).
[b] Values given as range for 3–7 rats.

Kostial et al. (1969a) have shown an increase in calcium absorption in lactating rats in vivo as well as in vitro. Absorption of ^{47}Ca in vivo (as percentage of administered dose) was increased twofold even in rats that were consuming a diet with an abnormally high calcium content (2.4% Ca, 1.1% P) (Kostial et al., 1969b). Their results in vitro, which were based on determination of the ratio of ^{45}Ca across the intestinal wall of inverted sacs of duodenum, suggested increased active transport by intestine from lactating rats. The specificity of the calcium absorption changes is well illustrated by the observation of Kostial et al. (1969a) that the concentration ratio was lower for ^{85}Sr than for ^{45}Ca even though the ratio for ^{85}Sr in duodenal sacs from lactating rats was higher than that for sacs from nonlactating rats.

We have confirmed the finding of increased calcium absorption in lactating rats in vivo and in vitro. In rats fed Purina Laboratory Chow (1.1% Ca, 0.8% P, and 5 IU of D_3 per gram of diet), we found that calcium absorption as percentage of intake was almost twice as high (30 vs 17%) in lactating as in nonlactating rats (Toverud et al., 1976). When a diet with 0.4% calcium and 0.4% phosphorus was used, there was a fourfold higher percentage of calcium absorption in the lactating rats (Table VI). In vitro we have shown that sacs of duodenum

TABLE VI

Net Calcium Absorption and Serum Calcium in
Lactating and Nonlactating Rats[a,b]

Groups	Body weight (gm)	Food intake (gm/day)	Net absorbed Ca (% of intake)	Serum Ca (mg/dl)
Experiment A				
Nonlactating +D	339 ± 6	19 ± 1	15 ± 3	9.8 ± 0.1
Lactating +D	345 ± 7	50 ± 1*	62 ± 4*	9.2 ± 0.1*
Experiment B				
Lactating +D	359 ± 13	56 ± 2*	68 ± 2*	8.7 ± 0.3*
Lactating −D	321 ± 11	41 ± 2	53 ± 2	4.1 ± 0.3

*Significantly different from nonlactating +D (experiment A) and lactating −D (experiment B) ($p < 0.01$).

[a] Modified from Toverud et al. (1978c).

[b] The +D diet contained 5 IU of vitamin D_3 per gram of diet, the −D diet contained no vitamin D, and both +D and −D diets contained 0.4% Ca and 0.4% P. The diets were introduced on day 4 of lactation. In experiment A absorption was studied during days 9–13 of lactation, and in experiment B, during days 23–27 of lactation while the mothers suckled new, 11-day-old pups. Blood samples were obtained on the final day of the absorption study. Each value is the mean ± SE of 5–7 rats.

from lactating rats achieved calcium concentration ratios of approximately 3 compared to ratios of 1 for similar sacs for nonlactating rats (Table VII).

It seemed reasonable to assume that vitamin D is required for the elevation of calcium absorption in lactation since the phenomenon of adaptation of calcium absorption to need (Haavaldsen et al., 1956) is vitamin D-dependent and 1,25-$(OH)_2D_3$ may be the postulated "endogenous factor." However, the results of our experiments indicate that vitamin D and circulating 1,25-$(OH)_2D_3$ cannot be the only factors responsible for the high efficiency of calcium absorption during lactation. True enough, as noted in the preceding section on vitamin D and shown in Table VI, serum 1,25-$(OH)_2D_3$ was high and serum calcium was normal in lactating rats fed a vitamin D-containing diet in which a greatly (fourfold) increased net calcium absorption was maintained. But, to our surprise, similar lactating rats deprived of vitamin D for 2 weeks, in which serum 1,25-$(OH)_2D_3$ was relatively low and serum calcium was very low (4.1 mg/dl), net calcium absorption was remarkably high, 3.5 times higher than in nonlactating controls. Net absorption was measured by calcium balance for a 3-day period after 21 days of lactation in rats suckling a second litter of 10-day-old pups. The unexpected high efficiency of calcium absorption in −D lactating rats was confirmed in vitro with everted gut sacs. These sacs developed very nearly the same high concentration ratios across the intestinal wall as did sacs from +D rats. Prior parathyroidectomy,

TABLE VII
CALCIUM TRANSPORT BY SACS OF INTESTINE *in Vitro*[a,b]

Intestinal segment	Ca concentration ratio, serosal: mucosal	
	Lactating rats	Nonlactating rats
Duodenum, segment 1	3.1 ± 0.3*	1.2 ± 0.3
Duodenum, segment 2	2.2 ± 0.2*	1.2 ± 0.2
Ileum	1.3 ± 0.05**	1.1 ± 0.06

*Significantly greater than nonlactating value ($p < 0.01$).
**Significantly greater than nonlactating value ($p < 0.025$).
[a] From Toverud *et al.* (1978a).
[b] Values are means ± SE of 10–13 sacs, each from a different rat. The small intestine was removed from nonfasted rats. Everted sacs of intestine, 4 cm long, were filled with 0.4 ml of incubation medium containing 0.4 mM Ca. The sacs were incubated at 37°C for 1 hour in 5 ml of this medium in flasks gassed with O_2. The rats were maintained on Purina Laboratory Chow containing 1.1% Ca, 0.8% P, and 5 IU of D_3 per gram of diet.

which should have reduced 1,25-$(OH)_2D_3$ production, did not significantly affect these ratios. The above results demonstrate that the enhanced calcium absorption during lactation does not require the large increase in serum 1,25-$(OH)_2D_3$ that occurs in vitamin D-fed lactating rats. However, the conclusion that vitamin D or 1,25-$(OH)_2D_3$ has no effect on calcium absorption in the lactating rat would not be warranted, since the data in our experiment (Table VI) did indicate somewhat lower (22%) net absorption of calcium in the vitamin D-deprived rats and since the mean calcium concentration ratios for duodenol sacs from −D rats were always numerically lower than those for sacs from +D rats, although the differences did not reach statistical significance (Toverud *et al.*, 1978a).

The high calcium absorption in the face of low circulating 1,25-$(OH)_2D$ in vitamin D-deprived lactating rats could be explained by the assumption that the intestinal content of 1,25-$(OH)_2D$ in these rats (not yet measured) is not reduced, in contrast to the serum level of 1,25-$(OH)_2D$. Favus *et al.* (1974) reported that the intestines of parathyroidectomized rats contained a normal amount of 1,25-$(OH)_2D_3$ in spite of the reduced level of 1,25-$(OH)_2D_3$ in the serum. On the other hand, Horst *et al.* (1978) have shown that blood levels and intestinal levels of 1,25-$(OH)_2D_3$ are well correlated at different ages in the nonlactating rat. Regardless of the detailed interpretation of the data in Table VI, it seems clear that a continual supply of dietary vitamin D is more important for serum calcium regulation than for intestinal absorption of calcium during lactation in the rat.

If vitamin D is not the only factor required for enhancement of calcium absorption in the lactating rat, what factor or factors are responsible for this phenomenon? Since there had been previous evidence to indicate that PTH can stimulate calcium absorption in vitamin D-deprived nonlactating rats (Toverud, 1964), we tested the hypothesis that PTH is the stimulating factor in D-deprived lactating rats. However, the results of our unpublished in vitro studies with gut sacs from parathyroidectomized, vitamin D-deprived lactating rats provided no support for this hypothesis. The fact that calcium absorption in these gut sacs in vitro was not reduced may have been because parathyroidectomy did not affect the intestinal level of $1,25\text{-}(OH)_2D_3$ despite reduction of serum $1,25\text{-}(OH)_2D_3$, as in the work of Favus et al. (1974) in nonlactating rats.

We subsequently suggested, but have not yet tested, the possibility that prolactin may be the factor in question (Toverud et al., 1978c), since prolactin administered to nonlactating rats has been shown to increase calcium absorption (Mainoya, 1975), and since prolactin blood levels are elevated at least in the first 2 weeks of lactation in the rat (Simpson et al., 1973). This hypothesis is indirectly supported by the recent demonstration that bromocriptine, an inhibitor of prolactin secretion and antagonist of prolactin action, caused a significant decrease in net calcium absorption in normal vitamin D-fed lactating rats (James et al., 1977). Other factors, including gastrointestinal hormones, should also be investigated.

D. Calcium Absorption in Lactating Ruminants

In a detailed study of calcium kinetics in lactating sheep fed ample amounts of calcium and vitamin D, Braithwaite et al. (1969) found the efficiency of calcium absorption (as percentage of intake) to be approximately 1.5 times that of nonlactating sheep. In early lactation (during the first 5 weeks), when the milk yield was high, the increase in calcium absorption was not sufficient to allow the sheep to remain in calcium balance. As would be expected, the rate of calcium removal from bone by resorption during these weeks was severalfold higher than in late lactation when the milk yield was low. Because of the persistently increased efficiency of calcium absorption throughout lactation and the reduced milk production the sheep were in positive calcium balance during the last 8–9 weeks of lactation. The efficiency of intestinal calcium absorption begins to increase in late pregnancy in ewes only after considerable loss of skeletal mineral has taken place. In late lactation the calcium absorption rate does not decrease until after skeletal mineral stores have been replenished (Braithwaite and Glascock, 1976). These observations are consistent with the concept of Nicolaysen and associates of a vitamin D-dependent "endogenous factor" that mediates an increase in intestinal calcium absorption when skeletal mineral stores are depleted (Haavaldsen et al., 1956). The recent demonstration of a marked increase in intestinal calcium absorption (as percentage of calcium ingested) in lactating ewes given daily injections of 1α-(OH)D$_3$ (5 μg/day) suggests that 1,25-(OH)$_2$D$_3$ (the biogenic metabolite of 1α-(OH)D$_3$) may be synonymous with the "endogenous factor" (Braithwaite, 1978). This suggestion is further supported by the observation that the treatment led to a decrease in bone resorption rate and prevention of the normal loss of bone mineral at peak lactation.

Lactating cows also generally absorb a higher proportion of dietary calcium than nonlactating cows. In one study fractional absorption (α) increased approximately twofold within the first 1–3 weeks of lactation, after which time it decreased toward the prepartum level (Ramberg et al., 1970). van't Klooster (1976) found the same increase in absorption of ^{45}Ca (as percentage of dose) during the first week of lactation; over this period calcium absorption was closely correlated with the daily amount of calcium secreted into the milk.

E. Calcium Absorption in Lactating Women

Macy et al. (1930) found negative net absorption of calcium in three women during the seventh month of lactation when they were consuming 2–4 gm of calcium daily and secreting from 0.5 to 1.3 gm of calcium in the milk daily. Two months after daily administration of 400–600 IU of vitamin D, net absorption of calcium had become positive and had increased to 20–50% of ingested calcium in two of the women. Similar net absorption values at high intake levels were observed by Donelson et al. (1931) in late lactation when it was thought that adequate amounts of vitamin D had been given. Liu et al. (1937) also found negative net absorption of calcium in four of five lactating women with calcium intakes less than 1 gm daily and severe hypocalcemia due to deficient intake of vitamin D. Net calcium absorption increased in all five women to 30–70% of ingested calcium after treatment with vitamin D (12,000 IU daily, as Vigantol). In another study, in which there was an intermediate calcium supply (1–2 gm of calcium daily) (Toverud and Toverud, 1931), net absorption of calcium as percentage of intake was in the range 42–67% for five women who secreted 180–260 mg of calcium in the milk daily; one subject absorbed far less calcium in spite of increased vitamin D intake. A similar study of women during the second trimester of pregnancy by the same investigators revealed calcium absorption percentages in the same range as for the five lactating women. In a more recent study of calcium balance and kinetic parameters in pregnant women (Heaney and Skillman, 1971), the absorption fraction, α, during the last 20 weeks of pregnancy was twice as high as the value determined for nonpregnant women. Thus, calcium absorption appears to be significantly increased well in advance of the last 2 months of pregnancy, during which time most of the skeletal mineral deposition in the fetus takes place. It is therefore quite possible that the net absorption values reported for mid pregnancy by Toverud and Toverud (1931), which were similar to those observed during lactation, reflected more efficient absorption than in nonpregnant or nonlactating women. It is pertinent to note that the daily amount of calcium transferred to the fetus during the last 2 months of pregnancy may exceed that secreted in the milk by most women. Therefore, there would be no need for a further increase in calcium absorption after parturition (during lactation) in order to maintain calcium balance.

Although less than ideal procedures were used in the lactation studies in the 1930s, such as short (4-day) metabolic periods, there can be little doubt that the marked and consistent changes seen after vitamin D treatment in most of the women in these studies implied a definite requirement for vitamin D for adequate calcium absorption in lactating women. Whether this requirement is greater in lactation than in nonlactation cannot be determined from these studies, since they did not include observations on age-matched nonlactating subjects on the same diet, nor did they include the effects of different dose levels of vitamin D.

Based on the work of Heaney and Skillman (1971), the adaptive increase in calcium-absorptive ability would be expected to take place some time before week 20 of pregnancy and to persist during lactation as long as milk production is heavy. However, data to support the latter view, namely that percentage calcium absorption is higher in lactating than in nonlactating women, are not available. The large variability in the amount of calcium absorbed from the gut and excreted in urine and milk, as illustrated in the studies discussed above, will make it difficult to show a clear-cut effect of lactation on calcium absorption in the human.

Two main differences should be noted between women and females of other species with regard to the need for an adaptive increase in calcium absorption during lactation. The need is relatively small in lactating women, since the additional calcium loss in the milk each day is usually no greater than the average daily loss of calcium in the urine, whereas, in cows, sheep, and rats calcium loss in the milk may be 10- to 100-fold greater than in urine (see further discussion in Section IV). In the rat the fetal calcium requirement is almost negligible compared to the calcium requirement of lactation (Spray, 1950), while in women daily fetal calcium requirement during the last 2 months of pregnancy usually exceeds the daily calcium requirement in lactation (Toverud and Toverud, 1931).

In summary, efficiency of calcium absorption during lactation is elevated in cows, sheep, and rats and, presumably, in women as well, although firm evidence for enhanced calcium absorption in lactating women is not available. The mechanism underlying this enhancement, at least in the rat, includes a nonspecific enhancement of absorption of nutrients in general, which appears to be related to intestinal hypertrophy and a calcium-specific phenomenon that is partly vitamin D-dependent and that also may be related to unknown humoral factors, such as prolactin. There is indirect evidence that in the rat the efficiency of calcium absorption is regulated according to calcium needs during lactation and that enhanced calcium absorption may persist after weaning to allow restoration of skeletal mineral deficiency incurred during lactation. Although it has been assumed that this adaptation process is vitamin D-dependent (mediated by elevated plasma and tissue levels of $1,25\text{-}(OH)_2D_3$), data to support this contention in the rat are not yet available.

IV. Urinary Calcium Excretion in Lactation

Urinary calcium output is generally determined by the amount of calcium absorbed, the serum calcium level, and the secretion rate or blood level of PTH (briefly reviewed by Sutton and Dirks, 1978). In man, high calcium intakes and, presumably, increased calcium absorption are associated with increased calcium loss in the urine (Davis et al., 1970; Peacock et al., 1967). This relationship has recently been demonstrated in patients with idiopathic hypercalciuria in whom increased intestinal calcium absorption is associated with increased urinary calcium excretion and a normal serum calcium level (Shen et al., 1977). The same study also showed that in both control and hyper-calciuric patients urine calcium was negatively correlated with serum PTH level. In rats, the separate effects of PTH and the serum calcium level are well illustrated by experiments of Talmage (1956), which showed that the immediate effect of parathyroidectomy was an increase in urine calcium (because of the absence of PTH-mediated tubular reabsorption of calcium), while the effect several hours later, after serum calcium had fallen, was a decrease to normal range because of the reduced filtered load of calcium. The role of vitamin D or $1,25\text{-}(OH)_2D_3$ in renal reabsorption of calcium is unclear, although evidence for a stimulating effect has been obtained (Haussler and McCain, 1977; Sutton and Dirks, 1978). Presumably, the influence of vitamin D status on urinary calcium excretion may depend more on the effects of $1,25\text{-}(OH)_2D_3$ on intestinal calcium absorption and the serum calcium level than on a direct effect on the kidney (Omdahl and DeLuca, 1973). For example, the patients of Shen et al. (1977) who showed elevated circulating $1,25\text{-}(OH)_2D$, experienced hypercalciuria presumably as a consequence of a demonstrated increase in intestinal calcium absorption.

In lactating rats, urinary calcium excretion appears to be less than that of pregnant or nonlactating rats. In the study of Fournier and Susbielle (1952) daily urinary calcium decreased from approximately 2 mg during pregnancy to negligible amounts during the second and third weeks of lactation whether the diet contained 0.83% or 0.22% calcium (Table V). The lower urinary loss of calcium during lactation is probably because of the lower serum calcium level (lower filtered load) and the presumed higher PTH blood level. The relative importance of the two determinants can be assessed only with para-thyroidectomized lactating rats maintained on a diet with sufficient calcium to prevent hypocalcemia (Boass et al., 1980). Regardless of the cause, the lower urinary calcium excretion during lactation would appear to be part of the general adaptation of the lactating animal to the demands of milk secretion. However, the contribution that the reduced calcium excretion makes to the calcium economy of the lactating rat on a normal diet is almost negligible. Based on the study of Fournier and Susbielle (1952) (Table V), a saving of 2 mg of calcium per day represents only 1–2% of the 120–140 mg of net absorbed calcium each day in lactating rats on diets with 0.4 to 1.2% calcium (Toverud et al., 1976; Boass et al., 1980). Since estimates of daily loss of calcium in the milk are in the range of 100–150 mg (Toverud et al., 1976), it is apparent that a urinary loss of even 2 mg of calcium per day (the value for nonlactating rats) would be of little importance. However, in rats on the low-calcium diet (0.22%) used by Fournier and Susbielle (1952) that had a net absorption of only 20–27 mg of calcium daily, the reduction in urinary calcium excretion from 2 mg to essentially zero was probably of some significance.

The role of vitamin D in urinary calcium excretion in lactation is uncertain, as it also is in nonlactation. Preliminary studies in our laboratories (Boass *et al.*, 1980) indicate no difference in urinary calcium between normal lactating rats and lactating rats on a vitamin D-free diet that developed severe hypocalcemia. Presumably any stimulating effect of vitamin D on renal reabsorption of calcium was counteracted by the reduction in filtered calcium load because of the hypocalcemia.

An interesting rebound increase in urinary calcium excretion after weaning was observed by Fournier and Susbielle (1952) in rats that consumed the diet with 0.83% calcium (Table V). By the second and third days after weaning urinary calcium excretion had risen from 1 to 10–16 mg per day. A return to the nonlactating baseline value of 2 mg was seen by day 4 after weaning. Since serum calcium levels were not determined in this study, the relationship of this rebound rise in urinary calcium excretion to a possible rise in the filtered load cannot be evaluated. However, we have recently reported a rebound rise in serum calcium 1–2 days after weaning in rats consuming a diet with 0.4% calcium (Pike *et al.*, 1979) (Table III). In a preliminary study (Boass *et al.*, 1980) a rise in urinary calcium excretion 1 and 2 days after weaning was indeed accompanied by a rise in serum calcium from 9.5 to 10.8 mg/dl. Since the serum calcium increase not only represents an increase in the filtered load of calcium, but also causes reduction in PTH secretion, we suggest that the rebound rise in urinary calcium is caused by a combination of increased filtered load of calcium and reduced PTH-mediated tubular reabsorption of calcium.

In lactating ewes, urinary calcium excretion appears to decrease to a level approximately one-third that of nonlactating ewes at the same time as the efficiency of calcium absorption from the intestine increases (Braithwaite *et al.*, 1969). This pattern of change is very similar to that shown for the rat by Fournier and Susbielle (1952). As was also pointed out for the rat, the amount of calcium lost in the urine in ewes is so small compared to that lost in the milk (less than 4% in the study of Braithwaite *et al.*, 1969) that the reduction in urinary calcium from the prepartum level makes a relatively small contribution to the overall calcium economy during lactation. Since serum calcium values were not reported in this study, one cannot relate the decreased urinary calcium excretion to a possible reduction in the filtered load of calcium. However, in a subsequent study of lactating ewes daily treatment with 5 μg of 1α-OH-D_3 resulted in a 20% increase in serum calcium and a three- to fourfold increase in urinary calcium excretion (Braithwaite, 1978). It is presumed that the increase in serum calcium was responsible for the increased urine calcium.

Braithwaite (1976) has expressed the opinion that urinary excretion in the cow is not much affected by the physiological state. However, Mayer *et al.* (1969a) and Ramberg *et al.* (1970, 1975) have reported decreased urinary calcium excretion in lactating cows, particularly during early lactation when the cows tend to be hypocalcemic and when increased blood levels of PTH have been found (Pickard *et al.*, 1975).

Lactating women may excrete relatively more calcium in the urine than lactating females of other species. Since more than 200 mg of calcium may be excreted in the urine and a comparable amount, and sometimes less, in the milk (Donelson *et al.*, 1931; Toverud and Toverud, 1931), it is obvious that even small changes in urine calcium can make important contributions to the calcium balance in lactating women. Urinary calcium loss was indeed lower during lactation in most women in both studies. A marked decrease was also seen in a group of 22 women studied for several weeks before and after parturition (Retallack *et al.*, 1977). In the studies of Liu *et al.* (1937) urinary calcium loss was rather low (mostly less than 70 mg/day) in the vitamin D-deficient, hypocalcemic women. As serum calcium rose in response to vitamin D treatment, urinary calcium also increased. In general, urinary calcium excretion in lactating women appears to be high relative to calcium secretion in the milk and highly variable within and between subjects.

In conclusion, it appears that urinary calcium excretion decreases during lactation in women, cows, ewes, and rats. Because of the already relatively small amount of calcium excreted in nonlactating animals, this decrease is of little importance for the calcium economy during lactation. However, in contrast to experimental animals, lactating women, who may lose as much calcium in the urine as in the milk, may benefit significantly from even a small reduction in urine calcium. The most important determinants of urinary calcium excretion during lactation seem to be filtered load of calcium and parathyroid hormone.

V. Calcium and Vitamin D in Milk

A. Calcium

The calcium content of milk from women, cows, and rats appears to remain relatively constant except when the lactating female has been subjected to multiple dietary deficiencies (see review by Toverud, 1963). Dietary deprivation of lactating rats of either calcium or vitamin D did not significantly affect the calcium content relative to the total milk solids (Table II), even though marked reductions in serum calcium and phosphorus occurred (Table VIII). The calcium to phosphorus ratios also remained remarkably constant in spite of fluctuations in the serum levels. These observations in the rat are in general agreement with those in the lactating cow (Reid, 1961), and in lactating women (Hytten and Thomson, 1961). A study of 60 women in India also revealed the lack of a correlation between dietary calcium intake (over the range 0.17–1.14 gm per day) and milk calcium concentration (Karmarkar and Ramakrishnan, 1960).

The mechanisms by which calcium is taken up by the mammary gland and the forms in which calcium exists in the milk have been reviewed by Baumrucker (1978). Hormonal influences on calcium uptake and distribution in milk have not yet been uncovered.

B. Vitamin D

Vitamin D in milk should probably be considered not so much a vitamin source as an alternative supply of a prohormone, the other prohormone source being cholecalciferol produced in the skin from UV irradiation of 7-dehydrocholesterol (Haussler and McCain, 1977). The

TABLE VIII

Phosphorus and Calcium: Phosphorus Ratios
in Serum and Milk from Rats[a,b]

Expt. No.	Group	Serum (mg/dl)		Serum Ca:P	Milk (mg/dl)		Milk Ca:P
		Ca	P		Ca	P	
22	+D	9.30 ± 0.13	6.31 ± 0.29	1.51 ± 0.07	262 ± 8	210 ± 3	1.25 ± 0.03
22	−D	5.74 ± 0.49	4.69 ± 0.30	1.29 ± 0.15	304 ± 11	241 ± 6	1.27 ± 0.03

[a] From Toverud (1963).

[b] The numbers are means ± SE. The serum calcium and milk calcium values are the same as those obtained on day 15 of lactation in experiment 22, Table II.

amount of exposure to the sun required for sufficient prohormone formation is evidently quite small. According to Johnson *et al.* (1968) the dose of UV radiation needed to cure rickets in children is approximately 5% of the dose needed to produce a mild sunburn.

Milk from rats fed a normal diet must contain enough vitamin D for normal skeletal growth of the pups, since the pups may be deprived of UV radiation in the wild and in many laboratories. While data on the D content of rat milk are not available, Weisman *et al.* (1976) in a preliminary study, found that 89% of the total vitamin D content of the mammary gland after injection of cholecalciferol to lactating rats was unchanged vitamin D_3, and 25-(OH)D_3 represented only 8% of the content. Using the same technique in rats, Mendelsohn and Haddad (1975) concluded that mostly cholecalciferol, and possibly a small amount of 25-(OH)D_3, were transferred in the milk to the pups. It seems reasonable to assume that most of the circulating 25-(OH)D_3 in suckling pups is endogenously produced, since the same investigators found evidence for 25-hydroxylation by the neonatal liver. However, the rate of hydroxylation or the supply of substrate must be low, because serum levels of 25-(OH)D_3 decreased during the first week of life and remained low until after weaning in normal rat pups (Mendelsohn and Haddad, 1975).

Total vitamin D content of rat milk is undoubtedly affected by the vitamin D status of the mother; data from our laboratory (Toverud *et al.*, 1979) show that vitamin D deprivation of the mother beginning on day 6 of pregnancy caused reductions in the serum 25-(OH)D_3 levels of the pups to 50% of the level of control pups by 8 days of age and to undetectable levels (< 0.25 ng/ml) at 15 and at 21 days of age. As would have been expected, evidence of vitamin deficiency begins to develop at age 15 days; by 21 days of age the pups displayed hypocalcemia, hypophosphatemia, reduced bone ash, and characteristic rachitic bone changes such as a widening of the hypertrophic cartilage zone, irregular line of calcification, and short, wide, and irregularly arranged bony trabeculae. It is thus clear that vitamin D deprivation of the pregnant rat will result in the development of vitamin D deficiency in the suckling pup evidenced in part by hypophosphatemia and the rachitic bone lesion, both of which are typical of infant rickets and neither of which can be obtained in the weaned rat unless they are deprived of dietary phosphate as well as vitamin D (Nicolaysen *et al.*, 1953; DeLuca, 1978). Paradoxically, when mother rats had been deprived of vitamin D for 8 months and showed undetectable circulating levels of 1,25-(OH)$_2$D, their 23-day-old pups did not show hypocalcemia relative to + D pups in a preliminary study by Halloran and DeLuca (1979), in which data on bone ash and histology were not provided.

Most reports indicate that human milk and cow milk contain such low amounts of vitamin D ($<$ 5 IU/100 ml) that either a dietary supplement of D or ample UV irradiation of skin is required for normal growth of the breastfed infant (Toverud et al., 1950; Vorherr, 1974). The finding of sulfoconjugates of cholecalciferol in milk (Sahashi et al., 1967; Lakdawala and Widdowson, 1977) suggests the possibility that the total D content of the milk is higher than previously thought. However, it is not certain that the sulfated form is active in the suckling rat pup or infant (Noff and Edelstein, 1978). The high incidence of rickets in infants who are exclusively breastfed and not given vitamin D supplements (Toverud et al., 1950) would indeed argue against the idea that the sulfated form is active. Increasing the intake of vitamin D does not appear to increase appreciably the D level in human milk (Drummond et al., 1939; Polskin et al., 1943) or in cow's milk (Payne and Manston, 1967). Administration of superphysiological daily doses of 40,000 IU of vitamin D for 10 days to lactating women increased the D content of the milk only to between 12 and 44 IU/100 ml (Polskin et al., 1943). A high dose of 25-(OH)D$_3$ to prevent bovine parturient paresis did not lead to detectable levels of 25-(OH)D$_3$ in the milk (Frank et al., 1977).

In lactating rats, consumption of a diet with a high content of vitamin D, 300 IU per gram of diet, has led to hypercalcemia in the 12-and 17-day-old suckling pups (serum calcium in the range 11–12 mg/dl), indicating that administration of superphysiological amounts of vitamin D or D metabolites resulted in some transfer into the milk (L. A. Dostal, A. Boass, and S. U. Toverud, unpublished experiments). Since the lactating rats showed hypercalcemia during the first week of lactation, the intake level of vitamin D (at least 20-fold higher relative to body weight than in the human study of Polskin et al., 1943) was presumably in the toxic range for the mother as well as the pups. It is thus clear that in the rat vitamin D activity in the milk may reflect the vitamin D intake during pregnancy and lactation, since both vitamin D deficiency and hypervitaminosis D can be induced in the suckling pups by appropriate manipulation of the mother's vitamin D intake. It will now be of interest to verify the presence of the excessive vitamin D activity in the milk and to examine the mechanism of the uptake and metabolism of vitamin D in the mammary gland. The suggestion that the vitamin D content of rat milk can be increased above the normal level should be of value in studies of vitamin D metabolism in the lactating mother as well as in the suckling pups.

VI. SKELETAL CALCIUM CONTENT

A. LACTATING RATS

Observations in several studies indicate that rats store skeletal calcium during pregnancy and suffer a net loss during lactation (Duckworth and Warnock, 1942–1943; Ellinger *et al.*, 1952). Even when a diet with an adequate calcium content (0.6–0.8%) is given, 15–25% of femur calcium may be lost (Kletzien *et al.*, 1932; Warnock and Duckworth, 1944; Spray, 1950). Consistent with this observation is the finding of a decreased calcium accretion rate in lactating compared to nonlactating rats (Blanusa *et al.*, 1971). In rats subjected to repeated pregnancies and lactations without intervening rest periods, mineral loss during lactation was made up during the subsequent pregnancy, since the mineral mass of femurs was just as high at the end of the third pregnancy as after the first. When the diet was essentially calcium free (0.04% calcium), the bone mineral level of the combined femur and tibia decreased by 40% over the 3-week lactation period, but even at that intake level 39% of the lost bone mineral was recovered during the subsequent pregnancy (Ellinger *et al.*, 1952). Rasmussen (1977) determined that bone loss in response to dietary calcium deprivation during lactation took place mostly in the metaphyses of tibias and femurs and to lesser extent on the endosteal surfaces of the diaphyses, and that bone resorption at these sites appeared to have been mediated by hypertrophic mononuclear cells. When vitamin D deprivation was added to calcium deprivation (0.05% calcium in the diet) total body calcium decreased 46% during 3 weeks of lactation compared to total calcium in rats receiving a diet with 1.03% calcium and 1.0 IU of D_3 per gram of diet (de Winter and Steendijk, 1975). Since none of the studies included dietary deprivation of vitamin D alone, the relative importance of vitamin D and dietary calcium for bone mineral conservation in the lactating rat cannot be assessed.

B. LACTATING WOMEN

Several recent studies indicate that lactating women consuming a "normal" diet (average in the United States and western Europe) show relatively little (4% or less) loss of bone mineral mass during lactation (Atkinson and West, 1970; Lamke *et al.*, 1977). However, interpretation of these findings is complicated by the fact that no information is given on the volume of milk secreted or on the dietary intake of calcium and vitamin D before and during lactation. Therefore, one cannot relate the bone loss either to calcium supply or to loss in the milk. It is obvious that the maintenance of calcium balance requires only minor adjustments in a woman who produces only 500 ml of milk each day (such as during the first postpartum month or for an extended period if the infant is only partially breastfed). The daily calcium loss in the milk in this case (150 mg), which is probably no greater than the calcium loss in the urine, can be compensated for by doubling of the calcium intake or by a small increase in efficiency of calcium absorption. In vitamin D-deficient women with inefficient calcium absorption, even a low rate of milk production is associated with a negative calcium balance (Liu *et al.*, 1937), which if continued for 3 months, could lead to loss of about 10% of skeletal mineral.

If lactation generally is accompanied by negative calcium balance and a net loss of 5-10% of skeletal mineral, one might expect a higher incidence of postmenopausal osteoporosis in women who have breast-fed three or four children. On the other hand, it is possible that such women represent a select group with a well developed ability to meet all nutritional demands of lactation including calcium, and that whatever calcium deficit occurs during lactation is made up, perhaps in excess, between lactations. The idea that the ability to breastfeed for long periods of time may be associated with ability to maintain a positive calcium balance is supported by the observation of Lamke *et al.* (1977) that women who nursed for less than 3 months showed a net loss of 4% in bone mineral mass while those nursing for 6 months showed no loss at either 3 or 6 months. Over a 3-month period after weaning the former group not only made up the loss of mineral incurred while lactating but achieved a net gain of bone mineral of 7%.

With increasing amounts of milk secretion the efficiency of calcium absorption becomes increasingly important for maintenance of calcium balance. This raises the question of the requirement for vitamin D during lactation, a question that cannot be answered with the available data, according to the joint FAO/WHO Expert Group of 1970 and the National Research Council, Food and Nutrition Board in 1974. However, both groups have acted on the assumption that the requirement for vitamin D is increased during lactation and have recommended a daily intake of 400 IU compared to either 100 IU or no dietary requirement for D for other adults. A recommendation of 800 IU of vitamin D (or the equivalent from sun exposure of the skin) for lactating women may appear to be more appropriate for the following reasons:

1. Vitamin D appears to be the most important determinant of calcium balance, particularly during lactation.
2. Efficiency of absorption and conversion of vitamin D to active metabolites may be reduced in certain individuals, as exemplified by patients on anticonvulsant therapy.
3. The loss of vitamin D in the milk may be greater than previously thought because of the presence of sulfoconjugates of vitamin D in the milk. This view is consistent with our observation of more rapid development of signs of vitamin D deficiency during lactation than during nonlactation in rats.
4. Studies in adult men have shown that the ability to adapt to a decrease in calcium intake (by increasing the efficiency of calcium absorption) is quite variable and that some individuals require weeks or months to reestablish a positive calcium balance (Malm, 1963); the relatively low vitamin D intake, 200 IU/day, may have contributed to lack of immediate adaptation.
5. There is no evidence that a daily intake of 800 IU of vitamin D causes any adverse effects in an adult woman. In fact, most women in the United States who spend several hours in the sun each week during the summer months and who receive 400 IU of vitamin D from dietary sources probably receive a total of more than 800 IU daily.

However, the question of the requirement of vitamin D during human lactation, as well as the importance of calcitonin and parathyroid hormone, will probably not be answered until studies can be made in women secreting large amounts of milk for several months, such as mothers nursing twins. In these women, changes in blood levels of calcium, phosphorus, and the calcium-regulating hormones should be accentuated and therefore easier to detect than they are in women producing less than 7 dl of milk daily. We predict that such studies will reveal changes that are at least qualitatively similar to the clear-cut changes seen in the lactating rat, such as the increased serum level of $1,25\text{-}(OH)_2D_3$. Such studies should also take into account the patients' previous intakes of calcium and vitamin D, particularly during early adolescence when skeletal mass is still increasing. Since the rate of the inevitable loss of bone mineral associated with the aging process appears to be inversely related to skeletal mass of the young adult, it is clear that the amount of lactational bone loss may also be related to the original state of the skeleton. Criteria for adequacy of vitamin D supply should be based not only on changes in bone mineral during and after lactation, but also on changes in the serum levels of calcium and phosphate. Based on the human studies of Liu *et al.* (1937) and our work with rats (Boass *et al.*, 1977), hypocalcemia may be the most sensitive indicator of vitamin D deficiency during lactation.

VII. CONCLUSIONS AND HYPOTHESES

In lactating animals that secrete relatively large amounts of calcium in the milk (manyfold greater loss of calcium in the milk than in the urine), a number of adaptive changes in calcium metabolism occur. Efficiency of calcium absorption from the intestine increases twofold or more, and, in the rat, absorption may remain elevated for some time after weaning if dietary calcium intake has been limited so that skeletal calcium stores are mobilized to meet the demands of milk secretion. Presumably, vitamin D and parathyroid hormone act in concert to mediate these changes. Vitamin D through its conversion to $1,25\text{-}(OH)_2D_3$ stimulates calcium absorption, and both parathyroid hormone and the vitamin D metabolite enhance skeletal calcium mobilization. Both hormones are also closely related to the serum calcium level. An elevated blood level of parathyroid hormone, which has been documented in lactating cows, is not only stimulated and maintained by a low serum calcium level, but may be required to prevent an excessive drop in serum calcium in response to the calcium drain into the milk. Elevated blood levels of $1,25\text{-}(OH)_2D_3$, which have been found in rats during the last 2 weeks of lactation and in lactating women 2–4 weeks postpartum, are also essential for normal calcium homeostasis and may contribute to the increased efficiency of intestinal calcium absorption. Parathyroid hormone is essential for maintaining the elevated $1,25\text{-}(OH)_2D_3$ level, presumably by serving as the most important stimulator of the 1-hydroxylase system in the kidney.

High circulating levels of calcitonin have been observed in lactating rats and sheep and in at least some lactating women. In the rat there is evidence that calcitonin is secreted in response to eating, that its peripheral effects are enhanced during lactation, and that its hypocalcemic effect helps to maintain serum calcium at a level approximately 10% lower than that of nonlactating rats.

A low normal serum calcium level would appear to be beneficial since it would tend to reduce the filtered load of calcium and thus reduce urinary loss of calcium. In fact, urinary excretion of calcium is reduced during lactation in several species. However, the reduction, which may amount to 70% of the urinary loss seen in the nonlactating state, contributes an almost negligible amount to the calcium economy during lactation, since milk calcium secretion may be 10- to 100-fold greater than urinary calcium output. The exception is the lactating woman who may excrete as much calcium in the urine as in the milk and who may therefore conserve a significant amount of calcium when urinary calcium excretion is reduced by, perhaps, 50% during lactation. Increased PTH-mediated renal reabsorption of calcium and decreased filtered load of calcium can explain the adaptive decrease in urinary calcium loss, at least in the lactating cow.

In order to facilitate further work on the hormonal interactions in calcium metabolism in lactation, we have formulated the following working hypothesis for the sequence of events and relationships seen in the lactating rat.

1. The rapid transfer of calcium to milk at the onset of lactation leads to mild hypocalcemia, which serves as a stimulus for increased PTH secretion.
2. The increased level of PTH stimulates the renal 1-hydroxylase system, which results in elevation of the circulating level of $1,25\text{-}(OH)_2D_3$.
3. Increased secretion of calcitonin in response to eating may be due to humoral factors that enhance the secretory responsiveness of calcitonin-secreting cells in the thyroid gland, such as $1,25\text{-}(OH)_2D_3$ or prolactin, which circulate at higher levels during lactation. Alternatively, postprandial hypersecretion of calcitonin could be due to intestinal hypertrophy and hyperfunction that cause increased secretion of the hypothetical calcitonin secretagogue of the rat intestine.
4. The increased calcitonin level helps to protect the skeleton against excessive calcium efflux and bone resorption.
5. A consequence of the action of calcitonin on bone is the maintenance of a relatively low serum calcium level, which then ensures a continued high rate of secretion of parathyroid hormone. Thus, we predict that the ability of the lactating rat to sustain the loss of more than 100 mg of calcium daily in the milk is based on a state of hypersecretion and integrated action of all three calcemic hormones—parathyroid hormone, calcitonin, and $1,25\text{-}(OH)_2D_3$.

ACKNOWLEDGMENTS

The authors gratefully acknowledge the wise counsel and enthusiastic support for their research given by Dr. Paul L. Munson. The senior author expresses particular appreciation to Dr. Munson for having introduced him to this field of research.

The authors also wish to acknowledge the collaboration of Drs. Cary W. Cooper, Mark R. Haussler, and D. I. Becker and of Mrs. Catherine Lane and the assistance of Mrs. Joan Berry in the preparation of the manuscript. The authors' research has been supported by Grants DE-02668 from the National Institute of Dental Research and RR-05333 from the Division of Research Facilities and Resources, National Institutes of Health.

REFERENCES

Atkinson, P. J., and West, R. R. (1970). *J. Obstet. Gynaecol. Br. Commonw.* **77**, 555.

Baumrucker, C. R. (1978). *In* "Lactation: A Comprehensive Treatise" (B. L. Larson and V. R. Smith, eds.), Vol 4, p. 463. Academic Press, New York.

Barton, B. A., Horst, R. L., Jorgensen, N. A., and DeLuca, H. F. (1977). *J. Dairy Sci.* **60**, Suppl. 1, 122.

Becker, D. I., Toverud, S. U., Ontjes, D. A., and Cooper, C. W. (1979). *J. Endocrinol. Invest.* **2**, 159.

Blahosova, A., Neradilova, M., Velicky, J., Tillbach, M., Marsikova, L., and Reischaur, R. (1974). *Endokrinologie* **63**, 122.

Blanusa, M., Harmut, M., Momcilovik, B., Durakovic, A., and Kostial, K. (1971). *Calcif. Tissue Res.* **7**, 299.

Blum, J. W., Mayer, G. P., and Potts, J. T., Jr. (1974). *Endocrinology* **95**, 84.

Boass, A., Toverud, S. U., McCain, T. A., Pike, J. W., and Haussler, M. R. (1977). *Nature (London)* **267**, 630.

Boass, A., Toverud, S. U., and Munson, P. L. (1980). In preparation.

Braithwaite, G. D. (1976). *J. Dairy Res.* **43**, 501.

Braithwaite, G. D. (1978). *Br. J. Nutr.* **40**, 387.

Braithwaite, G. D., and Glascock, R. F. (1976). *Bien. Rev. Natl. Inst. Res.*, p. 43.

Braithwaite, G. D., Glascock, R. F., and Riazuddin, S. (1969). *Br. J. Nutr.* **23**, 827.

Campbell, R. M., and Fell, B. F. (1964). *J. Physiol. (London)* **171**, 90.

Cooper, C. W., and Obie, J. F. (1978). *Proc. Soc. Exp. Biol. Med.* **157**, 374.

Cooper, C. W., Obie, J. F., and Hsu, W. H. (1976). *Proc. Soc. Exp. Biol. Med.* **151**, 183.

Cooper, C. W., Obie, J. F., Toverud, S. U., and Munson, P. L. (1977). *Endocrinology* **101**, 1657.

Cotes, P. M., and Cross, B. A. (1954). *J. Endocrinol.* **10**, 363.

Cowie, A. T., and Folley, S. J. (1945). *Nature (London)* **156**, 719.

Cramer, C. F. (1972). *In* "Methods and Achievements in Experimental Pathology; Nutritional Pathobiology" (E. Bajusz and G. Jasmin, eds.), p. 172. Karger, Basel.

Cripps, A. W., and Williams, V. J. (1975). *Br. J. Nutr.* **33**, 17.

Cushard, W. G., Jr., Creditor, M. A., Canterbury, J. M., and Reiss, E. (1972). *J. Clin. Endocrinol. Metab.* **34**, 767.

Davis, R. H., Morgan, D. B., and Rivlin, R. S. (1970). *Clin. Sci.* **39**, 1.

DeLuca, H. F. (1978). *In* "Handbook of Lipid Research" (D. J. Hanahan, ed.), Vol. II, p. 69. Plenum, New York.

de Winter, F. R., and Steendijk, R. (1975). *Calcif. Tissue Res.* **17**, 303.

Donelson, E., Nims, B., Hunscher, H. A., and Macy, I. G. (1931). *J. Biol. Chem.* **91**, 675.

Drummond, J. C., Gray, C. H., and Richardson, N. E. G. (1939). *Br. Med. J.* **2**, 757.

Duckworth, J., and Warnock, G. M. (1942–1943). *Nutr. Abstr. Rev.* **12**, 167.

Elias, E., and Dowling, R. H. (1976). *Clin. Sci. Mol. Med.* **51**, 427.

Ellinger, G. M., Duckworth, J., and Dalgarno, A. C. (1952). *Br. J. Nutr.* **6**, 235.

Fairney, A., and Weir, A. A. (1970). *J. Endocrinol.* **48**, 337.

FAO/WHO Expert Group Report (1970). FAO Nutrition Meetings Report Series, No. 47, Rome.

Favus, M. J., Walling, M. W., and Kimberg, D. V. (1974). *J. Clin. Invest.* **53**, 1139.

Fell, B. F., Smith, K. A., and Campbell, R. M. (1963). *J. Pathol. Bacteriol.* **85**, 179.

Filer, L. J., Jr. (1975). *Clinics Perinatol.* **2**, 353.

Fournier, P., and Susbielle, H. (1952). *J. Physiol. (Paris)* **44**, 123, 575.

Frank, F. R., Ogilvie, M. L., Koshy, K. T., Kakuk, T. J., and Jorgensen, N. A. (1977). *In* "Vitamin D: Biochemical, Chemical and Clinical Aspects Related to Calcium" (A. W. Norman *et al.*, eds), p. 577. de Gruyter, Berlin.

Fry, J. M., Curnow, D. H., Gutteridge, D. H., and Retallack, R. W. (1979). *J. Endocrinol.* **82**, 323.

Garel, J.-M., and Besnard, P. (1979). *Endocrinology* **104**, 1617.

Garel, J.-M., Care, A. D., and Barlet, J.-P. (1974). *J. Endocrinol.* **62**, 497.

Gray, T. K., and Munson, P. L. (1969). *Science* **166**, 512.

Haavaldsen, R., Mortensen Egnund, K., and Nicolaysen, R. (1956). *Acta Physiol. Scand.* **36**, 108.

Halloran, B. P., and DeLuca, H. F. (1979). *Science* **204**, 73.

Harding, J. D., and Cairnie, A. B. (1975). *Cell Tissue Kinet.* **8**, 135.

Harper, C., and Toverud, S. U. (1973). *Endocrinology* **93**, 1354.

Haussler, M. R., and McCain, T. A. (1977). *N. Engl. J. Med.* **297**, 974, 1041.

Heaney, R. P., and Skillman, T. G. (1971). *J. Clin. Endocrinol. Metab.* **33**, 661.

Hennessy, J. F., Wells, S. A., Jr., Ontjes, D. A., and Cooper, C. W. (1974). *J. Clin. Endocrinol. Metab.* **39**, 487.

Hilliard, C. J., Cooke, T. J. C., Coombes, R. C., Evans, I. M. A., and MacIntyre, I. (1977). *Clin. Endocrinol.* **6**, 291.

Horst, R. L., Eisman, J. A., Jorgensen, N. A., and DeLuca, H. F. (1977). *Science* **196**, 662.

Horst, R. L., DeLuca, H. F., and Jorgensen, N. A. (1978). *Metab. Bone Dis. Related Res.* **1**, 29.

Hughes, M. R., Baylink, D. J., Jones, P. G., and Haussler, M. R. (1976). *J Clin. Invest.* **58**, 61.

Hughes, M. R., Baylink, D. J., Gonnerman, W. A., Toverud, S. U., Ramp, W. K., and Haussler, M. R. (1977). *Endocrinology* **100**, 799.

Hytten, F. E., and Thomson, A. M. (1961). *In* "Milk: the Mammary Gland and Its Secretion" (S. K. Kon and A. T. Cowie, eds.), Vol. 2, p. 3. Academic Press, New York.

Jacobs, L. R., Polak, J., Bloom, S. R., and Dowling, R. H. (1976). *Clin. Sci. Mol. Med.* **50**, 14p.

James, M. F., Makeen, A. M., Foley, S., Stevens, J., and Robinson, C. J. (1977). *J. Endocrinol.* **75**, 53P.

Johnson, B. E., Daniels, F., and Magnus, I. A. (1968). *In* "Photophysiology" (A. C. Giese, ed.), Vol 4, p. 176. Academic Press, New York.

Kalu, D. N. (1978). *Horm. Metab. Res.* **10**, 72.

Kamoun, A., and Haberey, P. (1969) *Pathol. Bio.* **17**, 159.

Karmarkar, M. G., and Ramakrishnan, C. V. (1960). *Acta Paediat.* **49**, 599.

Kennedy, G. C., Pearce, W. M., and Parrot, D. M. W. (1958). *J. Endocrinol.* **17**, 158.

Kletzien, W. F., Templin, V. M., Steenbock, H., and Thomas, B. H. (1932). *J. Biol. Chem.* **97**, 265.

Komárková, A., Zahor, Z., and Czabanova, V. (1967). *J. Lab. Clin. Med.* **69**, 102.

Kostial, K., Gruden, N., and Durakovic, A. (1969a). *Calcif. Tissue Res.* **4**, 13.

Kostial, K., Durakovìc, A., Simonoviz, I., and Juvancic, V. (1969b). *Int. J. Radiat. Biol.* **15**, 563.

Kumar, R., Cohen, W. R., Silva, P., and Epstein, F. H. (1979). *J. Clin. Invest.* **63**, 342.

Lakdawala, D. R., and Widdowson, E. M. (1977). *Lancet* **1**, 167.

Lamke, B., Brundin, J., and Moberg, P. (1977). *Acta Obstet. Gynecol. Scand.* **56**, 217.

Lawson, D. E. M. (1978). *In* "Vitamin D" (D. E. M. Lawson, ed.), p. 167. Academic Press, New York.

Lewis, P. E., Rafferty, B., Shelley, M., and Robinson, C. J. (1971). *J. Endocrinol.* **49**, ix.

Littledike, E. T. (1976). *J. Dairy Sci.* **59**, 1947.

Liu, S., Su, C. C., Wang, C. W., and Chang, K. P. (1937). *Chin. J. Physiol.* **11**, 271.

MacIntyre, I., Colson, K. W., Robinson, C. J., and Spanos, E. (1977). *In* "Molecular Endocrinology" (I. MacIntyre and M. Szelke, eds.), p. 73. Elsevier/North-Holland Biomedical Press, Amsterdam.

Macy, I. G., Hunscher, H. A., McCosh, S. S., and Nims, B. (1930). *J. Biol. Chem.* **86**, 59.

Mainoya, J. R. (1975). *Endocrinology* **96**, 1158, 1165.

Malm, O. J. (1963). *In* "The Transfer of Calcium and Strontium across Biological Membranes" (R. H. Wasserman, ed.) p. 143. Academic Press, New York.

Marcus, C. S., and Lengemann, F. W. (1962). *J. Nutr.* **77**, 155.

Mayer, G. P., Ramberg, C. F., Jr., and Kronfeld, D. S. (1969a). *Clin. Orthop. Related Res.* **62**, 79.

Mayer, G. P., Ramberg, C. F., Kronfeld, D. S., Buckle, R. M., Sherwood, L. M., Aurbach, G. D., and Potts, J. T., Jr. (1969b). *Am. J. Vet. Res.* **30**, 1587.

Mendelsohn, M., and Haddad, J. G. (1975). *J. Lab. Clin. Med.* **86**, 32.

Munson, P. L., and Gray, T. K., (1970). *Fed. Proc. Fed. Am. Soc. Exp. Biol.* **29**, 1206.

Munson, P. L., Hirsch, P. F., and Tashjian, A. H., Jr. (1963). *Annu. Rev. Physiol.* **25**, 325.

National Research Council, Food and Nutrition Board (1974). *In* "Recommended Dietary Allowances," p. 54. Natl. Acad. Sci., Washington, D.C.

Nelson, D. H. (1979). *In* "Endocrinology" (L. J. DeGroot, G. F. Cahill, Jr., L. Martini, D. H. Nelson, W. D. Odell, J. T. Potts, Jr., E. Steinberger, and A. I. Winegrad, eds.), Vol. 2, p. 1179. Grune & Stratton, New York.

Nelson, M. M., and Evans, H. M. (1961). *In* "Milk: The Mammary Gland and Its Secretion" (S. K. Kon and A. T. Cowie, eds.), Vol. 2, p. 137. Academic Press, New York.

Neuenschwander, J., and Talmage, R. V. (1963). *Proc. Soc. Exp. Biol. Med.* **112**, 297.

Nicolaysen, R., Eeg-Larsen, N., and Malm, O. J. (1953). *Physiol. Rev.* **33**, 424.

Noff, D., and Edelstein, S. (1978). *Horm. Res.* **9**, 292.

Norman, A. W. (1978). *In* "Vitamin D" (D. E. M. Lawson, ed.), p. 93. Academic Press, New York.

Omdahl, J. L., and DeLuca, H. F. (1973). *Physiol. Rev.* **53**, 327.

Ota, K., Harai, Y., Unno, H., Sakanchi, S., Tomogane, H., and Yokoyama, A. (1974). *J. Endocrinol.* **62**, 679.

Payne, J. M., and Manston, R. (1967). *Vet. Rec.* **79**, 215.

Payne, P. F., and Wheeler, E. F. (1968). *Proc. Nutr. Soc.* **27**, 129.

Peacock, M., Hodgkinson, A., and Nordin, B. E. C. (1967). *Br. Med. J.* **3**, 469.

Peng, T.-C., and Garner, S. C. (1978). *Fed. Proc. Fed. Am. Soc. Exp. Biol.* **37**, Abstr. No. 3540, p. 887.

Perault-Staub, A. M., Staub, J. F., and Milhaud, G. (1974). *Endocrinology* **95**, 480.

Pickard, D. W., Care, A. D., Tomlinson, S., and O'Riordan, J. L. H. (1975). *J. Endocrinol.* **67**, 45P.

Pike, J. W., Toverud, S. U., Boass, A., McCain, T., and Haussler, M. R. (1977). *In* "Vitamin D: Biochemical, Chemical and Clinical Aspects Related to Calcium Metabolism" (A. W. Norman *et al.*, eds.), p. 187. de Gruyter, Berlin.

Pike, J. W., Parker, J. B., Haussler, M. R., Boass, A., and Toverud, S. U. (1979). *Science* **204**, 1427.

Pitkin, R. M. (1976). *Clin. Obstet. Gynecol.* **19**, 489.

Polskin, L. J., Kramer, B., and Sobel, A. E. (1943). *Fed. Proc., Fed. Am. Soc. Exp. Biol.* **2**, 68.

Ramberg, C. F., Jr., Mayer, G. P., Kronfeld, D. S., Phang, J. M., and Berman, M. (1970). *Am. J. Physiol.* **219**, 1166.

Ramberg, C. F., Jr., Kronfeld, D. S., and Wilson, G. D. A. (1975). *In* "Digestion and Metabolism in the Ruminant" (I. W. McDonald and A. C. I. Warner, eds.), p. 231. Univ. of New England Publishing Unit, Armidale, N.S.W., Australia.

Rasmussen, P. (1977). *J. Periodont. Res.* **12**, 491.

Reid, J. T. (1961). *In* "Milk: The Mammary Gland and Its Secretion" (S. K. Kon and A. T. Cowie, eds.), Vol. 2, p. 47. Academic Press, New York.

Retallack, R. W., Jeffries, M., Kent, G. N., Hitchcock, N. E., Gutteridge, D. H., and Smith, M. (1977). *Calcif. Tissue Res.* **22**, Suppl., 142.

Sahashi, Y., Suzuki, T., Higaki, M., and Asam, T. (1967). *J. Vitaminol. (Kyoto)* **13**, 33.

Schachter, D., and Rosen, S. M. (1959). *Am. J. Physiol.* **196**, 357.

Shayanfar, F., Head, H. H., Wilcox, C. J., and Thatcher, W. W. (1975). *J. Dairy Sci.* **58**, 870.

Shen, F. H., Baylink, D. J., Nielsen, R. L., Sherrard, D. J., Ivey, J. L., and Haussler, M. R. (1977). *J. Lab. Clin. Med.* **90**, 955.

Sherwood, L. M., Potts, J. T., Jr., Care, A. D., Mayer, G. P., and Aurbach, G. D. (1966). *Nature (London)* **209**, 52.

Simkiss, K. (1967). "Calcium in Reproductive Physiology." Reinhold, New York.

Simpson, A. A., Simpson, M. H. W., Sinha, Y. N., and Schmidt, G. H. (1973). *J. Endocrinol.* **58**, 675.

Smotherman, W. P., Wiener, S. G., Mendoza, S. P., and Levine, S. (1976). *Breast Feeding and the Mother, Ciba Found. Symp.* **45** [N.S.] p. 5.

Spanos, E., Pike, J. W., Haussler, M. R., Colston, K. W., Evans, I. M. A., Goldner, A. M., McCain, T. A., and MacIntyre, I. (1976). *Life Sci.* **19**, 1751.

Spray, C. M. (1950). *Br. J. Nutr.* **4**, 354.

Sutton, R. A. L., and Dirks, J. H. (1978). *Fed. Proc., Fed. Am. Soc. Exp. Biol.* **38**, 2120.

Talmage, R. V. (1956). *Ann. N. Y. Acad. Sci.* **64**, 326.

Talmage, R. V., Doppelt, S. V., and Cooper, C. W. (1975). *Proc. Soc. Exp. Biol. Med.* **149**, 855.

Taylor, T. G., Lewis, P. E., and Balderstone, D. (1975). *J. Endocrinol.* **66**, 296.

Toverud, G. (1926). *Norske Tannlegefor. Tidende* **36**, Suppl.

Toverud, K. U., and Toverud, G. (1931). *Acta Paediat.* **12**, Suppl. 2.

Toverud, K. U., Stearns, G., and Macy, I. G. (1950). *Bull. Natl. Res. Counc. (U.S.)* **123**, 59.

Toverud, S. U. (1963). *In* "The Transfer of Calcium and Strontium across Biological Membranes." (R. H. Wasserman, ed.), p. 341. Academic Press, New York.

Toverud, S. U. (1964). *Acta Physiol. Scand.* **62**, Suppl. 234, 1.

Toverud, S. U., Harper, C., and Munson, P. L. (1976). *Endocrinology* **99**, 371.

Toverud, S. U., Becker, D. I. Boass, A., Cooper, C. W., Hirsch, P. F., Ontjes, D. A., Peng, T.-C., and Ramp, W. K. (1978a). *In* "Endocrinology of Calcium Metabolism." (D. H. Copp and R. V. Talmage, eds.), p. 125. Excerpta Med. Found., Amsterdam.

Toverud, S. U., Cooper, C. W., and Munson, P. L. (1978b). *Endocrinology* **103**, 472.

Toverud, S. U., Boass, A., and Munson, P. L. (1978c). *U.S. Endocrine Soc. 60th Annu. Meeting*, Abstr. No. 318, p. 233.

Toverud, S. U., Boass, A., and Ramp, W. K. (1979). *U.S. Endocrine Soc. 61st Annu. Meeting*, Abstr. No. 757, p. 262.

van't Klooster, A. T. (1976). *Z. Tierphysiol. Tierernehr. Futtermittelk.* **37**, 169.

Vorherr, H. (1974). "The Breast: Morphology, Physiology and Lactation," p. 105. Academic Press, New York.

Wagner, W. C., and Oxenreider, S. L. (1972). *J. Anim. Sci.* **34**, 630.

Warnock, G. M., and Duckworth, J. (1944). *Biochem. J.* **38**, 220.

Wasserman, R. H., Fullmer, C. S., and Taylor, A. N. (1978). *In* "Vitamin D" (D. E. M. Lawson, ed.), p. 133. Academic Press, New York.

Weisman, S., Sapir, R., Harrell, A., and Edelstein, S. (1976). *Biochim. Biophys. Acta.* **428**, 388.

Subject Index

A

ACTH
  effects on neurons, 230
  endorphins and, 203–206
  hypothalamic control of release of, 125–128
  radioimmunoassays of, 118–121
  release of by extrahypothalamic CRF, 141–143
  secretion of
    circadian rhythm of, 121–123
    control by corticotropin-releasing factors, 111–152
    dynamic changes in, 115
  stress effects on, 129–131
ACTH-10
  effect on memory, 216–217
  effect on vigilance, 217
ACTH-like peptides
  in amnesia prevention, 197
  in amnesia reversal, 199–202
  effects on memory, 163
    in cognitively impaired, 215–219
    after hypophysectomy, 165
    mechanism and sites of action, 219–220
    neurochemistry, 227–231
    neurophysiology, 225–227
    in normal animals, 211–215
    after pituitary lobe ablation 172–175
Adenylcyclase, in intestine, vitamin D effects on, 54
African skin, UV light penetration into, 18–19
Aged animals, memory studies on, 179–180
Alcoholics, memory impairment in, vasopressin therapy, 217–218
Alkaline phosphatase/Ca-ATPase, in intestine, vitamin D effects on, 54–56
Amnesia
  pituitary peptide effects on, 181
    ACTH-like peptides, 197
    vasopressin-like peptides, 197–199
  reversal of, by peptides, 199–202

Androgens, inhibin interaction with, 279–280

B

Binding proteins, for vitamin D, 28–43
Blood, hypothalamic corticotropin-releasing factor in, 140–141
Bone, vitamin D effects on formation of, 3, 59–60
Brain, peptide-sensitive areas of, 222–227
Brush-border membrane proteins, properties and synthesis of, 51–52

C

Calcitonin effects on calcium metabolism in lactation, 309–314
Calcium
  homeostasis, vitamin D effects on, 3
  intestinal absorption of, 43–46
  in milk, 335
Calcium-binding protein properties and synthesis of, 47–51
Calcium metabolism, in lactation, hormonal control, 303–345
Cell transformation, epidermal growth factor-urogastrone role in, 100–103
Central nervous system (CNS), in activation of corticotropin-releasing factor, 112–113
Circadian rhythm, in ACTH secretion, 121–123
Cognitively impaired, peptide effects on, 215–219
Corticotropin-releasing factors (CRF)
  assays for, 132–143
    in vitro, 135–138
  CNS activation of, 112–113
  control of ACTH secretion, 111–152
  hypothalamic
    nature, 113–115
    peripheral blood, 138–143
  in peripheral blood, 123–125

Corticotropin-releasing factors (CRF),
  (*Cont.*)
  in tissue, 143–149
    regulation, 145–146
    significance, 147–150
    suppression, 146–147
Cortisol, radioimmunoassays of, 118–121
Cybernine, inhibin as possible, 296–298

D

7-Dehydrocholesterol
  in skin
    distribution in, 4–5
    factors affecting, 5
    UV light effects, 6
Diabetes insipidus, hereditary, memory
  deficits in, 176–179
1, 25-Dihydroxyvitamin D
  binding proteins for, 40–43
  receptors for, 42–43

E

Endorphins, 202–219
  ACTH and, 203–206
  effect on memory, 208–210
  vasopressin and, 207
Epidermal growth factor-urogastrone
  (EGF–URO)
  amino acid sequences of, 71
  biological actions of, 78–82
    in vitro, 79–82
    in vivo, 78–79
  biosynthesis, storage, and secretion of,
    75–78
  in cell transformation and tumorigen-
    esis, 100–103
  isolation and properties of, 72–75
    from man, 74–75
    from mouse, 72–74
  membrane receptor for, 83–97
    affinity labeling of, 91–97
    in liver and placental membranes, 87–
      91
  mitogenic action of, 85–87
  as possible hormone, 103–106
  structure-activity relationships of, 97–
    100

in various species, 104
Estrogens, inhibin interaction with, 279–
  280

F

Follicle-stimulating hormone (FSH)
  assay of inhibin using, 251
  gametogenesis and secretion of, 244–
    246
  inhibin effects on, 272
  in negative feedback, 294–296

G

G$_c$-protein
  amino acid composition of, 33
  isolation and properties of, 31–33
Gonadotropins
  inhibin effects on, 272
    kinetics, 274–279
    secretion, 282–287
Gonads, inhibin effects on, 270–271

H

Hippocampus, behavioral functions of,
  223–224
Hormone(s)
  in control of calcium metabolism in lac-
    tation, 303–345
  epidermal growth factor-urogastrone as
    possible, 103–106
Humans, epidermal growth factor-
  urogastrone of, 74–75, 77–78
Human chorionic gonadotropin (HCG), in
  inhibin assay, 251–254
Hydroxyvitamin D, binding proteins for,
  39–40
Hypophysectomy, effects on memory,
  amelioration by peptides, 165–170
Hypothalamopituitary axis, inhibin
  transport to, 293
Hypothalamus
  corticotropin-releasing factor of, 113–
    115
  inhibin effects on, 268–270
  lesions of, effect on ACTH secretions,
    128–132

I

Inhibin, 243–302
  amino acid composition of, 261
  biological properties of, 267–287
  definition of, 246
  detection and measurement of, 249–260
    by radioimmunoassay, 256–257
  effects on
    gonadotropin secretion, 282–287
    spermatogenesis, 280–282
  immune reactions of, 293
  interactions with androgen and estrogens, 279–280
  lack of carbohydrate in, 265–266
  mechanism of action of, 272–274
  molecular weight of, 261–264
  origin and transport of, 287–293
    in follicles, 290–291
    to hypothalamopituitary axis, 293
    in testes, 287–290, 291–292
  physicochemical and immunological properties of, 260–266
  as possible cybernine, 296–298
  possible roles of, 293–298
  receptors for, in gonadotrophs, 274
  sites of action of, 267–271
    gonads, 270–271
    hypothalamus, 268–270
    pituitary, 267–268
  sources and purification of, 246–249
    from ram rete testis fluid, 247–249
    from seminal plasma, 247
Intestine
  calcium absorption in, 43–46
    during lactation, 321–331
  changes in, during lactation, 321–322
  1,25-dihydroxyvitamin D binding proteins in, 40–43
  response to vitamin D of, 46–58
    enzyme activity, 54–56
  RNA synthesis in nuclei of, 52–53

K

Korsakoff's disease, vasopressin effects on, 217–218

L

Lactation
  hormonal control of calcium metabolism in, 303–345
    intestinal, 321–331
    urinary, 331–334
Learning
  active avoidance type, 158–161
  passive avoidance type, 161–162
Liver, receptor for epidermal growth factor-urogastrone, 87–91
Luteinizing hormone (LH), inhibin effect on secretion of, 296

M

Median eminence, tissue CRF and, 143–145
Membrane receptor, for epidermal growth factor-urogastrone, 82–97
Memory
  ACTH-10 effects on, 216–217
  active avoidance learning in, 158–161
  amelioration of behavioral deficits in, 165–182
    in amnesia, 181
    in diabetes insipidus, 176–179
    hypophysectomy, 165–170
    in old animals, 179–180
    after pituitary-lobe ablation, 170–176
  analysis of, 154–155
  assessment of, 158–162
  human and nonhuman, 157–158
  hypophysectomy effects on, 167–170
  opioid effects on, 207–210
  passive avoidance learning in, 161–162
  peptide effect on, 162–182
    in cognitively impaired, 215–219
    in normal subjects, 211–215
    sites of action and mechanisms, 219–231
  pituitary hormone and related peptide effects on, 153–241
  pituitary-lobe ablation effects on, 170–176
  processing in, 154–158
  storage and retrieval in, 157
  treatments affecting, 155–157

Mice, epidermal growth factor-
    urogastrone of, 72–74, 75–77
Milk, calcium and vitamin D in, 335–337

N

Neurons, ACTH effects on, 230

O

25-(OH)D$_3$-1-hydroxylase, inhibitor of,
    and vitamin D-binding protein, 38–39
Opioids, effect on memory, 207–210

P

Parathyroid hormone, effects on calcium
    metabolism in lactation, 305–309
Peptides, memory modulation by, 153–
    241
Peripheral blood
    corticotropin-releasing factor in, 123–
    125
    hypothalamic, 138–141
Phosphorus metabolism, vitamin D regu-
    lation of, 3
Pituitary inhibin effects on, 267–268
Pituitary cell cultures, inhibin assay by,
    254–255
Pituitary hormones, memory modulation
    by, 153–241
Pituitary lobes
    ablation of, effects on memory, 170–176
    incubated, inhibin assay by, 255–256
Placental membranes, receptor for epi-
    dermal growth factor-urogastrone in,
    87–91
Plasma, vitamin D metabolite binding
    proteins in, 28–39
Posterior thalamus, behavioral functions
    of, 222
Pre-vitamin D
    biological activity of, 10–11
    conversion to vitamin D, 7–9
    formation of, 6–7

R

Rete testis fluid, inhibin extraction from,
    247–249

RNA, synthesis of, in intestinal nuclei,
    52–53

S

Septal area (of brain), behavioral func-
    tions of, 222–223
Serum, calcium concentration in, during
    lactation, 305–321
Skeleton, calcium content of, during lac-
    tation, 335–337
Skin
    7-dehydrocholesterol in, 4–5
    lipids in, UV radiation effects on, 6
    sterol absorption by, 19–20
    UV light penetration into, 17–19
    vitamin D absorption of, 19
    vitamin D synthesis in, 9–10
    vitamin D in, 11–14
    synthesis, 9–10
Spermatogenesis, inhibin effects on,
    280–282
Sterols, cutaneous absorption of, 19–20
Stress, sensitization to, ACTH secretion
    and, 131–132

T

Testes, inhibin from, 287–290
Tumorigenesis, epidermal growth factor-
    urogastrone role in, 100–103

U

Ultraviolet light (UV)
    effect on 7-dehydrocholesterol in skin, 6
    penetration into skin, 17–19
    role in management of, in vitamin D de-
    ficiency, 26–27
    in vitamin D biosynthesis, 6–11
Urinary excretion of calcium, during lac-
    tation, 331–334

V

Vasopressin
    effect on cognitively impaired subjects,
    217–219
    effect on memory

mechanism and sites of action, 220–222
in normal humans, 215
endorphins and, 207
Vasopressin-like peptides
in amnesia prevention, 197–199
in amnesia reversal, 202
effect on memory, 163
after hypophysectomy, 170
in normal animals, 185–190, 194–196
after pituitary lobe ablation, 175–176
Vigilance
ACTH-10 effects on, 217
peptide effects on, 213–215
Vitamin D, 1–67
binding proteins for, 28–43
enzyme inhibitor and, 38–39
metabolite specificity, 37–38
species distribution, 36–37
in plasma, 28–39
biosynthesis of
factors affecting, 14–19
by irradiation, 6–11
pathway, 8

physical and environmental factors, 14–19
in skin, 9–10
in bone formation, 59–60
cutaneous absorption of, 19–21
deficiency of UV in management, 26–27
effects on calcium metabolism in lactation, 316–320
metabolism and function of, 1–67
pathway, 2
metabolites, binding proteins for, 28–43
in milk, 335–337
intestinal response to, 46–58
pre-vitamin D conversion to, 7–9
in skin, 11–14
storage in body, 21–26
sites, 21–23
UV effects on, 23–26
UV light in biosynthesis of, 6–11

W

Women, lactating, skeletal calcium content of, 338–341

Date Due

			UML 735